Advanced Pancreaticobiliary Endoscopy

Douglas G. Adler

Editor

Advanced Pancreaticobiliary Endoscopy

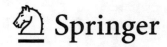 Springer

Editor
Douglas G. Adler
Salt Lake City, Utah
USA

Videos can also be accessed at http://link.springer.com/book/10.1007/978-3-319-26854-5

ISBN 978-3-319-80025-7   ISBN 978-3-319-26854-5   (eBook)
DOI 10.1007/978-3-319-26854-5

This Springer imprint is published by Springer Nature
The registered company is Springer International Publishing AG Switzerland

For my family

Preface

Therapeutic endoscopy is at the leading edge of gastroenterology today. Endoscopic procedures that are now performed on a routine basis have, in many cases, replaced surgeries that were in widespread use only a few years ago. The greatest areas of advancement have, without a doubt, come in the realm of pancreaticobiliary endoscopy. Endoscopic retrograde cholangiopancreatography (ERCP) and endoscopic ultrasound (EUS) are the dominant therapeutic modalities in gastroenterology, and this is very unlikely to change in the coming years. The treatment of pseudocysts or walled-off pancreatic necrosis is now primarily endoscopic with surgery being reserved for only a small subset of these patients, to give one such example. This trend will only continue as our tools, training, and technology continue to develop.

For many therapeutic endoscopists, the first few years after the completion of their training are marked by continuous growth and development, both in cognitive and technical terms. Early on, "bread and butter" cases (such as the treatment of small bile duct stones and uncomplicated bile leaks) are often very appealing as they allow the endoscopist to hone their skills in a relatively low-risk patient cohort. Over time, many therapeutic endoscopists master these basic skills and seek out and/or are called upon to perform more invasive, complex, and high-risk procedures. This can be an exciting, if challenging, transition.

Years ago, my first job after completing my advanced training required me to provide advanced endoscopic procedure services at two very large urban academic hospitals, 365 days a year, with no backup whatsoever. Although I was very well trained as a fellow, nothing could have prepared me for everything I encountered in those first few years in practice. I know that my own endoscopic development was a mixture of formal training, didactic learning, hard won boots-on-the-ground experience, and in more than a few cases I had to teach myself to do new and more complex procedures because there was simply no one else available. The proverbial buck stopped with me!

This book germinated out of the idea that an all-in-one guide to advanced pancreaticobiliary procedures would be both highly desirable and eminently useful to those who want to move out of the realm of routine ERCP and EUS and look for greater challenges. Another reason I put this book together was that I would have loved to have had something like it as a junior therapeutic endoscopist.

In this book, I have tried to cover the entire range of advanced pancreaticobiliary procedures. The book starts off with a discussion of advanced cannulation and sphincterotomy in ERCP and moves on to such topics as cholangioscopy and pancreatoscopy, ERCP to remove pancreatic duct stones, endoscopic ampullectomy, minor papilla interventions, interventional EUS for pancreaticobiliary duct access, fiducial placement, pancreatic fluid collection drainage, endoscopic necrosectomy, and many other advanced procedures. My goal is that this book can serve as a vital reference for just about any advanced pancreaticobiliary procedure and can help guide endoscopists to clinical success.

Each chapter covers a specific topic or set of related topics and is lavishly illustrated with endoscopic, ultrasonographic, and fluoroscopic images. Each chapter also is accompanied by one or more high-quality videos to further illustrate the tools and techniques discussed therein. These videos give this volume a multimedia dimension as readers can watch key procedures from start to finish as they are performed in real patients.

As you move forward in your own endoscopic career and undertake more advanced procedures, I hope that this volume becomes a well-worn resource for years to come.

Salt Lake City, UT   Douglas G. Adler

Contents

Contributors

Douglas G. Adler, M.D., F.A.C.G., A.G.A.F. Gastroenterology and Hepatology, Huntsman Cancer Center, University of Utah School of Medicine, Salt Lake City, UT, USA

Laura Alder Department of Gastroenterology, Advanced Endoscopy, Ochsner Medical Center, Ochsner Cancer Institute, New Orleans, LA, USA

Mayne Medical School, University of Queensland School of Medicine, Brisbane, QLD, Australia

Tyler M. Berzin, M.D., M.S. Division of Gastroenterology, Advanced Endoscopy Center, Beth Israel Deaconess Medical Center, Harvard Medical School, Boston, MA, USA

Kathryn R. Byrne, M.D. Gastroenterology and Hepatology, University of Utah, Salt Lake City, UT, USA

Brenna W. Casey, M.D., F.A.S.G.E. Interventional Gastroenterology, Endoscopic Training, Harvard Medical School, Boston, MA, USA

Natalie Danielle Cosgrove, M.D. Thomas Jefferson University, Philadelphia, PA, USA

Christopher J. DiMaio, M.D. The Dr. Henry D. Janowitz Division of Gastroenterology, Icahn School of Medicine at Mount Sinai, Mount Sinai Hospital, New York, NY, USA

Peter V. Draganov, M.D. Division of Gastroenterology, Hepatology, and Nutrition, University of Florida College of Medicine, Gainesville, FL, USA

Matthew E. Feurer, M.D., M.S. Division of Gastroenterology, Hepatology, and Nutrition, University of Florida College of Medicine, Gainesville, FL, USA

Norio Fukami, M.D., A.G.A.F., F.A.C.G. Division of Gastroenterology and Hepatology, Mayo Clinic Arizona, Scottsdale, AZ, USA

Eric Goldberg, M.D. Gastroenterology and Hepatology, University of Maryland, School of Medicine, Baltimore, MD, USA

Mariano Gonzalez-Haba, M.D. Center for Endoscopic Research and Therapeutics (CERT), University of Chicago Medicine, Chicago, IL, USA

Eric G. Hilgenfeldt, M.D. Division of Gastroenterology, Hepatology, and Nutrition, University of Florida College of Medicine, Gainesville, FL, USA

Matthew J. Hudson, M.D. Gastroenterology and Hepatology, Buffalo General Medical Center, Buffalo, NY, USA

Virendra Joshi, M.D., A.G.A.F. Tulane School of Medicine, New Orleans, LA, USA

University of Queensland School of Medicine, Brisbane, QLD, Australia

Department of Gastroenterology, Advanced Endoscopy, Ochsner Cancer Institute, Ochsner Medical Center, Jefferson, LA, USA

Vivek Kaul, M.D. Division of Gastroenterology and Hepatology, Strong Memorial Hospital, University of Rochester Medical Center, Rochester, NY, USA

Center for Advanced Therapeutic Endoscopy, URMC/Strong Memorial Hospital, Rochester, NY, USA

Raymond G. Kim, M.D. Gastroenterology and Hepatology, University of Maryland Medical Center, Baltimore, MD, USA

Shivangi T. Kothari, M.D. Division of Gastroenterology and Hepatology, University of Rochester Medical Center & Strong Memorial Hospital, Rochester, NY, USA

Center for Advanced Therapeutic Endoscopy, URMC/Strong Memorial Hospital, Rochester, NY, USA

Truptesh H. Kothari, M.D., M.S. Division of Gastroenterology and Hepatology, University of Rochester Medical Center & Strong Memorial Hospital, Rochester, NY, USA

Center for Advanced Therapeutic Endoscopy, URMC/Strong Memorial Hospital, Rochester, NY, USA

Anand R. Kumar, M.D., M.P.H. Center for Digestive Health, Drexel University, Philadelphia, PA, USA

Hahnemann University Hospital, Philadelphia, PA, USA

Linda S. Lee, M.D. Division of Gastroenterology, Hepatology and Endoscopy, Brigham and Women's Hospital, Boston, MA, USA

Alexander Lee, M.D. Division of Gastroenterology, Hepatology and Endoscopy, Brigham and Women's Hospital, Boston, MA, USA

Jay Luther, M.D. Clinical and Research Fellow, Gastrointestinal Unit, Massachusetts General Hospital, Boston, MA, USA

Meir Mizrahi, M.D. Division of Gastroenterology, Advanced Endoscopy Center, Beth Israel Deaconess Medical Center, Harvard Medical School, Boston, MA, USA

Jeffrey D. Mosko, M.D., F.R.C.P.C. Department of Medicine, University of Toronto, Toronto, ON, Canada

Mohamed O. Othman, M.B.Bch. Gastroenterology and Hepatology Section, Department of Internal Medicine, Baylor College of Medicine, Houston, TX, USA

Gulshan Parasher, M.D. Division of Gastroenterology and Hepatology, Department of Medicine, University of New Mexico School of Medicine, Albuquerque, NM, USA

Mansour A. Parsi, M.D., M.P.H. Center for Endoscopy and Pancreatobiliary Disorders, Department of Gastroenterology and Hepatology, Digestive Disease Institute, Cleveland Clinic, Cleveland, OH, USA

Douglas Pleskow, M.D. Division of Gastroenterology, Advanced Endoscopy Center, Beth Israel Deaconess Medical Center, Harvard Medical School, Boston, MA, USA

Thomas Queen, M.D. Division of Gastroenterology & Hepatology, University of New Mexico School of Medicine, Albuquerque, NM, USA

Waqar A. Qureshi, M.D. Gastroenterology and Hepatology Section, Department of Internal Medicine, Baylor College of Medicine, Houston, TX, USA

Brian P. Riff, M.D. The Dr. Henry D. Janowitz Division of Gastroenterology, Icahn School of Medicine at Mount Sinai, New York, NY, USA

Haroon Shahid, M.D. Thomas Jefferson University Hospital, Philadelphia, PA, USA

Ali Ahmed Siddiqui, M.D. Department of Gastroenterology, Thomas Jefferson University Hospital, Philadelphia, PA, USA

Uzma D. Siddiqui, M.D. Center for Endoscopic Research and Therapeutics (CERT), University of Chicago Medicine, Chicago, IL, USA

Pushpak Taunk, M.D. University of South Florida, Tampa, FL, USA

Jeffrey L. Tokar, M.D., F.A.S.G.E., A.G.A.F. Department of Medicine, Fox Chase Cancer Center, Philadelphia, PA, USA

About the Editor

Douglas G. Adler, M.D., F.A.C.G., A.G.A.F. received his medical degree from Cornell University Medical College in New York, NY. He completed his residency in internal medicine at Beth Israel Deaconess Medical Center/Harvard Medical School in Boston, MA. Dr. Adler completed both a general gastrointestinal fellowship and a therapeutic endoscopy/ERCP fellowship at Mayo Clinic in Rochester, MN. He then returned to the Beth Israel Deaconess Medical Center for a fellowship in endoscopic ultrasound.

Dr. Adler is currently a tenured Professor of Medicine and Director of Therapeutic Endoscopy at the University Of Utah School Of Medicine in Salt Lake City, UT. Dr. Adler is also the GI Fellowship Program Director at the University Of Utah School Of Medicine. Working primarily at the University Of Utah School Of Medicine's Huntsman Cancer Institute, Dr. Adler focuses his clinical, educational, and research efforts on the diagnosis and management of patients with gastrointestinal cancers and complex gastrointestinal disease, with an emphasis on therapeutic endoscopy. He is the author of more than 250 scientific publications, articles, and book chapters. This is Dr. Adler's fifth text on gastroenterology.

Cannulation and Sphincterotomy: Beyond the Basics

Kathryn R. Byrne and Douglas G. Adler

Introduction

Most ERCP procedures performed in the modern era are therapeutic in nature, with biliary procedures being, overwhelmingly, the most commonly performed. Selective cannulation and sphincterotomy are the cornerstones of successful ERCP procedures. Multicenter analysis has revealed that approximately 16 % of all ERCP procedures with native papilla anatomy have failed selective biliary cannulation [1]. Failure of biliary cannulation leads to delay of intended therapy and the need for a repeat procedure on a different date or the use of alternative therapeutic procedures. It is important to master the skill of biliary sphincterotomy using traditional techniques and to be familiar with more advanced sphincterotomy techniques.

This chapter reviews standard and advanced cannulation and sphincterotomy techniques.

Standard Cannulation Techniques

Once the duodenoscope has been advanced to the second portion of the duodenum, the "short position" is typically obtained by full rightward deflection of the lateral wheel, with upward deflection of the large wheel, and simultaneous

Electronic supplementary material: The online version of this chapter (doi:10.1007/978-3-319-26854-5_1) contains supplementary material, which is available to authorized users. Videos can also be accessed at http://link.springer.com/chapter/10.1007/978-3-319-26854-5_1.

K.R. Byrne, M.D.
Gastroenterology and Hepatology, University of Utah School of Medicine, Salt Lake City, UT, USA

D.G. Adler, M.D., F.A.C.G., A.G.A.F. (✉)
Gastroenterology and Hepatology, Huntsman Cancer Center, University of Utah School of Medicine,
30N 1900E 4R118, Salt Lake City, UT, USA
e-mail: Douglas.adler@hsc.utah.edu

withdrawal and clockwise torque of the shaft of the endoscope. This shortening maneuver places the endoscope shaft along the lesser curvature of the stomach and results in the duodenoscope being positioned underneath the papilla with the tip of the endoscope 1–3 cm from the ampulla itself (the "middle distance"). There are certain instances where a "long position" (wherein the shaft of the duodenoscope rests along the greater curvature of the stomach) is needed to obtain an improved alignment with the major papilla for cannulation, but this is usually if the short position gives a suboptimal position for cannulation and/or sphincterotomy.

In contrast to earlier eras, the modern practice of cannulation during ERCP almost always involves a sphincterotome, as opposed to a straight biliary catheter, to achieve biliary cannulation. This reflects, at least in part, the shift of ERCP from a diagnostic procedure to a therapeutic procedure.

There have been numerous studies demonstrating higher cannulation success rates with sphincterotomes versus straight biliary catheters, with no significant difference in rates of post-ERCP pancreatitis [2–5]. A prospective study demonstrated a biliary cannulation success rate of 82 % with a straight catheter, with a success rate of 97 % after the failed patients were crossed over to a sphincterotome and guidewire [3]. In another study, although the cannulation success rates between standard catheter (94 %) versus sphincterotome (97 %) were similar, the number of attempts needed to achieve biliary cannulation (12.4 attempts versus 2.8 attempts; $p=0.0001$) and mean time to achieve cannulation (13.5 min versus 3.1 min; $p=0.0001$) were significantly in favor of using a sphincterotome [2].

There are numerous different types of sphincterotomes, with the selection primarily dependent on the individual preference of the endoscopist. No single type of sphincterotome has been proven to be superior over other currently available devices. The differences between various types of sphincterotomes include the length of the cutting wire, the length and shape of the tip of the sphincterotome, and the number of lumens. Tapered tips, ultra-tapered tips, ball-shaped tips, and rounded sphincterotome tips are available. In addition, certain types of sphincterotomes have unique

D.G. Adler (ed.), *Advanced Pancreaticobiliary Endoscopy*, DOI 10.1007/978-3-319-26854-5_1

features such as the ability to rotate whereas other types of sphincterotomes have the ability to reverse-bow, which may be useful in patients with Billroth II anatomy.

The selection of a 0.025″ wire versus a 0.035″ wire is also dependent on the individual preference of the endoscopist. A prospective randomized trial comparing the two wires demonstrated that the wire diameter did not appear to affect primary cannulation success rate or post-procedure complication rates [6].

It should be stressed at the outset that a significant amount of time is needed to master the skill of biliary cannulation. A retrospective study involving a single operator demonstrated that biliary cannulation success rates on native papillary anatomy increased from 43 % at the beginning of training, with continued improvement to ≥80 % at the end of training, and then to >96 % as an independent operator, with very high levels of success being encountered after 350 procedures had been performed [7]. It is important to keep track of one's cannulation success (and failure) over time to determine appropriate progress, particularly with success in achieving biliary cannulation in patients with native papillary anatomy.

Guidewire Cannulation

The term "guidewire cannulation" refers to a set of techniques to obtain deep biliary or pancreatic duct access via the use of sphincterotomes/catheters and guidewires without the use of

contrast during the process of cannulation itself. If contrast injection is performed during cannulation, the term "guidewire cannulation" is not applicable (Fig. 1.1). Guidewire cannulation and other cannulation and sphincterotomy techniques are demonstrated in Video 1.1.

There are several different methods that can be used to perform guidewire-assisted biliary cannulation. Two techniques that utilize a single guidewire have been termed Single Wire Method #1 and Single Wire Method #2 by one of the authors (DGA). Single Wire Method #1 involves advancing the tip of the sphincterotome into the ampullary orifice (with physical contact between the tip of the sphincterotome and the ampulla) followed by gentle advancement of the guidewire into the ampulla, with simultaneous fluoroscopic evaluation to see if the desired duct has been accessed.

Single Wire Method #2 involves placing the tip of the sphincterotome in alignment with the ampullary orifice and the desired duct without making physical contact between the tip of the sphincterotome and the ampulla, and advancing the guidewire across the "air gap" and into the ampulla. This advancement of the guidewire is also performed under simultaneous fluoroscopic guidance to see if the desired duct has been accessed. In both Single Wire Methods 1 and 2, once the guidewire has been advanced into the desired duct, the sphincterotome is advanced over the wire, and injection of dye into the duct can commence.

Potential concerns of guidewire cannulation include creating a false passage/guidewire perforation and the possibility of causing pancreatitis via pancreatic trauma (i.e.,

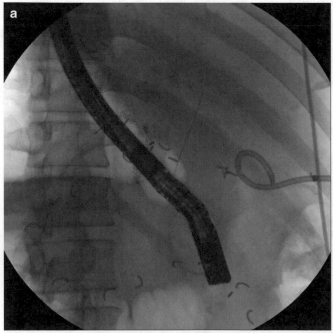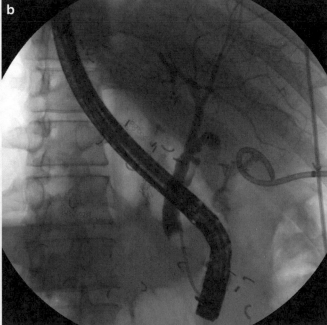

Fig. 1.1 Guidewire cannulation. (**a**) Fluoroscopic image of guidewire cannulation. This patient had a suspected bile leak following cholecystectomy. Note that a guidewire has been advanced into the CBD without the use of any contrast during cannulation. (**b**) Injection of contrast into the CBD is only performed after deep access is obtained. Bile can be seen extravasating into the gallbladder fossa at the region of the percutaneous drain

from a submucosal tear/perforation, ampullary trauma, or if the wire is forcefully advanced into a side branch of the pancreatic duct).

There have been numerous trials that have compared cannulation success rates and complication rates between guidewire cannulation versus traditional contrast-assisted cannulation techniques. Most of the data on this subject favors guidewire cannulation for improvement of cannulation success rates and minimizing complications such as post-ERCP pancreatitis. Several of the studies have also demonstrated decreased cannulation time and decreased fluoroscopy time by using guidewire cannulation instead of traditional contrast-assisted cannulation methods.

An early trial randomized 440 patients to traditional cannulation methods versus guidewire cannulation by a single endoscopist [8]. While both methods demonstrated similar cannulation success rates, there were higher rates of post-ERCP pancreatitis with the traditional cannulation method (eight cases of post-ERCP pancreatitis in the traditional methods group, zero cases of post-ERCP pancreatitis in the guidewire cannulation group).

High rates of deep biliary cannulation success and low rates of complications using guidewire cannulation were demonstrated in a large retrospective review of 822 consecutive ERCP procedures performed by a single, experienced operator [9]. Overall biliary cannulation success rate in this study was 801 of 822 patients (97 %), with 99 % of the successful cannulations performed with a dye-free method. Complications included mild post-ERCP pancreatitis in 11 patients (1.3 %) and guidewire perforation in 11 patients (1.3 %). None of the patients with guidewire perforation required surgery—these patients were treated conservatively with NPO status and antibiotics as needed.

Further positive studies regarding guidewire cannulation were demonstrated in a meta-analysis reviewing seven different randomized controlled trials involving 1383 patients [10]. There were overall increased rates of cannulation success and decreased rates of post-ERCP pancreatitis with guidewire cannulation versus traditional cannulation techniques using contrast-guided methods. The rates of post-ERCP pancreatitis were significantly decreased when guidewire cannulation was used (3.2 % versus 8.7 % with contrast-guided cannulation). However, two crossover studies within this meta-analysis did not demonstrate any significant difference in rates of post-ERCP pancreatitis between the two groups [11, 12].

A large prospective study with 400 patients comparing cannulation with wire-guided techniques versus traditional cannulation techniques showed similar cannulation success rates and similar rates of post-ERCP pancreatitis between the two groups [13]. This study did, however, demonstrate shorter cannulation times and decreased fluoroscopy times with wire-guided cannulation.

Double-Wire Cannulation

Attempts to obtain deep biliary cannulation occasionally result in repeated guidewire entry into the pancreatic duct. If this situation occurs, the endoscopist can consider using double-wire cannulation, also known as the two-wire technique. In this approach, the first wire can remain in place in the pancreatic duct as the sphincterotome is removed and then loaded with a second guidewire. With the first wire in place in the pancreatic duct, biliary cannulation can then be reattempted with the sphincterotome and the second wire (Fig. 1.2). In most cases, having the pancreatic duct wire in place will assist with successful biliary cannulation by helping to identify (both endoscopically and fluoroscopically) the pancreatic orifice and the angle of the pancreatic duct. This information often allows the endoscopist to extrapolate the likely position and angle of the bile duct. Access to the pancreatic duct also facilitates pancreatic duct stent placement during the case if needed.

Numerous studies have demonstrated that leaving a guidewire in the pancreatic duct while performing this technique is effective and, in general, does not lead to increased risk of post-ERCP pancreatitis [8, 14–17]. However, a multicenter randomized trial involving 166 patients demonstrated higher risk of post-ERCP pancreatitis when cannulation was achieved using the double-wire technique in comparison to standard techniques [18]. Given the potential concern of increased rates of post-ERCP pancreatitis when using the two-wire technique, the possibility of placing a prophylactic pancreatic duct stent when this cannulation technique is used has been formally evaluated by single prospective, randomized trial. This study demonstrated the benefit of placing a prophylactic pancreatic duct stent when the two-wire technique is used to decrease the rates of post-ERCP pancreatitis [19]. This trial randomized 70 patient cases in which the two-wire technique was used to obtain deep biliary cannulation to either prophylactic pancreatic stent or no stent and found the frequency of post-ERCP pancreatitis significantly lower in the stent group (2.9 % vs. 23 %, relative risk 0.13, confidence interval 0.016, 0.95). Still, the use of a pancreatic stent in patients undergoing cannulation via the two-wire technique is not universally performed and there is no hard-and-fast requirement for an endoscopist to do so.

Overall, the two-wire technique is thought to be both an effective and safe method for achieving deep biliary cannulation.

Use of a Pancreatic Duct Stent to Achieve Biliary Cannulation

The placement of a pancreatic duct stent to facilitate biliary cannulation has been employed for years and was first described in 1996 [20]. Placement of a pancreatic duct stent

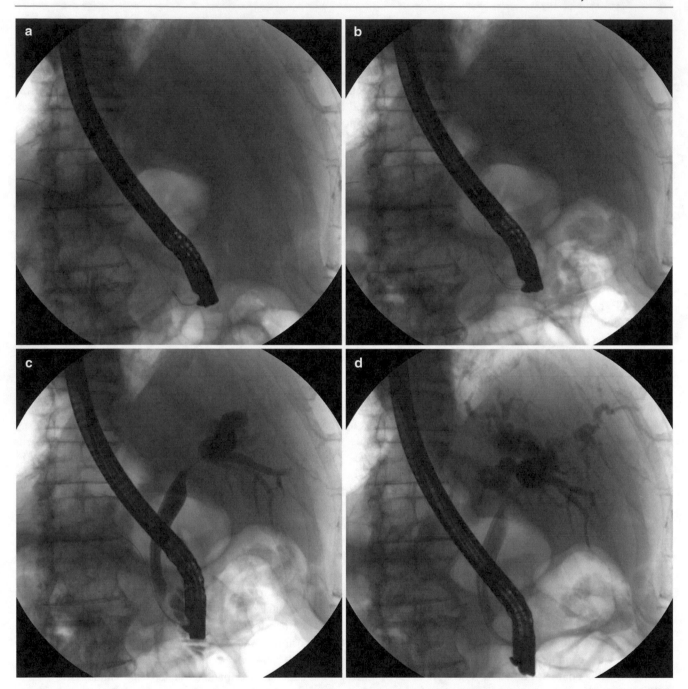

Fig. 1.2 The two-wire technique. (**a**) Fluoroscopic image of cannulation attempt resulting in pancreatic duct access. (**b**) Same patient as (**a**). The pancreatic wire has been left in place and a second wire has been loaded into the sphincterotome with deep biliary access obtained. (**c**) Contrast is injected only after deep biliary cannulation is obtained. Note the common hepatic duct stricture. The pancreatic duct wire is still in place. (**d**) A plastic biliary stent is now in place and the PD wire has been removed. No pancreatogram was obtained during the entire procedure

may not only help reduce rates of post-ERCP pancreatitis in cases where (intended or unintended) guidewire access to the pancreatic duct is obtained, but can also be used to facilitate biliary cannulation.

As with the two-wire technique, having a pancreatic duct stent in place can help straighten the ampulla, provide information about the angle and location of the pancreatic duct, and allow the endoscopist to extrapolate this

information to help determine the likely position and angle of the bile duct (Fig. 1.3).

An early retrospective study examining the success of pancreatic duct stent placement to facilitate biliary cannulation demonstrated successful biliary cannulation in 38 of the 39 patients (97.4 %) in which the technique was attempted [21]. Post-ERCP pancreatitis occurred in two patients and was reported to be mild in both. Of note, 23 patients (59 %)

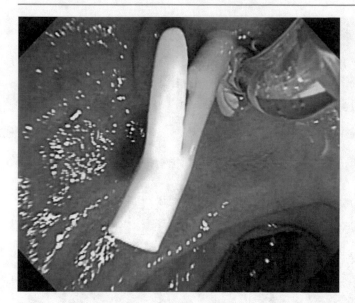

Fig. 1.3 Endoscopic image of biliary cannulation next to a previously placed pancreatic duct stent

in which the technique was successful did require a precut sphincterotomy over the pancreatic duct stent.

A large retrospective study including 2345 patients with native papillary anatomy demonstrated that 76 (4.9 %) cases used pancreatic duct stent placement to help achieve biliary cannulation [22]. Successful biliary cannulation was obtained in 71/76 (93 %) of the cases, with mild pancreatitis developing in only four of these patients (5.3 %). Of note, two of the four patients who developed post-ERCP pancreatitis had the pancreatic duct stent removed at the time of the procedure. The authors stated that the stents in these patients were only placed as an aid to cannulation and were removed after deep biliary access was obtained.

The efficacy of a pancreatic duct stent to facilitate bile duct cannulation was compared with the two-wire technique to facilitate bile duct cannulation in a prospective trial involving 87 patients with native papillary anatomy who were felt to have "difficult cannulations" [23]. The initial bile duct cannulation rates (within a time limit of 6 min) were overall relatively low but similar in both groups with a 38.1 % success rate in the pancreatic duct wire group and 51.9 % in the pancreatic duct stent group ($p=0.18$). If bile duct access was not obtained after 6 min, the endoscopist was allowed to perform precut sphincterotomy or other techniques to obtain cannulation. The overall cannulation success rate was 66.7 % in the pancreatic duct wire group and 90.7 % in the pancreatic stent group with overall complication rates similar between the two groups.

Overall, pancreatic duct stent placement to help facilitate biliary cannulation appears to be an effective technique that can also reduce the risk and severity of post-ERCP pancreatitis. No particular type of pancreatic duct stent (diameter, length, internal flaps versus not) has been demonstrated to be most advantageous for either efficacy or safety [19]. The choice of stent type is typically a preference of the endoscopist.

Biliary Sphincterotomy

Historically ERCP was commonly used as a diagnostic procedure; however noninvasive and less invasive procedures such as MRCP and EUS have replaced ERCP for many indications. Since ERCP in the modern era is primarily a therapeutic procedure, biliary sphincterotomy is a fundamentally important aspect of the procedure and a critical skill to master (Fig. 1.4).

Biliary sphincterotomy is most commonly performed in the context of treatment of choledocholithiasis, bile leaks, the facilitation of bile duct stent placement (in some cases), and cholangioscopy. Biliary sphincterotomy is also performed for the treatment of sphincter of Oddi dysfunction at some centers.

Despite the common practice of performing biliary sphincterotomy prior to placement of a self-expanding metal stent, sphincterotomy is generally not necessary in this situation especially if the stent is being placed in the context of pancreatic cancer, although to do so is not to be considered wrong or a violation of the standard of care.

A retrospective review of 104 subjects undergoing SEMS placement demonstrated technical success in all cases of stent placement without performing sphincterotomy [24]. Post-sphincterotomy bleeding was associated with biliary sphincterotomy prior to SEMS placement ($p=0.001$). Another trial randomized 200 patients with unresectable pancreatic cancer to endoscopic sphincterotomy (ES) or non-ES prior to SEMS placement for malignant biliary obstruction [25]. Results did not show any benefit of ES prior to SEMS placement as ES did not affect the incidence of adverse events (bleeding, perforation, pancreatitis), SEMS patency, or patient survival times.

The primary contraindication to biliary sphincterotomy is the presence of coagulopathy. In patients with known or suspected coagulopathy, coagulation studies should be obtained prior to the procedure and corrected if sphincterotomy is planned. It is not necessary to check coagulation studies in all patients prior to ERCP, although some centers do this routinely. Although biliary sphincterotomy is not believed to increase the risk of bleeding complications in patients taking aspirin, it is generally recommended that antiplatelet agents such as clopidogrel be held for 7 days prior to sphincterotomy. A large prospective case-controlled study involving 308 patients who underwent endoscopic sphincterotomy demonstrated that ASA and NSAIDs did not increase the rates of post-sphincterotomy hemorrhage [26].

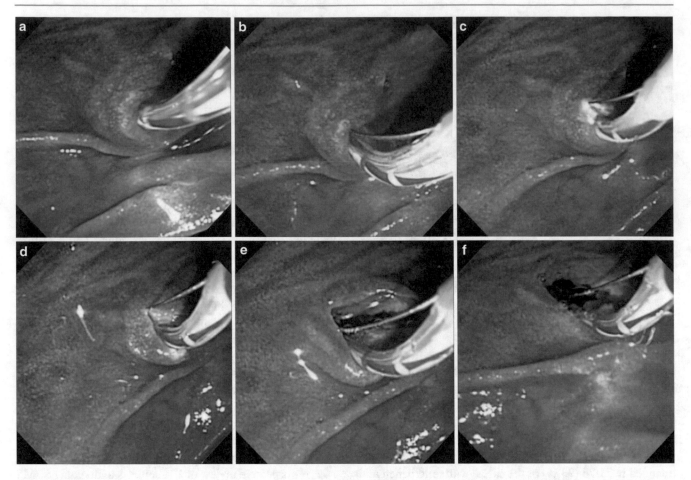

Fig. 1.4 Images (**a**) through (**f**) show the sequence of a typical biliary sphincterotomy. Note the 11 o'clock orientation during the sphincterotomy

Biliary sphincterotomy can be performed by using either pure-cutting current or mixed or blended cutting and coagulation electrosurgical current. Many endoscopists have strong personal preferences regarding current and generator settings used during sphincterotomy based on personal experience.

There have been numerous studies evaluating the effect of different current types on complication rates (pancreatitis, post-sphincterotomy bleeding), and the topic is somewhat controversial. Several early studies demonstrated that pure-cut electrocautery appeared to be safer than blended current, with decreased rates of post-ERCP pancreatitis with pure cut and no difference in bleeding rates [27, 28]. However, a meta-analysis including 804 total patients analyzed complication rates between the two current types and found pure current to be associated with more episodes of bleeding (mostly mild bleeding), with no significant difference in rates of pancreatitis between the two groups [29]. It is fair to say that endoscopists should use a type of current that they are comfortable and familiar with, but that pure cut likely increases the risks of minor GI bleeding.

Precut Papillotomy

The general term "precut" refers to any incision into the ampulla that is made *prior to obtaining deep ductal access with a guidewire*. The term "precut" is thought to originate in 1980 when the method of precut papillotomy with a sphincterotome was described [30]. There is significant confusion in the literature and between physicians regarding interchanging the terms of different types of precut techniques. Some use the term "needle knife sphincterotomy" interchangeably with the term "precut papillotomy" although in practice these may be two very different techniques. The Mayo Clinic Precut Sphincterotomy Classification System has divided the techniques into three categories: precut papillotomy (PP), precut fistulotomy (PF), and transpancreatic precut sphincterotomy (TPS) [31].

It is preferred to obtain selective biliary cannulation with standard techniques such as wire-guided cannulation and possibly use of the two-wire technique or a pancreatic duct stent to help facilitate biliary cannulation. If traditional cannulation techniques fail to achieve selective biliary cannulation, and the patient has an appropriate indication/urgency for biliary or pancreatic access to be obtained, then precut papillotomy is a technique that may be attempted.

In modern practice, most precut papillotomies are performed with a needle knife sphincterotome and not a standard biliary sphincterotome. A typical precut papillotomy is performed by inserting the tip of a needle knife sphincterotome into the upper portion of the papillary orifice and then cutting in the cephalad (upward) direction, tracking along the intraduodenal portion of the common bile duct. Many different techniques to do this simple maneuver exist, with some favoring multiple small incisions while others preferring to make longer, deeper incisions to expedite the process and potentially cause less tissue injury and swelling. Some physicians make shallow cuts while others make deeper cuts; again, the technique is nonstandardized and personal preferences generally dictate practice.

In general, the goal of a precut papillotomy/needle knife sphincterotomy is not to do a complete sphincterotomy, but rather to allow access to the desired duct (usually the common bile duct) (Fig. 1.5). Once access to the desired duct has been obtained and a guidewire has been advanced and deep access established, the needle knife can be exchanged for a standard sphincterotome and the sphincterotomy can be completed in a standard fashion.

All types of precut sphincterotomy are generally regarded as higher risk techniques that should only be performed by an experienced endoscopist (Fig. 1.6). In some situations (cholangitis, a known obstructing stone, clinically significant bile leak, etc.) needle knife sphincterotomy is warranted if standard techniques fail. If the case is more elective in nature, the endoscopist can consider aborting the procedure, asking a colleague for assistance, trying again on a different day, or referring the patient to a tertiary center before performing a precut papillotomy.

Potential complications from precut sphincterotomy include pancreatitis, perforation, hemorrhage, and cholangitis. A patient can develop more than one complication, of note, i.e., perforation and pancreatitis, even in expert hands. The complication rates from precut sphincterotomy do not necessarily decease with the level of experience of the endoscopist. An analysis of 253 consecutive patients undergoing precut sphincterotomy by a single endoscopist demonstrated that although the cannulation success rate increased over time, the complication rate did not decrease [32].

There have been numerous studies demonstrating increased rates of complications with precut sphincterotomy than with traditional cannulation techniques, including cholangitis, perforation, bleeding, and post-ERCP pancreatitis. The increased rates of post-ERCP pancreatitis with precut sphincterotomy may not be related to the technique itself, however, rather the numerous attempts that were made at cannulation prior to attempting precut sphincterotomy. The

multiple cannulation attempts being performed prior to the precut maneuver may have already set the state for, or even caused, an adverse event, i.e., pancreatitis. The trauma from repeated cannulation attempts causes papillary edema which can lead to impaired drainage of the pancreas. Several studies have demonstrated that the increased rates of post-ERCP pancreatitis with precut sphincterotomy are more likely related to the increased number of attempts at cannulation rather than the precut sphincterotomy itself [33, 34].

Precut Fistulotomy (PF)

Precut fistulotomy is an alternative, and equally valid, type of precut technique. This is used most commonly to achieve biliary access. The method typically involves using a needle knife sphincterotome to access the bile duct from a starting point that is above the ampullary orifice. Using the needle knife to dissect the intraduodenal portion of the common bile duct, the operator can proceed in either a caudal or a cephalad direction from the starting point. There is no consensus on which direction is best to choose when performing a precut fistulotomy. The potential advantage of this technique over precut papillotomy is avoiding thermal injury to the pancreatic orifice. As with precut fistulotomy, the goal, in general, is not to perform a complete sphincterotomy but rather to obtain access so that the sphincterotomy can be extended and completed with a standard sphincterotome. That having been said, if the sphincterotomy can be completed with the needle knife sphincterotome, it is not wrong to do so.

Although there have not been many studies comparing the various types of precut sphincterotomy techniques, precut fistulotomy is generally believed to have high rates of technical success and low complication rates when performed by experienced endoscopists. In a study of 88 consecutive patients undergoing precut fistulotomy, deep bile duct cannulation was achieved in 85/88 patients (96.5 %). There was 1 case (1.1 %) of mild post-ERCP pancreatitis [35].

Few studies have directly compared precut papillotomy versus precut fistulotomy. One prospective randomized study of 103 total patients (74 patients in the fistulotomy group, 79 patients in the papillotomy group) comparing the two techniques demonstrated successful bile duct cannulation in 91 % of patients in the precut fistulotomy group and 89 % of patients in the precut papillotomy group [36]. Post-ERCP pancreatitis was found in zero patients in the fistulotomy group and 7.59 % of patients in the papillotomy group ($p < 0.05$), with no difference in rates of other adverse events.

A retrospective comparison of 139 consecutive patients undergoing biliary sphincterotomy using precut techniques analyzed differences in outcomes between three different groups, precut fistulotomy, precut papillotomy, and precut

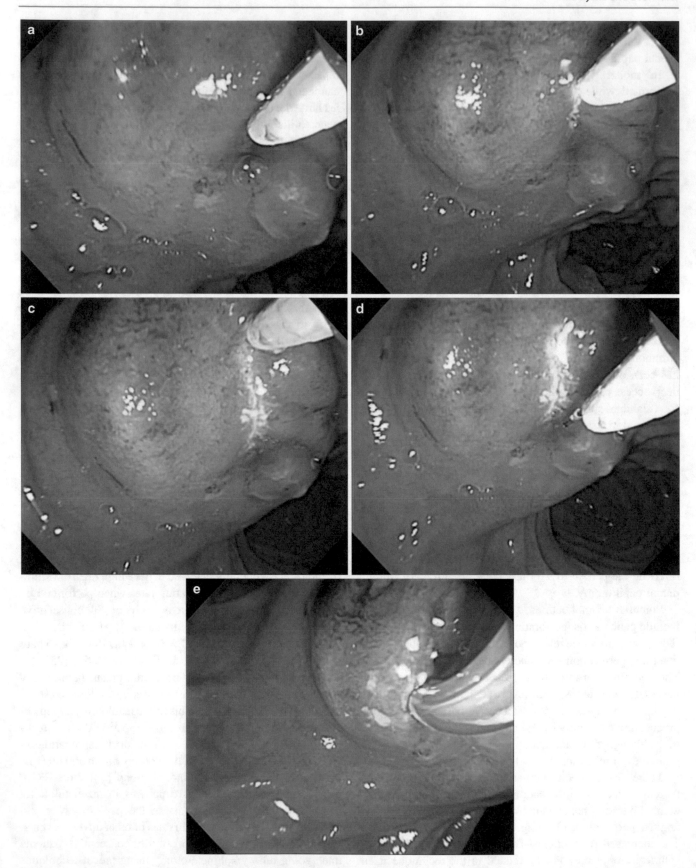

Fig. 1.5 Needle knife sphincterotomy. (**a–d**) Endoscopic series showing a short-segment needle knife sphincterotomy in a patient with an edematous ampulla. (**e**) Deep access to the bile duct is obtained

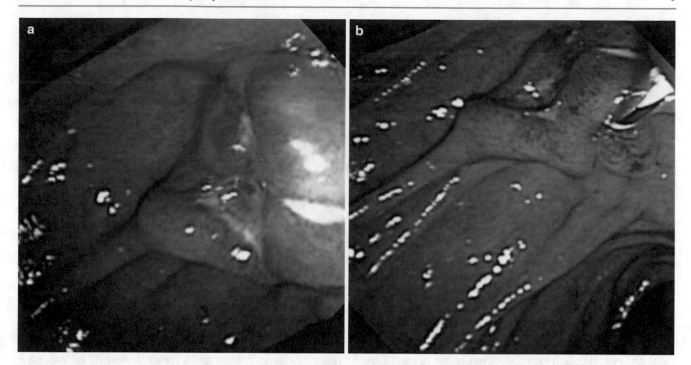

Fig. 1.6 Consequence of failed needle knife sphincterotomy attempt. (**a**) Ulcerated and inflamed major papilla after failed needle knife sphincterotomy attempt referred to our institution for repeat papillotomy with frequent pancreatic duct stent placement ERCP. (**b**) After biliary cannulation is achieved, it is clear that the prior needle knife sphincterotomy attempt was in the wrong tissue plane

[37]. Achieving biliary cannulation was successful in 95.5 %, 95.7 %, and 89.6 % at initial ERCP and 100 %, 97.8 %, and 95.6 % after a second ERCP. The number of complications was not significantly different between the three groups. There was a lower incidence of post-ERCP pancreatitis when a precut fistulotomy was used compared to the other techniques; however this difference was not statistically significant.

Transpancreatic Precut Sphincterotomy

The technique of performing transpancreatic precut sphincterotomy (TPS) to obtain biliary cannulation was initially described by Goff in 1995 [38–40]. In contrast to the two previously described methods of precut sphincterotomy, the TPS is performed with a standard sphincterotome rather than a needle knife sphincterotome. The technique is used to obtain deep biliary access when standard techniques have been unsuccessful. This technique can be particularly useful if repeated attempts at biliary cannulation result in the passage of the guidewire into the pancreatic duct.

With the standard sphincterotome inserted superficially into the pancreatic duct (over a wire deep in the pancreatic duct), the technique is performed by orienting the sphincterotome towards the 11 o'clock position (towards the presumed location of the bile duct) and making an incision through the septum. This should allow trans-septal access to the bile duct. Selective biliary cannulation can then be reattempted with the standard sphincterotome once biliary access has been achieved or a biliary orifice has been created. A potential advantage of this technique over the other types of precut techniques is that it does not require exchange of the standard sphincterotome for a needle knife sphincterotome.

A prospective study of 116 patients undergoing pancreatic precut sphincterotomy after standard cannulation methods failed analyzed success rates and complication rates of this technique [41]. In 85 % of cases (99 out of 116 patients) immediate biliary access was achieved after pancreatic precut sphincterotomy. There were complications in 12 % of cases (14 patients) including post-sphincterotomy bleeding (2.6 %), pancreatitis (8 %; mild in 8 cases, moderate in 1 case), and retroperitoneal perforation (1.7 %; 2 cases, both managed conservatively).

Comparison Between Different Precut Techniques

Several studies have analyzed success rates and complication rates between the different types of precut sphincterotomy techniques. A retrospective review of 2903 consecutive ERCPs with native papillary anatomy was performed in which 283 patients had failed biliary cannulation with standard cannulation techniques and precut techniques were performed [42]. Of the 274 patients included in the final analysis, precut papillotomy was performed in 129 cases (47.1 %), precut fistulotomy in 78 patients (28.5 %), and transpancreatic sphincterotomy in 67 cases (24.5 %). There were no significant differences found between the initial and eventual biliary cannulation success rates. Post-ERCP pancreatitis occurred in 27 cases (20.9 %) in the precut papillotomy group, 2 cases (2.6 %) in the precut fistulotomy group, and 15 cases (22.4 %) in the transpancreatic sphincterotomy group, with the difference statistically favoring the PF group. The overall rates of post-ERCP pancreatitis are higher than typically expected; however they are unusually low in the precut fistulotomy group. A possible explanation for the low rates of pancreatitis in this group is not introducing thermal injury at the level of the papilla.

It has been suggested that early precut sphincterotomy, rather than prolonged cannulation attempts using standard techniques, may help reduce rates of post-ERCP pancreatitis [43]. A meta-analysis of six randomized controlled trials with a total of 966 subjects compared cannulation success rates and complication rates between the use of early precut attempts (using a variety of different techniques) and persistent standard techniques [42]. The definition of "early precut" varied somewhat between the six different trials and ranged from immediate precut attempted to a range of 5–12 min of attempted cannulation using standard techniques prior to attempting a precut technique. Several of the trials also performed precut if there were three unintended pancreatic duct cannulations performed—a relatively low number, especially if dye-free guidewire cannulation techniques are employed. Overall cannulation success rates were 90 % in both groups (OR 1.20; 95 % CI 0.54–2.69). Post-ERCP pancreatitis occurred in 2.5 % of patients in the early precut group and 5.3 % in the persistent attempt group (OR 0.47; 95 % CI 0.24–0.91). The overall complication rates were similar, 5.0 % in the early precut group and 6.3 % in the persistent attempt group (OR 0.78; 95 % CI 0.44–1.37). Although it would be helpful to have further studies on this topic, this data suggests that if standard cannulation techniques are not successful within a short period of time, it may be advisable to proceed with a precut technique.

Cannulation and Sphincterotomy in Patients with Billroth II Anatomy

The classic Billroth II operation consists of an antrectomy and creation of a gastrojejunostomy with an end-to-side anastomosis with an afferent limb (leading to the major and minor papillas) and an efferent limb (leading to the distal small bowel). Now rarely performed, the operation was once in widespread use, mostly to treat peptic ulcer disease. In patients with Billroth II anatomy, the major papilla is located within the afferent limb at or near the end of the duodenal stump. Most patients with Billroth II anatomy have a major papilla that is endoscopically accessible. In rare cases, the afferent limb is too long to be easily reached or the gastrojejunostomy and/or the small bowel limbs are too severely angulated to allow endoscope passage to the ampulla. Patients with Billroth II anatomy present numerous different challenges to performing a successful ERCP.

Either a duodenoscope or a straight-viewing endoscope (typically a colonoscope, an enteroscope, or a balloon-enteroscope) can be used to perform ERCP in patients with Billroth II anatomy, although it is the author's preference to use a duodenoscope when possible given the advantages the elevator provides during the procedure. Advantages to using a colonoscope, enteroscope, etc., include forward viewing during intubation of the gastrojejunostomy and the afferent limb, while disadvantages include a lack of an elevator, limited accessories, and limited ability to orient a sphincterotome.

A prospective, randomized trial compared the success rates and complication rates between the use of a side-viewing duodenoscope and a forward-viewing endoscope in 45 patients with Billroth II anatomy who required ERCP with sphincterotomy [44]. Cannulation success rates were 68 % (15 of 22 patients) in the duodenoscope group and 87 % (20 of 23 patients) in the forward-viewing endoscope group. The cannulation failures in the duodenoscope group resulted in more serious complications including jejunum perforation during insertion ($n=4$), long afferent loop ($n=1$), severe abdominal pain during procedure ($n=1$), and failure to enter the afferent loop ($n=1$), while cannulation failures in the front-viewing endoscope group included long afferent loop ($n=2$) and inability to cannulate despite reaching the papilla ($n=1$). Successful sphincterotomy was performed in 80 % of the patients in the duodenoscope group and 83 % of the patients in the forward-viewing endoscope group.

Identification of the afferent limb from the efferent limb can sometimes present a challenge. The afferent limb can be attached to the stomach on either the greater or the lesser curvature; thus it may not be apparent prior to traversing each lumen to discover which the desired limb is. Often, a trial-and-error approach is undertaken (regardless of endoscope type selected) in evaluating the two limbs and working to identify the afferent limb. Depending on the angulation of the entry, the afferent limb may be difficult to traverse with any endoscope.

In patients with Billroth II anatomy, the endoscopic image of the ampulla is inverted compared to the view in patients with normal anatomy. Thus, the bile duct orifice is typically found at approximately the 5 o'clock position on the ampullary face. If a duodenoscope is utilized, the major papilla is typically found near the 12 o'clock position of the duodenum. The duodenoscope should then be withdrawn away from the major papilla as this position favors bile duct cannulation. The middle distance is still favored in this situation. With the lumen of the small intestine in view straight ahead, the bile duct typically angles straight ahead/ slightly to the right.

The choice of cannulation device is dependent on the preference of the endoscopist and a straight biliary catheter, a catheter bent into an S shape, an inverted standard sphincterotome, or a Billroth II papillotome are typically used. The Billroth II papillotome (Cook Medical, Inc., Winston Salem, NC) is designed with the cutting wire oriented in the opposite direction of a standard sphincterotome. As mentioned above, most commercial sphincterotomes, especially ones designed to rotate, can be spun into an inverted position for both cannulation and sphincterotomy (Fig. 1.7).

Biliary sphincterotomy can be accomplished in Billroth II patients by many techniques. When using a Billroth II papillotome or an inverted sphincterotome, it should be recognized that since the cut is being performed in the inverted position, a modification of standard techniques is required. This usually involves relaxation of the elevator and slight insertion of the endoscope during the actual

sphincterotomy as compared to tension on the elevator accompanied by a small withdrawal as would be performed in normal anatomy.

Another option is to perform the sphincterotomy with a needle knife sphincterotome over a previously placed biliary stent. A straight plastic biliary stent is inserted in the bile duct over a wire. A sphincterotomy can then subsequently be performed using a needle knife sphincterotome, guiding the direction of the incision based on the location of the stent. The biliary stent can then be removed and the procedure completed.

A Billroth II papillotome can be used to perform biliary sphincterotomy. If this papillotome is used, the device is pushed forward over the guidewire, and then the papilla is cut along the 5–6 o'clock position.

Performing biliary sphincterotomy is technically challenging in patients with Billroth II anatomy compared with patients with normal anatomy, and may be associated with increased risks. A randomized trial including 34 patients with retained bile duct stones and prior Billroth II gastrectomy were randomized to either endoscopic sphincterotomy or endoscopic balloon

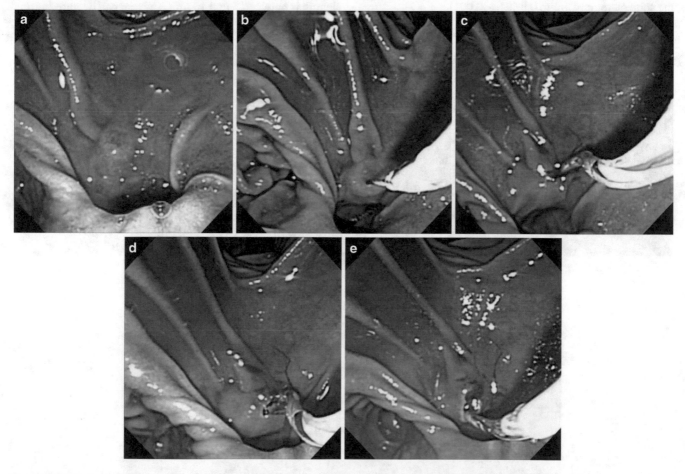

Fig. 1.7 Sphincterotomy using an inverted sphincterotome in a patient with Billroth II anatomy. (**a**) Ampulla in a patient with Billroth II anatomy next to a duodenal diverticulum. (**b**) Deep biliary access is obtained using Single Wire Technique #2. (**c–e**) Biliary sphincterotomy is performed using an inverted sphincterotome

dilation [45]. The patients in the endoscopic sphincterotomy group underwent sphincterotomy with a needle knife sphincterotome after placement of a biliary stent. Three patients in the endoscopic balloon group had early complications (two with fever, one with mild pancreatitis) in comparison with seven patients (three with bleeding, two with fever, one with perforation, one with respiratory complications) in the endoscopic sphincterotomy group ($p=0.27$). In comparison to patients with normal anatomy, patients with prior Billroth II gastrectomy had significantly increased risk of bleeding after endoscopic sphincterotomy (17 % versus 2 %, RR$=7.25$, $p<0.05$).

Of note, endoscopic papillary balloon dilation without first performing a biliary sphincterotomy is no longer a standard practice in the West. This is primarily based on a controlled, multicenter study of 237 patients randomized to either papillary balloon dilation or sphincterotomy (117 patients in the dilation group, 120 patients in the sphincterotomy group) for indication of choledocholithiasis [46]. The rates of overall morbidity were 17.9 % in the balloon group and 3.3 % in the sphincterotomy group ($p<0.001$). There were also two deaths in the balloon group and none in the sphincterotomy group. The rate of pancreatitis in the balloon group was 15.4 % and in the sphincterotomy group 0.8 % ($p<0.001$).

Pancreatic Sphincterotomy

Although not performed as frequently as biliary sphincterotomy, there are numerous reasons to perform pancreatic sphincterotomy and it is important to be familiar with the potential indications and available endoscopic techniques.

Potential indications for pancreatic sphincterotomy include removal of pancreatic stones in patients with chronic pancreatitis, treatment of a pancreatic pseudocyst with transpapillary drainage, treatment of pancreatic strictures secondary to either benign or malignant disease, and treatment of pancreatic sphincter of Oddi dysfunction.

There are two primary methods of performing pancreatic sphincterotomy: use of a standard sphincterotome and the use of a needle knife over a previously placed pancreatic duct stent. When using a standard sphincterotome, the guidewire is first inserted into the main pancreatic duct with placement typically confirmed by performing a limited or complete pancreatogram. The sphincterotome is then used to make an incision with similar technique as a biliary sphincterotomy except directed towards the right to the 1–2 o'clock position (Fig. 1.8). The typical incision length is between 5 and 10 mm. Current can be pure-cutting

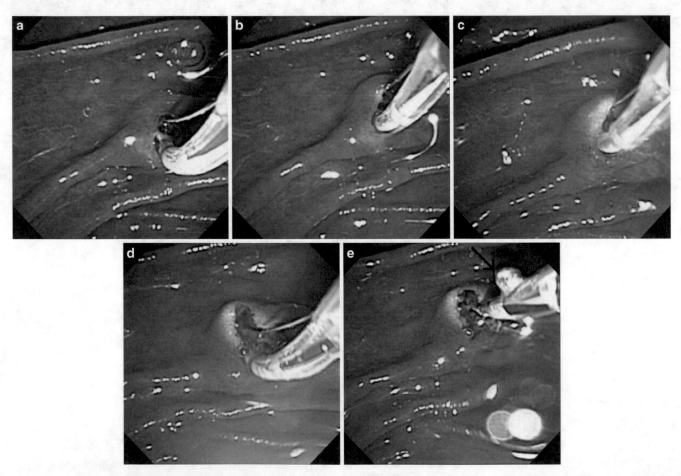

Fig. 1.8 Pancreatic sphincterotomy. (**a**) 1 o'clock orientation for a typical pancreatic sphincterotomy in a patient with chronic pancreatitis. (**b–d**) Series of images demonstrating a typical pancreatic sphincterot-

omy. Note the difference in orientation from a biliary sphincterotomy. (**e**) After the pancreatic sphincterotomy is complete, a pancreatic duct stone (*arrow*) spontaneously passes to the duodenum current or mixed current. Typically a pancreatic duct stent is placed following pancreatic sphincterotomy to help prevent pancreatitis from the edema following pancreatic sphincterotomy, although this is not a universal practice.

An alternative technique to performing pancreatic sphincterotomy is to initially place a pancreatic duct stent and perform a needle knife sphincterotomy over the stent. After placement of a pancreatic duct stent, a needle knife sphincterotome is used to make an incision along the plane of the pancreatic sphincter, using the stent as a guide. As with the sphincterotome technique, the length of the incision is usually between 5 and 10 mm.

There are also variations in opinion of which sphincterotomy technique to use. A survey of 14 expert endoscopists at nine different US centers demonstrated that six of the endoscopists "always" or "often" use the sphincterotome technique, while seven "always" or "often" use the needle knife over the stent technique [47]. Eight of the 14 physicians always performed biliary sphincterotomy prior to attempting pancreatic sphincterotomy and almost all endoscopists placed a pancreatic duct stent after sphincterotomy. Overall, there is no consensus on which type of pancreatic stent to use and how long to leave it in place.

Potential early complications from pancreatic sphincterotomy are similar to those secondary to biliary sphincterotomy and include bleeding, pancreatitis, and perforation. Possible late complications (>3 months) from pancreatic sphincterotomy include proximal pancreatic duct strictures and papillary stenosis.

Conclusion

Mastering selective biliary cannulation and sphincterotomy is an essential component of performing successful ERCP. If selective biliary cannulation is unsuccessful using traditional techniques, there are numerous alternative methods to help achieve cannulation that the advanced endoscopist should be familiar with. Since ERCP has transitioned from a diagnostic procedure historically to primarily a therapeutic procedure in the modern area, sphincterotomy is a vital aspect of the procedure and a critical skill to master.

Video Legend

Video 1.1 The accompanying video to this chapter demonstrates a variety of cannulation and sphincterotomy techniques in the setting of both normal and challenging anatomic variants.

References

1. Williams EJ, Ogollah R, Thomas P, Logan RF, Martin D, Wilkinson ML, Lombard M. What predicts failed cannulation and therapy at ERCP? Results of a large-scale multicenter analysis. Endoscopy. 2012;44(7):674–83.

2. Schwacha H, Allgaier HP, Deibert P, Olschewski M, Allgaier U, Blum HE. A sphincterotome-based technique for selective transpapillary common bile duct cannulation. Gastrointest Endosc. 2000;52(3):387–91.

3. Cortas GA, Mehta SN, Abraham NS, Barkun AN. Selective cannulation of the common bile duct: a prospective randomized trial comparing standard catheters with sphincterotomes. Gastrointest Endosc. 1999;50(6):775–9.

4. Karamanolis G, Katsikani A, Viazis N, Stefanidis G, Manolakopoulos S, Sgouros S, Papadopoulou E, Mantides A. A prospective cross-over study using a sphincterotome and a guidewire to increase the success rate of common bile duct cannulation. World J Gastroenterol. 2005;11(11):1649–52.

5. Laasch HU, Tringali A, Wilbraham L, Marriott A, England RE, Mutignani M, Perri V, Costamagna G, Martin DF. Comparison of standard and steerable catheters for bile duct cannulation in ERCP. Endoscopy. 2003;35(8):669–74.

6. Halttunen J, Kylänpää L. A prospective randomized study of thin versus regular-sized guide wire in wire-guided cannulation. Surg Endosc. 2013;27(5):1662–7.

7. Verma D, Gostout CJ, Petersen BT, Levy MJ, Baron TH, Adler DG. Establishing a true assessment of endoscopic competence in ERCP during training and beyond: a single-operator learning curve for deep biliary cannulation in patients with native papillary anatomy. Gastrointest Endosc. 2007;65(3):394–400.

8. Lella F, Bagnolo F, Colombo E, Bonassi U. A simple way of avoiding post-ERCP pancreatitis. Gastrointest Endosc. 2004;59(7):830–4.

9. Adler DG, Verma D, Hilden K, Chadha R, Thomas K. Dye-free wire-guided cannulation of the biliary tree during ERCP is associated with high success and low complication rates: outcomes in a single operator experience of 822 cases. J Clin Gastroenterol. 2010;44(3):e57–62.

10. Cheung J, Tsoi KK, Quan WL, Lau JY, Sung JJ. Guidewire versus conventional contrast cannulation of the common bile duct for the prevention of post-ERCP pancreatitis: a systematic review and meta-analysis. Gastrointest Endosc. 2009;70(6):1211–9.

11. Bailey AA, Bourke MJ, Williams SJ, Walsh PR, Murray MA, Lee EY, Kwan V, Lynch PM. A prospective randomized trial of cannulation technique in ERCP: effects on technical success and post-ERCP pancreatitis. Endoscopy. 2008;40(4):296–301.

12. Katsinelos P, Paroutoglou G, Kountouras J, Chatzimavroudis G, Zavos C, Pilpilidis I, Tzelas G, Tzovaras G. A comparative study of standard ERCP catheter and hydrophilic guide wire in the selective cannulation of the common bile duct. Endoscopy. 2008;40(4):302–7.

13. Kawakami H, Maguchi H, Mukai T, Hayashi T, Sasaki T, Isayama H, Nakai Y, Yasuda I, Irisawa A, Niido T, Okabe Y, Ryozawa S, Itoi T, Hanada K, Kikuyama M, Arisaka Y, Kikuchi S, Japan Bile Duct Cannulation Study Group. A multicenter, prospective, randomized study of selective bile duct cannulation performed by multiple endoscopists: the BIDMEN study. Gastrointest Endosc. 2012; 75(2):362–72.

14. Maeda S, Hayashi H, Hosokawa O, Dohden K, Hattori M, Morita M, Kidani E, Ibe N, Tatsumi S. Prospective randomized pilot trial of selective biliary cannulation using pancreatic guide-wire placement. Endoscopy. 2003;35(9):721–4.

15. Draganov P, Devonshire DA, Cunningham JT. A new technique to assist in difficult bile duct cannulation at the time of endoscopic retrograde cholangiopancreatography. JSLS. 2005;9(2):218–21.

16. Belverde B, Frattaroli S, Carbone A, Viceconte G. Double guide-wire technique for ERCP in difficult bile cannulation: experience with 121 cases. Ann Ital Chir. 2012;83(5):391–3.

17. Kramer RE, Azuaje RE, Martinez JM, Dunkin BJ. The double-wire technique as an aid to selective cannulation of the common bile duct during pediatric endoscopic retrograde cholangiopancreatography. J Pediatr Gastroenterol Nutr. 2007;45(4):438–42.

18. Herreros de Tejada A, Calleja JL, Díaz G, Pertejo V, Espinel J, Cacho G, Jiménez J, Millán I, García F, Abreu L, UDOGUIA-04

Group. Double-guidewire technique for difficult bile duct cannulation: a multicenter randomized, controlled trial. Gastrointest Endosc. 2009;70(4):700–9.

19. Ito K, Fujita N, Noda Y, Kobayashi G, Obana T, Horaguchi J, Takasawa O, Koshita S, Kanno Y, Ogawa T. Can pancreatic duct stenting prevent post-ERCP pancreatitis in patients who undergo pancreatic duct guidewire placement for achieving selective biliary cannulation? A prospective randomized controlled trial. J Gastroenterol. 2010;45(11):1183–91.

20. Slivka A. A new technique to assist in bile duct cannulation. Gastrointest Endosc. 1996;44(5):636.

21. Goldberg E, Titus M, Haluszka O, Darwin P. Pancreatic-duct stent placement facilitates difficult common bile duct cannulation. Gastrointest Endosc. 2005;62(4):592–6.

22. Coté GA, Ansstas M, Pawa R, Edmundowicz SA, Jonnalagadda SS, Pleskow DK, Azar RR. Difficult biliary cannulation: use of physician-controlled wire-guided cannulation over a pancreatic duct stent to reduce the rate of precut sphincterotomy (with video). Gastrointest Endosc. 2010;71(2):275–9.

23. Coté GA, Mullady DK, Jonnalagadda SS, Keswani RN, Wani SB, Hovis CE, Ammar T, Al-Lehibi A, Edmundowicz SA, Komanduri S, Azar RR. Use of a pancreatic duct stent or guidewire facilitates bile duct access with low rates of precut sphincterotomy: a randomized clinical trial. Dig Dis Sci. 2012;57(12):3271–8.

24. Banerjee N, Hilden K, Baron TH, Adler DG. Endoscopic biliary sphincterotomy is not required for transpapillary SEMS placement for biliary obstruction. Dig Dis Sci. 2011;56(2):591–5.

25. Hayashi T, Kawakami H, Osanai M, Ishiwatari H, Naruse H, Hisai H, Yanagawa N, Kaneto H, Koizumi K, Sakurai T, Sonoda T. No benefit of endoscopic sphincterotomy before biliary placement of self-expandable metal stents for unresectable pancreatic cancer. Clin Gastroenterol Hepatol. 2015;13(6):1151–8.e2.

26. Onal IK, Parlak E, Akdogan M, Yesil Y, Kuran SO, Kurt M, Disibeyaz S, Ozturk E, Odemis B. Do aspirin and non-steroidal anti-inflammatory drugs increase the risk of post-sphincterotomy hemorrhage--a case-control study. Clin Res Hepatol Gastroenterol. 2013;37(2):171–6.

27. Elta GH, Barnett JL, Wille RT, et al. Pure cut electrocautery current for sphincterotomy causes less post-procedure pancreatitis than blended current. Gastrointest Endosc. 1998;47:149–53.

28. Stefanidis G, Karamanolis G, Viazis N, et al. A comparative study of postendoscopic sphincterotomy complications with various types of electrosurgical current in patients with choledocholithiasis. Gastrointest Endosc. 2003;57:192–7.

29. Verma D, Kapadia A, Adler DG. Pure versus mixed electrosurgical current for endoscopic biliary sphincterotomy: a meta-analysis of adverse outcomes. Gastrointest Endosc. 2007;66(2):283–90.

30. Siegel JH. Precut papillotomy: a method to improve success of ERCP and papillotomy. Endoscopy. 1980;12(3):130–3.

31. Davee T, Garcia JA, Baron TH. Precut sphincterotomy for selective biliary duct cannulation during endoscopic retrograde cholangiopancreatography. Ann Gastroenterol. 2012;25(4):291–302.

32. Harewood GC, Baron TH. An assessment of the learning curve for precut biliary sphincterotomy. Am J Gastroenterol. 2002;97(7):1708–12.

33. Bailey AA, Bourke MJ, Kaffes AJ, Byth K, Lee EY, Williams SJ. Needle-knife sphincterotomy: factors predicting its use and the relationship with post-ERCP pancreatitis (with video). Gastrointest Endosc. 2010;71(2):266–71.

34. Manes G, Di Giorgio P, Repici A, Macarri G, Ardizzone S, Porro GB. An analysis of the factors associated with the development of complications in patients undergoing precut sphincterotomy: a prospective, controlled, randomized, multicenter study. Am J Gastroenterol. 2009;104(10):2412–7.

35. Ayoubi M, Sansoè G, Leone N, Castellino F. Comparison between needle-knife fistulotomy and standard cannulation in ERCP. World J Gastrointest Endosc. 2012;4(9):398–404.

36. Mavrogiannis C, Liatsos C, Romanos A, Petoumenos C, Nakos A, Karvountzis G. Needle-knife fistulotomy versus needle-knife precut papillotomy for the treatment of common bile duct stones. Gastrointest Endosc. 1999;50(3):334–9.

37. Abu-Hamda EM, Baron TH, Simmons DT, Petersen BT. A retrospective comparison of outcomes using three different precut needle knife techniques for biliary cannulation. J Clin Gastroenterol. 2005;39(8):717–21.

38. Goff JS. Long-term experience with the transpancreatic sphincter pre-cut approach to biliary sphincterotomy. Gastrointest Endosc. 1999;50(5):642–5.

39. Goff JS. Common bile duct pre-cut sphincterotomy: transpancreatic sphincter approach. Gastrointest Endosc. 1995;41(5):502–5.

40. Akashi R, Kiyozumi T, Jinnouchi K, Yoshida M, Adachi Y, Sagara K. Pancreatic sphincter precutting to gain selective access to the common bile duct: a series of 172 patients. Endoscopy. 2004;36(5):405–10.

41. Kahaleh M, Tokar J, Mullick T, Bickston SJ, Yeaton P. Prospective evaluation of pancreatic sphincterotomy as a precut technique for biliary cannulation. Clin Gastroenterol Hepatol. 2004; 2(11):971–7.

42. Katsinelos P, Gkagkalis S, Chatzimavroudis G, Beltsis A, Terzoudis S, Zavos C, Gatopoulou A, Lazaraki G, Vasiliadis T, Kountouras J. Comparison of three types of precut technique to achieve common bile duct cannulation: a retrospective analysis of 274 cases. Dig Dis Sci. 2012;57(12):3286–92.

43. Cennamo V, Fuccio L, Zagari RM, Eusebi LH, Ceroni L, Laterza L, Fabbri C, Bazzoli F. Can early precut implementation reduce endoscopic retrograde cholangiopancreatography-related complication risk? Meta-analysis of randomized controlled trials. Endoscopy. 2010;42(5):381–8.

44. Kim MH, Lee SK, Lee MH, Myung SJ, Yoo BM, Seo DW, Min YI. Endoscopic retrograde cholangiopancreatography and needle-knife sphincterotomy in patients with Billroth II gastrectomy: a comparative study of the forward-viewing endoscope and the side-viewing duodenoscope. Endoscopy. 1997;29(2):82–5.

45. Bergman JJ, van Berkel AM, Bruno MJ, Fockens P, Rauws EA, Tijssen JG, Tytgat GN, Huibregtse K. A randomized trial of endoscopic balloon dilation and endoscopic sphincterotomy for removal of bile duct stones in patients with a prior Billroth II gastrectomy. Gastrointest Endosc. 2001;53(1):19–26.

46. Disario JA, Freeman ML, Bjorkman DJ, Macmathuna P, Petersen BT, Jaffe PE, Morales TG, Hixson LJ, Sherman S, Lehman GA, Jamal MM, Al-Kawas FH, Khandelwal M, Moore JP, Derfus GA, Jamidar PA, Ramirez FC, Ryan ME, Woods KL, Carr-Locke DL, Alder SC. Endoscopic balloon dilation compared with sphincterotomy for extraction of bile duct stones. Gastroenterology. 2004;127(5):1291–9.

47. Alsolaiman M, Cotton P, Hawes R, et al. Techniques of pancreatic sphincterotomy: lack of expert consensus. Gastrointest Endosc. 2004;59:AB210.

Endoscopic Management of Large and Difficult Common Bile duct Stones

Thomas Queen and Gulshan Parasher

Introduction

Cholelithiasis or gallstone disease affects over 20 million people in the United States at an annual cost of 6.2 billion dollars [1–3]. In addition, cholelithiasis and complications related to cholelithiasis necessitate surgical intervention in a large number of patients with approximately 700,000 cholecystectomies performed annually [4, 5]. Amongst those individuals, who undergo cholecystectomy for symptomatic gallbladder disease, approximately 10–15 % are found to have common bile duct stones (choledocholithiasis) [4, 5]. This translates to 70,000–100,000 patients per year requiring further intervention for biliary stones, many of whom will require more than one treatment [4, 5].

Biliary sphincterotomy and stone extraction by ERCP have traditionally been the standard treatment for most patients with common bile duct (CBD) stones [6–8]. Following endoscopic biliary sphincterotomy, approximately 85–90 % of biliary stones can be extracted successfully using a simple balloon catheter or stone retrieval basket [9, 10]. However, in approximately 10–15 % of patients, extraction of bile duct stones by ERCP may be challenging [5]. Difficulties with stone extraction in these patients may be related to large bile duct stones, impacted stones (Fig. 2.1a–d), intrahepatic stones, associated biliary strictures, and challenging access due to surgically altered anatomy (Table 2.1) [5, 6, 10].

Electronic supplementary material: The online version of this chapter (doi:10.1007/978-3-319-26854-5_2) contains supplementary material, which is available to authorized users. Videos can also be accessed at http://link.springer.com/chapter/10.1007/978-3-319-26854-5_2

T. Queen, M.D.
Division of Gastroenterology & Hepatology, University of New Mexico School of Medicine, Albuquerque, NM, USA

G. Parasher, M.D. (✉)
Division of Gastroenterology & Hepatology, Department of Medicine, University of New Mexico School of Medicine, Albuquerque, NM, USA
e-mail: gparasher@salud.unm.edu

The patient's overall medical condition often also poses challenges for biliary stone extraction [10].

This chapter describes management of large and difficult common bile duct stones, review of existing literature along with description of various techniques such as mechanical lithotripsy, electrohydraulic lithotripsy, laser lithotripsy, extracorporeal shock wave lithotripsy (ESWL), and endoscopic papillary balloon dilation-assisted stone removal.

Endoscopic Approaches to Large and Difficult Biliary Stones

Biliary stones can range from 1 mm to greater than 30 mm in diameter; however stones as large as 7 cm have been described in patients with a markedly dilated CBD (Fig. 2.2) [6, 11]. Stones measuring less than 10 mm in diameter are commonly removed intact using balloon and/or stone retrieval basket, after endoscopic biliary sphincterotomy [6, 10]. The rate of successful extraction of biliary stones decreases with increasing stone size [10]. In order to reduce the risk of stone impaction, biliary stones with a diameter greater than 20 mm usually require fragmentation prior to removal [11, 12].

If conventional methods for stone extraction fail, mechanical lithotripsy, electrohydraulic lithotripsy, laser lithotripsy, extracorporeal shock wave lithotripsy, and endoscopic large papillary balloon dilation (used alone or in combination) have been shown to improve the success rate in large biliary stone extraction. Surgical removal of large stones by open common bile duct exploration is rarely required.

In general, identification of patients with large and difficult stones prior to attempting stone extraction is helpful in achieving higher success rate and minimizing unnecessary complications. When treating patients with large common bile duct stones, we adhere to several core principles:

1. Attempts should be made to review prior patient imaging studies and prior endoscopic records including transabdominal ultrasound, magnetic resonance cholangiopan-

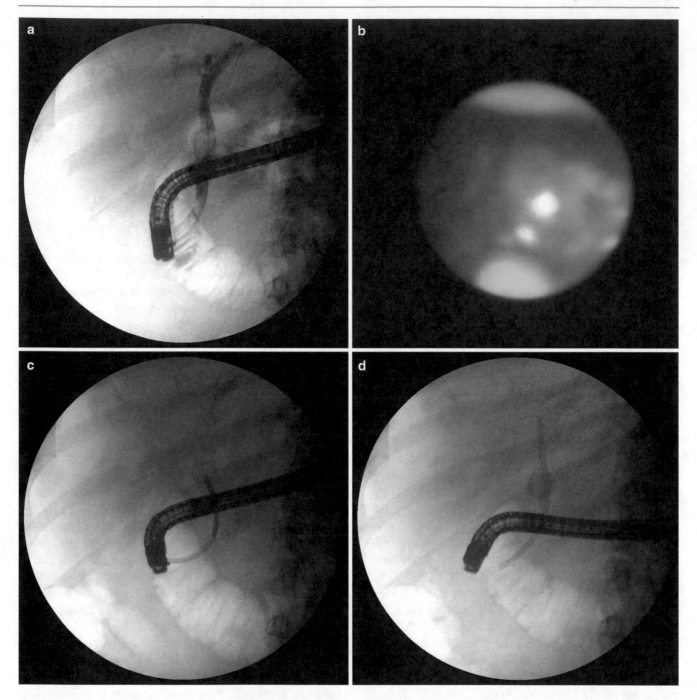

Fig. 2.1 Representative difficult common bile duct stone. (**a**) Cholangiogram showing a large, tightly impacted stone in the mid-common bile duct. A balloon catheter and basket could not be advanced proximal to the stone to retrieve it. (**b**) Cholangioscopic view of laser lithotripsy to fragment the stone from below. (**c**) A tunnel was created through the stone using holmium laser. (**d**) A plastic stent was placed through the tunnel with the intention of a repeat procedure few weeks later

creatography (MRCP), endoscopic ultrasound (EUS), and endoscopic retrograde cholangiopancreatography (ERCP) results. This is helpful in reviewing the anatomy, planning the procedure, achieving higher success rates, and meeting patient expectations. In the case of patients who have undergone prior ERCP without success, it is often helpful to see what maneuvers have been previously utilized in an attempt to clear the duct of stones.

2. If local expertise for above-mentioned techniques is not available, referring these cases to a tertiary center with expert pancreaticobiliary endoscopists should be considered, especially in nonemergent cases.

Table 2.1 Difficult CBD stones

1. Large size >15 mm
2. Multiple large stones >10, stacked stones in nondilated duct
3. Impacted and adherent stones
4. Unusual shape
5. Stones proximal to strictures
6. Unusual locations—intrahepatic stones, cystic duct stones, stones in bile duct diverticulum
7. Anatomical alterations Large periampullary diverticulum Sigmoid shaped and narrow distal CBD with large stone Postsurgical anatomy—Billroth 2 anatomy and Roux-en-Y gastrojejunostomy and gastric bypass surgery

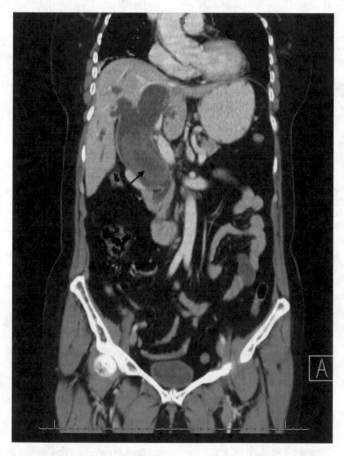

Fig. 2.2 CT scan image of a 7 cm long stone (*arrow*) identified in a very dilated common bile duct

3. Performing an informed consent that includes a detailed description of techniques, potential adverse events, expected outcomes, and the possible need for requirement for repeat procedures.
4. General anesthesia (GA) is generally used for ERCPs involving difficult stone extraction.
5. Finally, it is important to perform procedure with well-trained nurses and ancillary staff familiar with the equipment and technical aspects of the procedure.

Endoscopic Techniques for Management of Large and Difficult Biliary Stones

Mechanical Lithotripsy (ML)

First described by Riemann et al. in 1982, ML has been used to fragment large or difficult to remove biliary stones in order to facilitate easy extraction from the bile duct [12, 13]. ML has become one of the most common techniques for stone fragmentation since it is easily available, economical, and relatively simple to perform [3, 6, 10]. Removal of intact stones up to 3 cm can be achieved when an adequate biliary sphincterotomy is performed and a mixed stone retrieval/lithotripsy device such as a Trapezoid stone basket (Boston Scientific, Natick, MA, USA) is used (Fig. 2.3). Many stones cannot be removed intact and require some form of lithotripsy. The most commonly performed technique is mechanical lithotripsy.

A mechanical lithotripter is comprised of a wire basket, metal sheath, and crank/handle which enables mechanical retraction of the wire basket into the metal sheath [13]. In general, there are two different designs of mechanical lithotripters: devices that can be passed through the endoscope ("through-the-scope") and devices that can be used only after the endoscope has been removed from the patient (out-of-the-scope or salvage device) [11, 13]. The type of lithotripter used depends on whether the procedure is performed on an elective basis or emergent basis for basket impaction [11].

The through-the-scope lithotripter (Fig. 2.4a, b) is comprised of an integrated three-layer system with a large basket, inner plastic sheath, and outer metal sheath that is inserted through the accessory channel in the duodenoscope [5, 14]. Initial cannulation of the bile duct and subsequent stone capture are performed by using the plastic sheath and basket [14]. After the stone is captured within the basket, the metal sheath is then gradually advanced to the level of the stone [5, 11]. The handle is then used to apply tension to the wires resulting in tightening of the basket wires by mechanical retraction [14]. The force of the mechanical retraction generated by the crank handle crushes the captured stone within the basket (Fig. 2.4c) [14].

In the context of biliary stone extraction, the term "impaction" refers to the inability for a stone/basket complex to be removed from the duct (usually due to distal stones or strictures or an insufficiently large biliary sphincterotomy). Sometimes a stone can be captured but not completely crushed, resulting in a stone that is now "trapped" inside the basket and cannot be released.

Biliary stone and/or basket impaction is rare, although this can occur even during routine extraction of smaller biliary stones [11, 14]. An impacted stone/basket complex represents an urgent situation, and several techniques and

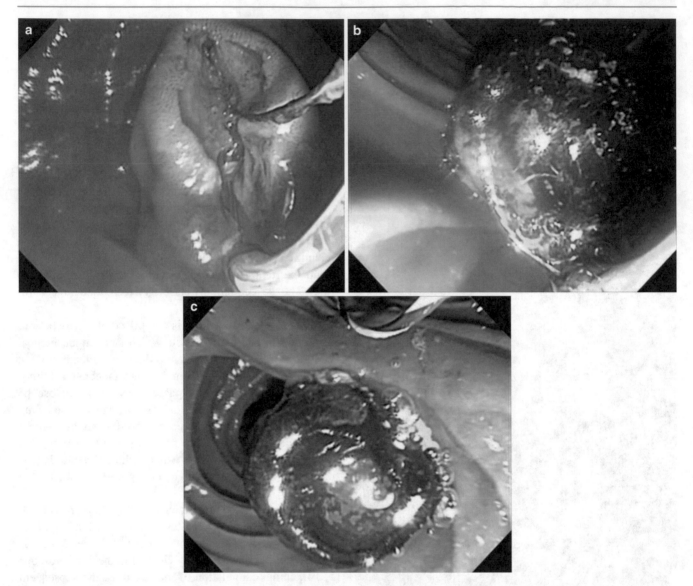

Fig. 2.3 Intact removal of a large bile duct stone. (**a**) ERCP revealed a 3 cm stone. A generous biliary sphincterotomy was performed. (**b**) The stone is captured and removed in one piece using a 3 cm Trapezoid basket. (**c**) The stone is released in the duodenum. No lithotripsy was required in this case. (Images courtesy Douglas G. Adler MD)

approaches have been developed to deal with this potential hazard.

The first-line therapy in cases of impaction involves the use of a salvage device or out-of-the-scope lithotripter. The purpose of using this device is not so much to crush the stone but rather to liberate the basket from the stone so that the basket can be removed from the patient. In practice, these devices will often break both the basket (allowing removal) and crush the stone simultaneously (Fig. 2.5a) [5, 14].

When using an emergency device, the handle of the basket and outer plastic sheath is physically detached from the rest of the device, usually with a wire cutter. This allows the duodenoscope to be withdrawn from the patient. At this point, the basket/stone complex will still be in the CBD and the wires from the basket device, now stripped of their sheath and handle, will be coming out of the patient's mouth. The wires of the basket are then threaded through the metal sheath of the lithotripter and affixed to the axle of the crank. Under fluoroscopic guidance, a spiral metal sheath is advanced over the basket wires by turning the handle. As the sheath is advanced over the wires, it passes down through the esophagus, stomach, and duodenum and eventually works its way up the common bile duct to the level of the stone/basket complex (Fig. 2.5b). At this point, usually under fluoroscopic guidance, the sheath is advanced further. As the sheath is advanced at the level of the stone/basket complex, the stone will be crushed, the basket will collapse, and the basket wires may break. Any of these events will result in the ability to, at the very least, remove the impacted basket from the patient. Once the stone is

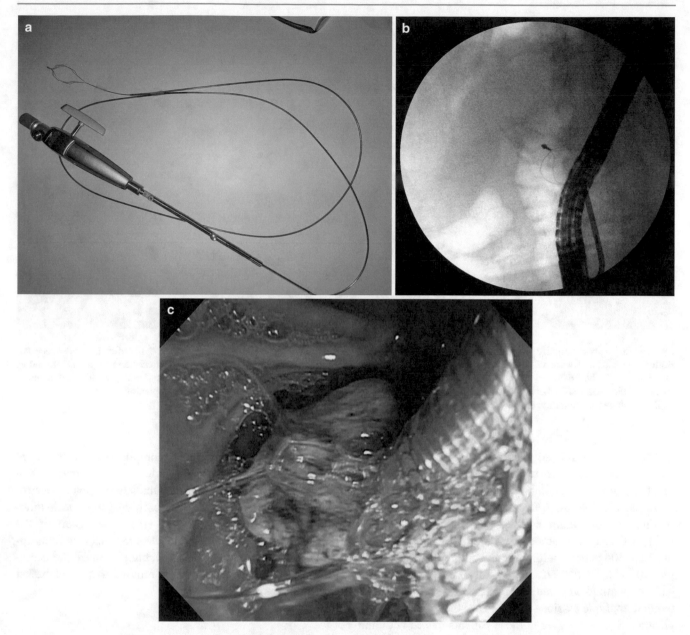

Fig. 2.4 (**a**) A through-the-scope mechanical lithotripter with its associated basket and inner plastic sheath. The outer metal sheath is seen attached to a cranking handle. After capturing the stone the metal sheath is advanced, collapsing the basket and fragmenting of the stone. (**b**) Fluoroscopic view showing the metal sheath and a captured stone in mid-CBD. (**c**) Endoscopic image demonstrating the retrieval of large stone fragments in lithotripter basket after mechanical lithotripsy has been performed

crushed against the metal sheath, the broken basket and stone fragments are removed [5, 13, 14].

Overall, ML is successful in 79–92 % of patients with difficult biliary stones; however, approximately 20–30 % of the patients require more than one lithotripsy session [3, 13, 15–18]. In a retrospective study of 162 patients by Cipolletta et al., the size of the stone was the only factor that significantly affected the success of bile duct clearance [19]. The overall stone clearance rate was 84 %; however, the cumulative probability of bile duct clearance ranged from >90 % for stones with a diameter <10 mm to 68 % for stones >28 mm in diameter ($P<0.02$) [19].

Conversely, a subsequent prospective study by Garg et al. demonstrated that stone size alone was not an important predictive factor unless considered together with the diameter of the bile duct itself [17]. The study concluded that the only important predictive factor for ML failure was stone impaction in the bile duct, with either the inability to pass the basket proximal to the bile stone or failure of the basket to open fully so that the stone in question could be captured [17].

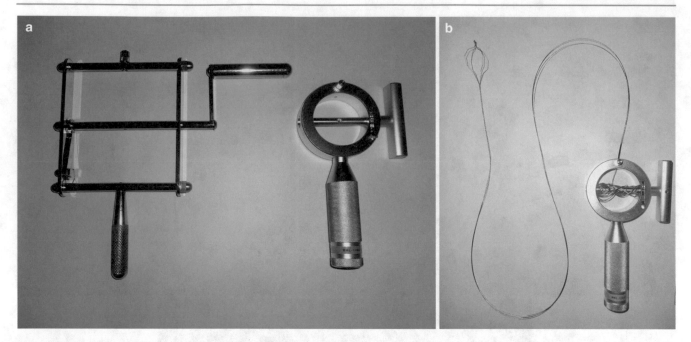

Fig. 2.5 (a) The two currently available emergency lithotripter devices. Both are similar and work via the same principle—they can allow a metal sheath to be advanced over an impacted basket. Once fully advanced, the impacted basket and its attendant stone are crushed. This facilitates stone fragmentation and basket removal. (b) Emergency lith- otripter device attached to a retrieval basket after the endoscope has been removed from the patient. Manual cranking of the handle causes tension on the basket wires, resulting in disintegration of the stone or basket wires freeing the basket from impaction

Complications related to ML are generally uncommon and mild in severity. In two large retrospective series, the incidence of reported complications from ML ranges from 6 to 13 %, with bleeding and post-ERCP pancreatitis representing the most common adverse outcome [3, 15, 17]. In a study by Chang et al., stone extraction by ML was successful in 272 of 304 patients with difficult common bile duct stones (90 %) [15]. Of the 272 successfully treated patients, 211 patients required only one session of ML whereas 61 patients required multiple sessions of ML. The study found the complication rate was higher in those patients treated with multiple sessions of ML when compared to those successfully treated with a single session. Complications included in this study included cholangitis 1.4 %, pancreatitis 3.3 %, and delayed bleeding 0.4 %. In contrast, of the 61 patients requiring multiple sessions of mechanical lithotripsy, 9.8 % had post-procedure cholangitis, 19.6 % had pancreatitis, and 14.7 % had delayed bleeding [15]. This likely reflects that patients requiring multiple procedures required more aggressive maneuvers that were more likely to be associated with complications.

Basket impaction occurs rarely (0.8–5.9 %) but has been a subject of study given the potential danger to the patient [20]. In a multicenter, retrospective study of over 600 patients that evaluated complications during ML (such as wire fracture, broken baskets, and basket impaction), basket impaction occurred in 3.6 % of cases [20]. The authors found that the vast majority of the technical complications that occurred during ML could be managed without surgical intervention by utilizing alternative lithotripsy modalities such as electrohydraulic lithotripsy (EHL), extracorporeal shockwave lithotripsy (ESWL), laser lithotripsy (LL), extension of the sphincterotomy, or use of out-of-the-scope salvage lithotriptor [20]. Using these additional techniques make the necessity for surgical intervention to remove a trapped basket exceptionally rare [3].

Electrohydraulic Lithotripsy (EHL)

EHL was used initially by the Soviet Union as an industrial tool for the fragmentation of rocks and minerals [21]. In the 1970s, EHL's technology was extrapolated for the treatment biliary stones [11, 21]. When compared with other modalities for the treatment of difficult biliary stones, EHL appears to be effective, compact, portable, and relatively inexpensive [3, 11]. In the United States, EHL is commonly used in tertiary academic centers that have expertise in the endoscopic management of complex biliary disorders [11]. EHL is used when conventional methods of stone extraction and ML are unsuccessful [22].

EHL consists of two main components: a bipolar lithotripsy probe and a charge generator [11, 13, 21]. The charge generator produces a series of sparks which are conducted

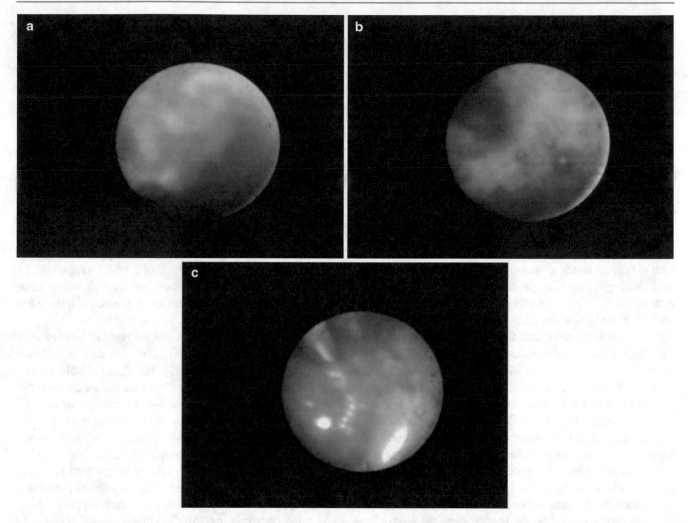

Fig. 2.6 Electrohydraulic lithotripsy. (**a**) Cholangioscopic view of a large stone in the common bile duct. (**b**) EHL at the moment of shockwave creation. Note the EHL probe at 10 O'clock. (**c**) Stone fragments visualized immediately after shockwave creation. Note the EHL probe at 10 o'clock. (Images courtesy Douglas G. Adler MD)

from the electrode tip into an aqueous medium, creating hydraulic shock waves [5, 11, 13]. The energy from the shock waves is transmitted to and through the adjacent stones, resulting in their fragmentation (Fig. 2.6) [5, 11]. During the procedure, continuous saline irrigation of the bile duct is necessary to assure visualization and removal of the stone fragments. Saline also provides a medium for shock wave energy transmission [13]. If the bipolar probe is deployed near the duct wall or away from stone, the hydraulic shock waves could cause inadvertent injury or perforation of the bile duct [5, 11]. In addition, contact between the probe and the bile duct walls can potentially result in a delayed biliary stricture. In practice, EHL often involves the probe touching the bile duct walls at least transiently during operation, and in most cases this does not result in any appreciable bile duct injury.

EHL can be performed under direct visualization by peroral cholangioscopy (POCS) or by using centering balloons or basket catheters with fluoroscopic guidance [3, 11]. The

drawback to only using fluoroscopic guidance is the inability to confirm correct positioning of the bipolar probe with only two dimensional imaging [11, 23]. Direct visualization by POCS is almost always preferred over fluoroscopic guidance in order to avoid damage to the bile duct wall and has largely superseded fluoroscopic guidance alone as a delivery technique. In current practice, EHL without POCS is rarely ever used [6, 23].

Initially, POCS used a mother-daughter scope assembly, in which a thin caliber daughter fiberoptic cholangioscope was inserted through the working channel of the mother duodenoscope [10, 24]. The original daughter fiberoptic cholangioscopes had technical limitations due to suboptimal image quality, small instrument channel, and lack of water and air irrigation channels [10, 24]. The subsequent development of the video/electronic cholangioscopes significantly improved the image quality and allowed the incorporation of narrow band imaging [10, 24, 25]. Despite the improvement in image quality, mother-daughter POCS still has many limitations [10, 24].

Mother-daughter POCS can be labor intensive as it requires considerable manual dexterity, and, depending on the type of cholangioscope used, may require two experienced operators to perform the procedure [10, 24]. Additionally, older cholangioscopes were fragile, easily damaged when inserted into the duodenoscope, and required frequent, costly repairs [6, 13, 24]. These cholangioscopes had poor maneuverability in the bile duct due to limited dual directional (up-down) scope tip movements [10, 24]. However, many of these limitations were negated with the introduction of the Spyglass direct visualization system (Boston Scientific, Natick, MA, USA) in 2005 [24, 26, 27].

The original Spyglass direct visualization, still in widespread use, system is a semi-disposable, single-operator per oral cholangioscopy (or pancreatoscopy) apparatus that is attached directly onto the duodenoscope (Video 2.1) [10, 24, 26, 27]. It contains a Spy Scope access and delivery catheter, Spyglass optical probe, and Spy Bite biopsy forceps [24]. The device has separate channels for the Spyglass optical probe and therapeutic intervention accessories and dual irrigation [24]. Unlike mother-daughter POCS, it only requires one operator and does not require a separate image processer, light source, and water-air pump [24]. In addition, the Spy Scope's ability for four-way tip deflection allows for significantly improved maneuverability in the bile duct when compared to the previous generation POCS [6, 10, 24]. The second generation Spyglass system, released in March of 2015, provides a much higher resolution, digital image with an integrated cholangioscope that requires no assembly or pre-focusing whatsoever.

Using a mother-daughter POCS system, EHL has an 85–98 % success rate of complete ductal clearance of stones with a complication rate of 2–9 %. Reported complications included pancreatitis, cholangitis, and hemobilia. Perforation of the bile duct is a serious risk; however, rarely it occurs (less than 1 %) [10, 28–32].

In a recent retrospective study of 13 patients using spyglass-guided EHL, bile duct clearance after EHL was achieved in 100 % of the patients [33]. 46.1 % of the patients had one stone, 38.5 % had two stones, and 15.4 % had three or more stones. 30.8 % of the patients had intrahepatic duct stones. 76 % of patients required only one ERCP to achieve duct clearance while 7.7 % required two ERCPs and 15.4 % required three ERCPs to clear the common bile duct. Only one patient (7.7 %) had adverse effects (cholangitis) from Spyglass-guided EHL and was treated with broad-spectrum antibiotics [33]. In summary cholangioscope-guided EHL is an effective treatment option for bile duct stones with an acceptable risk profile .

Laser Lithotripsy (LL)

LL was first described by Lux et al. in 1986 [34]. LL works on the principle of pulsed laser energy directed on the biliary stone at a particular wavelength resulting in a wave-mediated fragmentation [5, 11, 34]. A high-power density laser light is directed onto the stone creating a plasma composed of a gaseous collection of free electrons and ions that generate compressive and tensile waves [13]. These waves induce cavitation bubble formation with resultant shattering of the biliary stone [13]. LL is used as an alternative to EHL for biliary stones and is typically reserved for use in patients who have failed duct clearance by standard techniques such as endoscopic sphincterotomy with balloon/basket extraction and ML. Some prefer LL over EHL given the targeted and focused energy delivery during LL with less potential for bile duct trauma [35]. However, the cost of initial setup (approximately $100,000) can be a limiting factor when compared to EHL [3, 11, 35].

Since its inception in 1986, several types of laser systems have been utilized. Different lasers can deliver different energy, power, wavelength, and pulse width [35]. Short-wave length LL including coumarin (504 nm), rhodamine-6G (595 nm), neodymium (Nd):yttrium-aluminum-garnet (YAG) (1064 nm), and alexandrite:YAG (750 nm) are very effective in stone fragmentation (80–95 % success rate). These devices have been found to have a morbidity rate as high as 23 % [13, 35–41]. Short-wave LL results in deeper tissue penetration and can cause significant thermal effects, potentially resulting in bile duct perforation and hemobilia [35].

Currently, holmium (Ho):YAG lithotripsy has become the preferred choice for LL of biliary stones. Many of the positive attributes of Ho:YAG are due to its wavelength (2140 nm), which is near the wave length of water (1940 nm), making it very safe for stone fragmentation in an aqueous solution [35]. When compared to Nd:YAG, the tissue penetration of Ho:YAG is much more shallow (0.5 mm versus 5 mm, respectively) but with similar desirable coagulation effects of Nd:YAG [35].

Using a portable 100-W generator, Ho:YAG creates high-energy pulses of about 500–1000 mJ [13, 35, 42]. The Ho:YAG LL system consists of laser delivery fibers up to 4 m long and 200, 365, 550, or 1000 μm in diameter [13, 35]. The fibers fit through the working channels of currently available choledochoscopes and pancreatoscopes (Video 2.1) [13]. LL of bile duct stones is generally performed under direct visualization using cholangioscopes, similar to EHL in order to prevent bile duct injury [13]. LL is usually followed by ML and balloon extraction of stones once they have been fragmented.

A study of the Ho:YAG LL system by Weickert et al. included 20 patients who underwent cholangioscope-guided LL for choledocholithiasis when conventional methods failed [43]. Biliary stones were cleared in 19 out of the 20 patients. Fifteen patients required only 1 session, 4 patients required 2 sessions, and 1 patient required 3 sessions. No adverse events or serious complications were noted in this series at 30-day follow-up [43].

In the largest multicenter study of the Ho:YAG LL system to date, that included 69 patients, 97 % (67/69 patients) achieved complete ductal clearance [35]. LL failed in 2 of the 69 patients; both of these patients ultimately required surgery. Biliary stones were located in the extrahepatic biliary ducts in 82 %, intrahepatic ducts in 12 %, and the cystic duct in 6 % of the patients. 74 % of the patients achieved biliary duct clearance with one endoscopic session. In the study, the overall adverse event rate of the Ho:YAG LL system was 4.1 %. One patient had mild post-ERCP pancreatitis and two patients experienced minor bleeding thought to be arising from the bile duct wall. The study concluded that the Ho:YAG LL system was effective and safe in the treatment for patients with difficult to manage biliary stones [35].

Direct Peroral Cholangioscopy-Guided EHL or LL

When EHL or LL is required, most centers use the Spyglass direct visualization cholangioscope for guidance during lithotripsy. Recently there has been some literature regarding the use of ultraslim upper endoscopes for direct visualization and guidance during EHL or LL. Several versions of this approach exist, but all essentially involve the advancement of an ultraslim upper endoscope directly into the bile ducts. The technique is known as "direct peroral cholangioscopy" (DPOC) [6, 24]. The advantages of the ultraslim endoscope include a four-way tip deflection for improved steerability, high-resolution digital image quality, and a 2 mm working channel (which is large enough to accommodate EHL or LL devices) [6, 44, 45]. In addition, some ultraslim scopes have the ability to perform narrow band imaging (NBI) allowing for better identification of malignant lesions [23].

The challenge of using an ultraslim endoscope for DPOC is navigating the scope into the bile duct [24]. In most cases, ultraslim endoscopes can only be used after biliary sphincterotomy as the diameter of the ultraslim is usually 5–6 mm—far too wide to pass through a native papilla with ease [46]. Thus, a preliminary ERCP with a sphincterotomy and guidewire placement into the bile duct is required prior to ultraslim cannulation [24]. The technique is not always successful and it can be difficult to pass the endoscope into the bile duct even over a wire. Impediments to this approach include J-shaped stomachs, postsurgical anatomy, and large periampullary or duodenal diverticula [6, 45].

In most DPOC cases, a stiff 0.035-in. diameter guidewire is secured into the biliary tree via an initial ERCP procedure. The standard duodenoscope is removed over the wire and the ultrathin endoscope is advanced over the wire, which still terminates in the bile duct. This is followed by advancement of the ultraslim scope over the guidewire under direct endoscopic and fluoroscopic visualization [24]. The ultraslim scope is advanced through the stomach and duodenum and into the ampulla of Vater [24]. Looping of the ultraslim scope can occur even when the guidewire is in place. The use of an overtube to prevent looping often helps to increase the chance of successful DPOC procedure.

In a case study of 12 patients by Choi et al., overtube-balloon-assisted DPOC was performed successfully in 83.3 % of the patients (10 of 12 patients) [47]. Furthermore, in a prospective study by Moon et al., the feasibility and success rate of DPOC using an ultraslim anchored via an intraductal balloon was assessed and compared to the use of the traditional guidewire method [45]. In this study, 21 patients, including 3 patients in whom guidewire-based access approaches failed, underwent intraductal balloon-guided DPOC. This technique was performed as follows: a 0.025-in. diameter guidewire was placed into a branch of the intrahepatic duct after biliary sphincterotomy. The ultraslim endoscope is advanced over a 5 F balloon catheter into the duodenum and subsequently into the bile duct. After the balloon catheter was successfully directed into a branch of the intrahepatic duct by the guidewire, the balloon was inflated to anchor it to the duct. Under fluoroscopic guidance the ultrathin scope was advanced over the balloon catheter into the common bile duct. The anchoring balloon increases the chance of successful ductal intubation, but limits movement and tip deflection once the endoscope is in the bile duct. In the study by Moon, success rate when using intraductal balloon-guided DPOC was 95.2 % (20/21 patients, $P < 0.05$) versus 45.5 % (5/11 patients) in the traditional wire-guided DPOC patients. After DPOC, the authors successfully used LL, EHL, and forceps biopsies under direct visualization. The study did not observe any procedure-related complications [45].

The limiting factor of DPOC as a technique is the challenge of getting the ultraslim scope into the biliary tree, even when using the aforementioned techniques. Once the ultraslim endoscope is introduced into the bile duct, EHL and LL have been found to have a high success rate for biliary stones unable to be extracted by traditional methods. A small study of 18 patients using DPOC-guided EHL or LL after traditional methods and ML failed found the success rate for biliary clearance using DPOC of 88.9 % (16/18 patients) [48]. The study found that the patients required an average of 1.6 treatment sessions for biliary clearance. No procedure-related complications were observed [48].

Overall, possible complications of using the POC system include cholangitis, pancreatitis, hemobilia, and bile leakage [49, 50]. In addition, DPOC has potential for a rare and fatal complication of an air embolism [6, 51]. However, this potentially fatal complication can be markedly reduced by minimizing air insufflation and using CO_2 for insufflation instead of air [6].

Extracorporeal Shock Wave Lithotripsy

Initially used for urolithiasis, extracorporeal shock wave lithotripsy (ESWL) represents another additional modality in the management for biliary stones not amenable to traditional extraction [3]. During ESWL, high-pressure shock waves are generated outside the body in a water medium by water spark gap (electrohydraulic), or electromagnetic membrane technologies [11, 13]. These shock waves are focused by external transducers to the designated target [11]. Once the shock waves arrive at the focus point (the biliary stone), changes in acoustic impedance from soft tissue to the stone result in shearing forces that result in fragmentation [3, 11].

ESWL is usually assisted by fluoroscopy or ultrasound guidance [5]. When using fluoroscopy, placement of a nasobiliary tube for contrast instillation is required as most biliary stones are radiolucent and are not well visualized [11]. General anesthesia (GA) is typically recommended to minimize patient movement during the procedure [5].

With ESWL, the reported fragmentation rates of stones in the common bile duct have ranged from approximately 71 to 95 % [3, 32, 52–55]. Most of the patients require 1–3 sessions, leading to a final ductal clearance rate of approximately 70–90 % [3, 32, 52–58].

Complications from ESWL, including cholangitis, hematuria, hemobilia, and transient arrhythmias, arise in approximately 10–35 % of the patients [3, 32, 52–55, 59]. Newer ESWL devices have improved focusing abilities and may decrease both patient discomfort during the procedure and collateral tissue injury [3].

A study of 125 patients comparing ESWL to EHL by Adamek et al. showed no difference in ductal clearance rates [32]. Approximately 78.5 % (62 of 79 patients) achieved biliary duct clearance with ESWL versus 74 % (38 of 46 patients) in the EHL group. However, when using combined treatment including ESWL, EHL, and intracorporeal LL the overall success rate increased to 94 % (118 patients) [32].

When comparing ESWL to LL, LL has a higher rate of ductal clearance. In a study of 34 patients by Jakobs et al., complete stone fragmentation was achieved in 52.4 % (9 of 17 patients) of the ESWL group and in 82.4 % (14 of 17 patients) in the LL group [53]. In a subsequent study of 60 patients by Neuhaus et al., bile duct clearance was achieved in 73 % (22 of 30 patients) of the ESWL patients and in 97 % (29 of 30 patients) in the intracorporeal LL patients ($P<0.05$) [52].

Currently ESWL is rarely performed for the management of biliary stones in the United States [11]. Cholangioscope-guided EHL or LL for difficult biliary stone management is preferred over ESWL given the decreased number of treatment sessions, less complications, and overall higher success rates in patients requiring stone removal [11].

Endoscopic Papillary Balloon Dilation (EPBD) Combined with Biliary Sphincterotomy

The use of large diameter (12–20 mm) dilation balloons for biliary sphincter dilation after endoscopic sphincterotomy was first reported in 2003 by Ersoz et al. [60]. EPBD is an effective alternative to fragmentation techniques for the extraction of difficult or large common bile duct stones. Theoretically EPBD minimizes the complications associated with other modalities, and reduces the procedure time as well as the radiation exposure to the patient [60–62].

The procedure first requires a preliminary endoscopic retrograde cholangiogram confirming the presence of a dilated bile duct and large biliary stones [60–63]. A biliary sphincterotomy is performed over the guidewire toward the 1 o'clock position; some proponents of EPBD perform on a limited sphincterotomy while others perform a complete sphincterotomy before dilation [61–63]. Next, an exchange is performed and a large controlled radial expansion (CRE) dilation balloon is advanced over the guidewire. The size of the balloon is chosen in accordance with the size of the biliary stone and the diameter of the bile duct, although typical balloon diameters used when performing EPBD range from 10 to 18 mm. The dilation balloon is positioned across the papilla of Vater with much of the balloon within the distal portion of the common bile duct [63]. After adequate positioning, the balloon should be slowly inflated under endoscopic and fluoroscopic guidance to recommended pressure (Fig. 2.7a) [63]. As dilation continues, the waist of the balloon will gradually disappear. Once this occurs the balloon should be kept in place for at least an additional 30 s (overall dilation time should be in between 1 and 1.5 min, although the ideal amount of time required is unknown) [63]. After dilation, the balloon should be deflated until it is completely flat and withdrawn from the endoscope (Fig. 2.7b). The guidewire should be left in place to facilitate access in case of any adverse event occurs. Additionally, fluoroscopy should be used to ensure that there is no free air in the abdomen. Adverse events such as perforation can occur if the stone is incarcerated in between the bile duct wall and dilation balloon [63]. Stones should be pushed above the dilation balloon under fluoroscopic guidance prior to inflation of the balloon [63]. Following balloon sphincteroplasty, stone

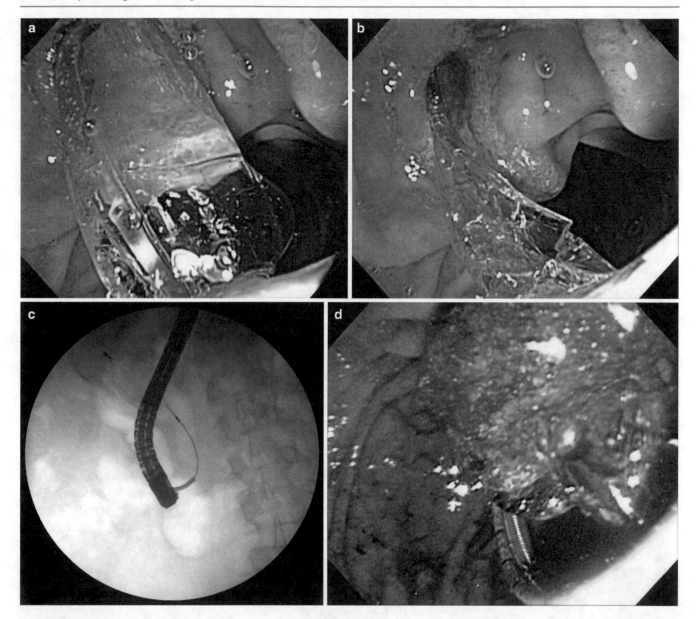

Fig. 2.7 (**a**) Endoscopic view of EPBD with a 12 mm CRE balloon. (**b**) Patulous biliary orifice following EPBD. (**c**) Fluoroscopic view of basket removal of large stone following EPBD. (**d**) Endoscopic image demonstrating retrieval of large stone fragments after EPBD

extraction balloons or retrieval baskets can be used to remove stones through the generous distal CBD and ampullary orifice (Fig. 2.7c, d). EPBD results in dilation of the bile duct and ampullary orifice for several minutes, and can be repeated as needed during the procedure.

The first study of this technique was reported by Ersoz et al. in 2003 and used large diameter balloons (12–20 mm) after endoscopic sphincterotomy in 58 patients in whom standard endoscopic sphincterotomy and extraction techniques had failed. Forty of the patients had square, barrel shaped and/or large stones (>15 mm) and 18 of the patients had associated biliary strictures [60]. The overall stone clearance rate was 88 % with only 7 % of the patients requiring

ML. 16 % of patients experienced complications [10, 60]. Complications included pancreatitis, cholangitis, and bleeding without the need for surgery [60].

Subsequent studies of EPBD with endoscopic sphincterotomy have shown high rates of successful biliary stone extraction (94–100 %) with a relatively low complication rates (0–17 %) [10, 60, 64–74]. In the largest randomized prospective study to date, 200 consecutive patients with choledocholithiasis were treated with either endoscopic sphincterotomy with EPBD (12–20 mm balloon diameter) or endoscopic sphincterotomy alone [68]. The study found similar outcomes in terms of overall successful stone removal (97 vs. 98 %), large (15 mm) stone removal (94 vs. 97 %), and the use of ML (8 vs. 9 %) [68]. Complications were similar between the two groups (5 vs. 7 %) with no differences in the rate of post-procedure pancreatitis (4 %) [68]. The study concluded that based on similar stone clearance rates and complication rates, EPBD with endoscopic sphincterotomy is an effective and safe tool for stone removal when compared to endoscopic sphincterotomy and stone extraction [68].

Originally there was concern for post-procedure pancreatitis due to EPBD causing inflammation/edema around the papilla from mechanical pressure and intramucosal hemorrhage [6]. In recent studies it does not appear that there is a higher risk of post-procedure pancreatitis when EPBD is performed in conjunction with endoscopic sphincterotomy [10]. The mechanism behind the protective effect of the endoscopic sphincterotomy is that it provides both room and a direction for the biliary ductal balloon to expand into, away from the pancreatic sphincter orifice. EPBD is thus almost always performed in conjunction with endoscopic sphincterotomy in the United States and Europe.

Special Situations with Difficult Biliary Stone

Mirizzi Syndrome

Mirizzi syndrome is an uncommon and atypical presentation of gallstone disease in which common hepatic duct obstruction is caused by an extrinsic compression from an impacted stone in the cystic duct or Hartmann's pouch of the gallbladder [3, 6, 75–77]. McSherry et al. classified Mirizzi syndrome into two variants based on ERCP findings [6, 78]. Type I Mirizzi syndrome involves external compression of the common hepatic duct or common bile duct by a stone impacted in the cystic duct or Hartmann's pouch (Fig. 2.8a, b). Type I is subdivided into type IA (cystic duct still present) or type IB (cystic duct obliterated). Type II–IV variants of Mirizzi syndrome results when a stone erodes into the cystic duct wall and produces a cholecysto-choledochal fistula into the common hepatic duct or common bile duct. Type II refers to a fistula that involves one third of the common hepatic duct diameter, type III involves a fistula that involves between one third and two thirds of the common hepatic duct diameter, and a type IV refers to a fistula that involves more than two thirds of the common hepatic duct diameter.

Endoscopic management of Mirizzi syndrome can be technically challenging and is associated with varying success. In most cases, the offending stone cannot be removed endoscopically as it is lodged in the cystic duct or the gallbladder. Accordingly, surgical intervention is the mainstay of therapy for Mirizzi syndrome and is usually required for definitive treatment. Historically, ERCP was used to diagnose Mirizzi syndrome and temporarily relieve the biliary obstruction through endoscopic stenting prior to definitive surgical management [3]. In some cases, ERCP can allow access to the stone through the cystic duct or a fistulous tract. In these cases, endoscopic stone removal can be performed.

Although surgery is still the mainstay of therapy, studies evaluating the utility of ESWL for patients with Mirizzi syndrome showed varying success with only 56–83 % of patients having complete ductal clearance [3, 6, 79, 80]. A recent study by Tsuyuguchi et al. evaluated the treatment outcomes

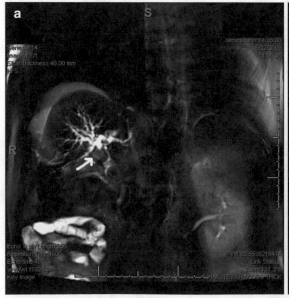
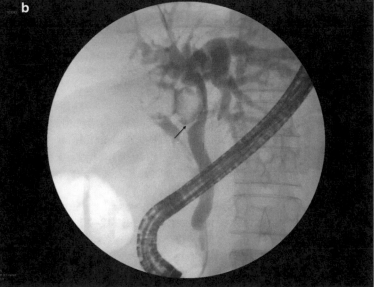

Fig. 2.8 Mirizzi syndrome. (**a** and **b**) MRCP and subsequent ERCP showing a type 1 Mirizzi syndrome with common hepatic duct compression from large cystic duct stones (*arrow*) resulting in obstructive jaundice in this patient

of POCS EHL and LL in 122 consecutive patients with difficult biliary stones (including 53 patients with Mirizzi syndrome) after long-term follow-up [6, 81]. Three patients had type I Mirizzi syndrome, 50 patients had type II Mirizzi syndrome, 50 patients had impacted stones, and 19 patients had large stones. The study demonstrated successful stone removal in 96 % of the patients with Mirizzi syndrome (96 % in type II Mirizzi syndrome, 0 % in type I Mirizzi syndrome) and 100 % of patients with impacted and large stones [6, 81]. Accordingly, when compared to type I Mirizzi syndrome, it appears that type II Mirizzi syndrome patients are more amenable to endoscopic therapy [6]. Future developments including ultraslim cholangioscope-guided EHL or LL in the cystic duct may provide vital option for more patients with Mirizzi syndrome.

Intrahepatic Choledocholithiasis

Intrahepatic choledocholithiasis or hepatolithiasis is defined as the presence of stones in the intrahepatic ducts [6] (Fig. 2.9a). Intrahepatic stones are commonly seen with biliary strictures in the setting of primary sclerosing cholangitis, oriental cholangiohepatitis, parasitic infections, postoperative biliary strictures, and recurrent cholangitis [3, 6, 10, 82–85]. Complications of intrahepatic stones include acute ascending cholangitis, benign intrahepatic strictures, lobar atrophy, secondary biliary cirrhosis (a.k.a. secondary sclerosing cholangitis), and cholangiocarcinoma [3].

Therapeutic options for intrahepatic stones include surgical resection (hepatectomy), percutaneous transhepatic catheter drainage, percutaneous cholangioscopy, lithotripsy via cholangioscopy performed percutaneously through a T-tube tract or a transhepatic tract, or via POCS lithotripsy. The main treatment for intractable intrahepatic stones is surgical resection of the afflicted segment of liver [10, 86]. Surgical resection plays the primary role in therapy as nonoperative treatment is frequently associated with stone recurrence and the potential risk of cholangiocarcinoma [12, 86]. Surgery should be reserved for patients who have failed less invasive approaches, those with an acceptable functional status, and unilateral stone disease (particularly if lobar atrophy and/or biliary strictures are also present) [3, 86, 87].

As previously stated, LL/EHL is an alternative to surgery when there are intrahepatic stones in multiple segments or the patient is not a good surgical candidate due to the presence of one or more comorbidities [10]. When transhepatic LL/EHL is performed in patients with intrahepatic duct stones, several studies have shown a complete clearance rate of 80–85 % with a major complication rate of 0–2.1 % [10, 82, 88–90]. Reported complications from transhepatic LL/EHL in this setting included septic shock, hemobilia, liver lacerations, intra-abdominal abscess, and disruption of the

transhepatic biliary drainage tract [10, 82, 88–90]. Long-term follow-up of patients showed recurrence of stones and/or cholangitis in 35–63 % of the patients related mostly to intrahepatic strictures [10, 82, 88–90].

While percutaneous LL/EHL is an alternative to surgery, it is invasive, painful, and time-consuming [10]. The creation and dilation of the percutaneous transhepatic tract usually requires 2 weeks to perform [10, 91].

ERCP can play an important role in the assessment of the biliary anatomy; however, the role of POCS lithotripsy for therapy of intrahepatic stones is somewhat limited (Fig. 2.9b, c) [88]. POCS lithotripsy for intrahepatic stones can be technically challenging and is associated with high rates of recurrent stones [3]. In a study of 36 patients, the rate of complete intrahepatic stone removal was 64 % (23 of 36 patients) with POCS lithotripsy [3, 92]. The frequent causes of failure in this series were attributed to the inability to access stones located in the left inferolateral and right posteroinferior segments due to sharp angulations [3, 92].

Surgically Altered Anatomy

Prior surgical reconstruction in the upper GI tract can present additional challenges in the management of patients with biliary stones requiring ERCP [3]. A standard duodenoscope can be used in patients who have undergone a gastroduodenal anastomosis (Billroth I surgery) without difficulty, although this situation can be more difficult than in patients with normal anatomy [10]. However, in patients who have undergone gastrojejunal anastomosis (Billroth II) or Roux-en-Y gastrojejunostomy/hepaticojejunostomy surgeries, ERCP by conventional methods can be quite challenging. Billroth II and Roux-en-Y reconstructive surgery results in a longer segment of small bowel to traverse when attempting to reach the major papilla, as well as an inverted approach to the papilla when it is within reach [93]. Additional techniques are often required for these patients.

Billroth II Anatomy

Patients with Billroth II anatomy are not immune to choledocholithiasis, and ERCP in these patients is not infrequently warranted. ERCP in patients with Billroth II anatomy can be challenging due to difficulty in identifying the afferent limb, advancing the scope through the limb to the major papilla, as well as cannulating and performing therapeutic maneuvers from an inverted position once the major papilla is reached [93].

Duodenoscopes are frequently preferred over the therapeutic gastroscopes or colonoscopes for Billroth II patients [93]. In most patients with Billroth II anatomy, the major papilla can be reached with a duodenoscope. However, getting the duodenoscope in the correct orientation and identifying the afferent

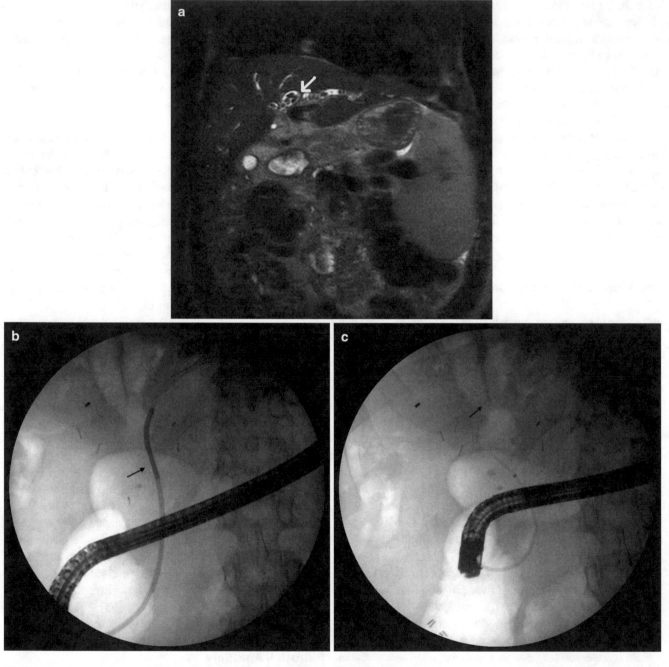

Fig. 2.9 Intrahepatic stones. (**a**) MRCP demonstrating multiple large and small intrahepatic stones (*arrow*) in multiple intrahepatic ducts. (**b**) Fluoroscopic images showing ERCP with cholangioscope-guided laser lithotripsy for intrahepatic stones. (**c**) After multiple session of laser lithotripsy, the duct has been cleared of stones

limb can be difficult due to the side-view optics inherent to duodenoscopes [93]. Several techniques have been proposed to help facilitate successful endoscopy in this situation. Applying external compression and changing the position of the patient (often from prone to left lateral decubitus position) may be helpful when advancing the endoscope [93]. Fluoroscopic guidance during insertion helps with proper orientation and ensures correct advancement of the duodenoscope toward the papilla. The use of a gastroscope or a colonoscope to map out the "lay of the land" prior to duodenoscope insertion is helpful in identifying any unexpected anatomic variations as delineating the afferent from the efferent limb. Once the afferent limb is identified, it can be marked in several ways. A guidewire can be left in place; India ink tattooing or endoclip placement at the site of the anastomosis can all help in easy identification of the afferent limb prior to duodenoscopy [93, 94].

Once the major papilla has been reached and when using a duodenoscope, biliary cannulation should be attempted toward the 5 o'clock position (reverse angle approach) [93]. Cannulation can be performed using the endoscope's elevator with or without guidewires for biliary access [93]. Dedicated papillotomes such as reverse papillotome and sphincterotomes that have the capacity to rotate are useful in both cannulation and sphincterotomy. In addition, straight biliary cannulas can be pushed against the duodenal wall in order to improve trajectory to the biliary duct by creating a "reverse" angulation [93].

When using a therapeutic gastroscope or a colonoscope in Billroth II patients, a transparent cap on the tip of the endoscope can be used to allow better visualization of the papilla and to optimize the angle of approach for cannulation [27, 93, 95].

When used in patients with Billroth II anatomy, both duodenoscopes and therapeutic gastroscopes can allow successful cannulation to be achieved in approximately 90 % of patients [3, 96, 97]. In patients with Billroth II anatomy and choledocholithiasis, biliary sphincterotomy is almost always performed. Once the papilla has been reached, given its orientation, endoscopic sphincterotomy can be performed by using a rotatable papillotome, reverse papillotome, or needle-knife catheter after placement of a biliary stent [3] (Fig. 2.10). EPBD can be used along with or independently of endoscopic sphincterotomy for stone removal in patients with large or difficult stones, although in practice most perform EPBD after biliary sphincterotomy. EPBD alone has been shown to be an effective treatment for patients with biliary stones and Billroth II anatomy [3, 98].

The overall success rate for removal of biliary stones in patients with Billroth II anatomy is high (85–92 %) [3, 96, 98, 99]. However, the rate of complications is higher with Billroth II patients during endoscopic therapy than those with normal anatomy [3]. Complications include post-sphincterotomy bleeding (as high as 17 % of patients) and perforations (up to 5 % of patients) [3, 98, 100].

Roux-en-Y Anatomy

Roux-en-Y bowel reconstructions are becoming increasingly common, and patients with these postsurgical reconstructions frequently require ERCP for treatment of choledocholithiasis. Techniques for removing stones endoscopically in these patients are similar to those in patients with normal anatomy, but the issue in these patients becomes one of endoscopic access.

The length of the afferent (roux) limb in these patients varies tremendously, based on the height of the patient, weight of the patient, indication for surgery, and type of surgery performed. As a rule, if biliary access can be achieved with a duodenoscope this should be the instrument of choice. If a duodenoscope cannot reach the desired location, forward-viewing endoscopes come into play as the instruments of choice when performing ERCP.

In patients with Roux-en-Y hepaticojejunostomy (RYHJ) and Roux-en-Y gastrojejunostomy (RYHJ) anatomy, duodenoscopes sometimes lack the length and maneuverability to reach the hepatocojejunostomy or the major papilla [3, 99]. Early studies of ERCP using duodenoscopes for patients

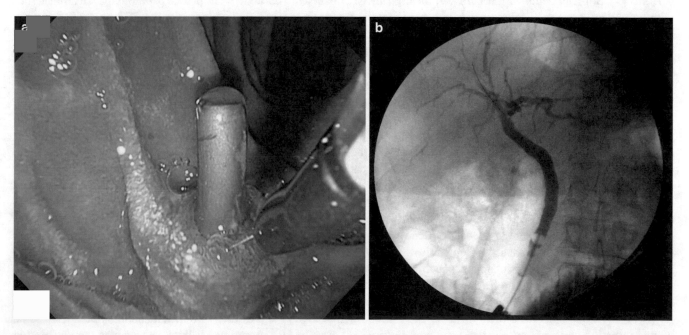

Fig. 2.10   Choledocholithiasis in a patient with Billroth II anatomy. (**a**) Endoscopic view of inverted papilla in a patient with Billroth II gastrojejunostomy and needle-knife sphincterotomy over a stent in 5 o' clock direction. (**b**) Fluoroscopic view of cholangiogram with a balloon extraction of stone in the same patient

with Roux-en-Y reconstructive surgeries demonstrated a poor success rate (33 %) primarily due to failure to reach the biliary orifice [93, 99]. Consequently, push enteroscopy (using a colonoscope or enteroscope) and deep enteroscopy techniques (spiral or single and double-balloon enteroscopy) have been used with varying degree of success (62–100 %) in reaching the hepaticojejunostomy or the major papilla in patients with Roux-en-Y reconstructions [3, 93, 101–110].

Biliary cannulation can be challenging when using endoscopes with forward-viewing optics (such as a colonoscope or enteroscope) as the papilla cannot be viewed *en face* [10]. Several studies have reported a cannulation rate of 70–80 % in Roux-en-Y patients with a native papilla when using forward-viewing instruments [3, 108, 111]. Techniques for stone removal are comparable to those utilized in patients with Billroth II anatomy once biliary cannulation has been achieved [3]. In addition, like Billroth II patients, Roux-en-Y gastrojejunostomy and hepaticojejunostomy patients have increased risk of perforation (up to 5 %) [3, 104].

If cannulation in Roux-en-Y and Billroth II anatomy patients is unsuccessful, stone extraction can be performed by PTCS LL/EHL or surgical interventions [10]. PTCS LL/EHL appears to be relatively safe and effective rescue therapy but can be technically difficult and, at times, impossible in the absence of dilated biliary duct [10, 112–115].

Patients who have undergone Roux-en-Y gastric bypass jejunojejunostomy (RYGB) typically have a longer roux and biliopancreatic limbs when compared to patients with RYGJ and RYHJ reconstructions, making access to, and cannulation of, the biliary orifice potentially more challenging to perform [3]. Some patients with RYGB can undergo ERCP with a duodenoscope or a colonoscope, but some can only have their major papilla accessed via a standard enteroscope or a balloon-assisted enteroscope depending on the length of the roux limb.

Studies using balloon-assisted enteroscopy in patients with RYGB have shown mixed results with regard to cannulation success rates when compared to RYHJ and RYGJ patients [3, 106, 108]. However, because of the unique anatomy of RYGB (intact antroduodenal pathway to the bile duct), transgastric endoscopic approaches such as endoscopic, radiologic, or surgical gastrostomy followed by subsequent access and dilation of the tract for 3–4 weeks can allow a duodenoscope to pass to the major ampulla [3, 116, 117]. Another option includes laparoscopy-assisted ERCP with creation of a laparoscopic gastrostomy with intraoperative passage of the duodenoscope through a laparoscopic trocar. This procedure has been associated with a high rate of success for common bile duct stone extraction; however, it has complication rates up to 13 % (including wound infection, gastrostomy site leak, and perforation) [3, 118–121].

Endoscopic Ultrasound (EUS) Guided Procedures

In some patients, standard ERCP techniques will fail to provide access to the biliary tree in patients with choledocholithiasis. The use of EUS as a means to access the biliary tree when ERCP alone has failed can be helpful in this situation [10]. Two EUS-based techniques that are currently being employed to access the bile ducts include the EUS-ERCP rendezvous (EUS-RV) technique and EUS-guided antegrade (EUS-AG) technique [10].

The idea behind the EUS-RV technique is as follows: a transduodenal puncture of the bile duct under EUS guidance is performed with a 19 gauge needle [10, 122–124]. Once access to the bile duct has been achieved, a guidewire is advanced under fluoroscopic guidance through the needle and directed down through the distal common bile duct, across the papilla, and into the duodenum [10]. While keeping the guidewire in place, the needle and subsequently the echoendoscope itself are withdrawn over the wire. A duodenoscope can then be advanced next to the wire, and when the duodenum has been reached cannulation next to the existing wire is often a simple matter [10]. At this point, standard biliary sphincterotomy and stone extraction techniques can be used.

EUS-RV can be highly successful based on limited data. In a retrospective study by Dhir et al., EUS-RV was performed in patients with distal bile duct obstruction in whom selective cannulation of the bile duct at ERCP failed after five attempts with a guidewire and sphincterotome [123]. The outcomes of EUS-RV were compared with those in a historical cohort of patients who underwent precut papillotomy. Treatment success was significantly higher for the EUS-guided RV (57 out of 58 patients) than for those undergoing precut papillotomy (130 out of 144 patients). There was no significant difference in the rate of procedural complications between the EUS and precut papillotomy techniques (3.4 % vs. 6.9 %).

In patients with an endoscopically inaccessible papilla (such as in patients with surgically altered anatomy or gastric outlet obstruction at the level of the apex of the duodenal bulb), EUS-RV is not a viable option [10]. In these patients, the EUS-AG technique can be utilized for stone extraction [10, 125, 126]. Using this technique, the left intrahepatic bile duct is accessed with a 19 gauge EUS FNA needle (usually in a transgastric manner) after which a guidewire is inserted through the needle into the left intrahepatic duct. The guidewire is then advanced through the bile ducts in an antegrade fashion into the duodenum under fluoroscopic guidance [10]. Using a dilation catheter, the puncture tract is dilated with a biliary dilation balloon and antegrade papillary balloon dilation is performed in an attempt to provide a sufficient ampullary opening for stone passage [10]. A retrieval balloon catheter can then be used to push the stone(s) out into the duodenum [10].

Although intriguing, this technique has only been used to remove bile duct stones in a small number of patients to date. In a study of six patients with previous Roux-en-Y anastomosis, tract dilation, anterograde balloon sphincteroplasty, and stone extraction were successful in 67 % (four out of six) of the patients [126]. Anterograde sphincteroplasty failed in two patients due to an inability to advance the transhepatic dilation catheters [126]. However, both patients subsequently underwent successful rendezvous ERCP using double-balloon enteroscopy. Five patients in the study did not experience any complications from EUS-AG. One patient developed a subcapsular hepatic hematoma which was managed conservatively [126]. EUS-AG offers a technically challenging alternative with limited success and requires a high level of endoscopic proficiency.

Endoscopic Biliary Stenting for Biliary Stones

In some patients, biliary sphincterotomy to allow stone extraction presents an unacceptably high risk. Patient who cannot stop anticoagulation or antiplatelet medications, the very elderly, and those who cannot tolerate a prolonged ERCP are some of these patients [6, 10]. If a patient cannot undergo biliary sphincterotomy, the placement of one or more endoscopic biliary stents can be used as a temporary or permanent measure to treat biliary stone disease. This approach is sometimes selected for patients who are poor candidates for not only emergent surgery but also future elective therapy [10].

The goal of endoscopic stenting in these patients is to prevent acute cholangitis and maintain patency of the biliary tree [127]. This approach will, in general, not provide a path to duct clearance although a small subset of patients can have spontaneous clearance of the biliary tree secondary to long-term stenting (possibly owing to the mechanical fracturing and passage of stones via long-term abrasive effects of the stents themselves).

In a study by Di Giorgio et al., plastic stent exchange at a defined interval of every 3 months was prospectively compared with stent exchange "on demand" with the acute onset of symptoms in patients who could not undergo biliary sphincterotomy [6, 127]. The study concluded that the rate of cholangitis was significantly lower in the group with elective stent exchanges every 3 months ($P=0.03$) [6, 127].

Biliary stenting is required for patients in between multiple treatment sessions for stone clearance, most commonly patients undergoing repeated session of EHL and LL with a large stone burden or if duct clearance cannot be achieved during ERCP. It is thought that the mechanical grinding of the stones against the biliary stents increases stone fragmentation, reduces the size of the biliary stones, and creates space around and between the stones, potentially facilitating extraction during follow-up ERCP [6].

The combination of oral dissolution agents ursodeoxycholic acid (60 mg daily) and 300 mg of terpene preparation daily for 6 months with biliary stenting has been shown to be superior to endoscopic stents alone for the clearance of bile duct stones, although this is rarely used in clinical practice [6, 128].

Patients with biliary stones and extrahepatic biliary duct strictures may also benefit from long-term endoscopic stenting, such as in patients with duct-to-duct anastomotic strictures and stones after an orthotopic liver transplant [5]. In these patients, dilation of the anastomotic stricture combined with one or more rounds of endoscopic stent placement may allow proximal stones to be successfully removed. Throughout the period that the stricture is being dilated, the biliary stents alleviate biliary obstruction and prevent cholangitis [5].

Conclusion

Biliary ductal stones are typically treated with endoscopic sphincterotomy followed by balloon or basket extraction. In patients with large biliary stones, intrahepatic stones, impacted stones, or those with surgically altered anatomy, stone extraction presents many additional challenges. If standard methods for stone extraction fail in these situations, other modalities such as ML, EHL, LL, ELPD, and ESWL or a combination of these has been shown to improve the success rate of stone extraction.

EPBD, most commonly performed with endoscopic biliary sphincterotomy, can be used for the extraction of difficult or large common bile duct stones. EPBD reduces the procedure time as well as the radiation exposure to the patient. Impacted stones (such as in Mirizzi syndrome) and intrahepatic biliary stones create challenges in endoscopic stone extraction. Although there has been some data supporting endoscopic therapy, the mainstay of therapy for Mirizzi syndrome is surgical intervention. Similarly, intrahepatic stones should be treated with surgical intervention (surgical resection) if endoscopic approaches fail, although PTCS LL/EHL can be used as an alternative to surgery when there are intrahepatic stones in multiple segments or if patients are good surgical candidate.

Billroth II and Roux-en-Y reconstructions can also cause challenges in the management of patients with choledocholithiais. The technical challenges of endoscopic intervention include difficulties in identifying the desired limb, advancing the scope through the limb to the papilla, and performing ERCP from an inverted position. When cannulation is not successful in Roux-en-Y patients, stone extraction can be performed by laparoscopic surgery assisted ERCP or PTCS LL/EHL. EUS-based approaches to accessing the bile duct in patients with stones are promising but are still in development.

For those patients with extrahepatic strictures, old age, severe cholangitis, or other serious medical comorbidities endoscopic biliary stents can be used as a temporary measure before endoscopic stone extraction or as definitive treatment for patients who are poor candidates for future therapy.

Video Legend
Video 2.1 Laser lithotripsy utilized in the fragmentation of a large biliary stone.

References

1. Everhart JE, Khare M, Hill M, Maurer KR. Prevalence and ethnic differences in gallbladder disease in the United States. Gastroenterology. 1999;117(3):632–9.
2. Everhart JE, Ruhl CE. Burden of digestive diseases in the United States part I: overall and upper gastrointestinal diseases. Gastroenterology. 2009;136(2):376–86. doi:10.1053/j.gastro.2008.12.015. Epub 2009 Jan 3. Review.
3. ASGE Standards of Practice Committee, Maple JT, Ikenberry SO, Anderson MA, Appalaneni V, Decker GA, Early D, Evans JA, Fanelli RD, Fisher D, Fisher L, Fukami N, Hwang JH, Jain R, Jue T, Khan K, Krinsky ML, Malpas P, Ben-Menachem T, Sharaf RN, Dominitz JA. The role of endoscopy in the management of choledocholithiasis. Gastrointest Endosc. 2011;74(4):731–44. doi:10.1016/j.gie.2011.04.012. Erratum in: Gastrointest Endosc. 2012;75(1):230–230.e14.
4. Ko CW, Lee SP. Epidemiology and natural history of common bile duct stones and prediction of disease. Gastrointest Endosc. 2002;56(6 Suppl):S165–9. Review.
5. McHenry L, Lehman G. Difficult bile duct stones. Curr Treat Options Gastroenterol. 2006;9(2):123–32.
6. Trikudanathan G, Arain MA, Attam R, Freeman ML. Advances in the endoscopic management of common bile duct stones. Nat Rev Gastroenterol Hepatol. 2014;11(9):535–44. doi:10.1038/nrgastro.2014.76. Epub 2014 May 27. Review.
7. Classen M, Demling L. Endoscopic sphincterotomy of the papilla of vater and extraction of stones from the choledochal duct (author's transl). Dtsch Med Wochenschr. 1974;99(11):496–7. German.
8. Kawai K, Akasaka Y, Murakami K, Tada M, Koli Y. Endoscopic sphincterotomy of the ampulla of Vater. Gastrointest Endosc. 1974;20(4):148–51.
9. Seitz U, Bapaye A, Bohnacker S, Navarrete C, Maydeo A, Soehendra N. Advances in therapeutic endoscopic treatment of common bile duct stones. World J Surg. 1998;22(11):1133–44. Review.
10. Yasuda I, Itoi T. Recent advances in endoscopic management of difficult bile duct stones. Dig Endosc. 2013;25(4):376–85. doi:10.1111/den.12118. Epub 2013 May 8. Review.
11. Trikudanathan G, Navaneethan U, Parsi MA. Endoscopic management of difficult common bile duct stones. World J Gastroenterol. 2013;19(2):165–73. doi:10.3748/wjg.v19.i2.165. PubMed Central PMCID: PMC3547556, Review.
12. Riemann JF, Seuberth K, Demling L. Clinical application of a new mechanical lithotripter for smashing common bile duct stones. Endoscopy. 1982;14(6):226–30.
13. DiSario J, Chuttani R, Croffie J, Liu J, Mishkin D, Shah R, Somogyi L, Tierney W, Song LM, Petersen BT. Biliary and pancreatic lithotripsy devices. Gastrointest Endosc. 2007;65(6):750–6. Epub 2007 Mar 26. Review.
14. Leung JW, Tu R. Mechanical lithotripsy for large bile duct stones. Gastrointest Endosc. 2004;59(6):688–90.
15. Chang WH, Chu CH, Wang TE, Chen MJ, Lin CC. Outcome of simple use of mechanical lithotripsy of difficult common bile duct stones. World J Gastroenterol. 2005;11(4):593–6. PubMed Central PMCID: PMC4250818.
16. Vij JC, Jain M, Rawal KK, Gulati RA, Govil A. Endoscopic management of large bile duct stones by mechanical lithotripsy. Indian J Gastroenterol. 1995;14(4):122–3.
17. Garg PK, Tandon RK, Ahuja V, Makharia GK, Batra Y. Predictors of unsuccessful mechanical lithotripsy and endoscopic clearance of large bile duct stones. Gastrointest Endosc. 2004;59(6):601–5.
18. Shaw MJ, Mackie RD, Moore JP, Dorsher PJ, Freeman ML, Meier PB, Potter T, Hutton SW, Vennes JA. Results of a multicenter trial using a mechanical lithotripter for the treatment of large bile duct stones. Am J Gastroenterol. 1993;88(5):730–3.
19. Cipolletta L, Costamagna G, Bianco MA, Rotondano G, Piscopo R, Mutignani M, Marmo R. Endoscopic mechanical lithotripsy of difficult common bile duct stones. Br J Surg. 1997;84(10):1407–9.
20. Thomas M, Howell DA, Carr-Locke D, Mel Wilcox C, Chak A, Raijman I, Watkins JL, Schmalz MJ, Geenen JE, Catalano MF. Mechanical lithotripsy of pancreatic and biliary stones: complications and available treatment options collected from expert centers. Am J Gastroenterol. 2007;102(9):1896–902. Epub 2007 Jun 15.
21. Harrison J, Morris DL, Haynes J, Hitchcock A, Womack C, Wherry DC. Electrohydraulic lithotripsy of gall stones--in vitro and animal studies. Gut. 1987;28(3):267–71. PubMed Central PMCID: PMC1432697.
22. Swahn F, Edlund G, Enochsson L, Svensson C, Lindberg B, Arnelo U. Ten years of Swedish experience with intraductal electrohydraulic lithotripsy and laser lithotripsy for the treatment of difficult bile duct stones: an effective and safe option for octogenarians. Surg Endosc. 2010;24(5):1011–6. doi:10.1007/s00464-009-0716-8. Epub 2009 Oct 23.
23. Yoo KS, Lehman GA. Endoscopic management of biliary ductal stones. Gastroenterol Clin North Am. 2010;39(2):209–27, viii. doi:10.1016/j.gtc.2010.02.008. Review.
24. Monga A, Ramchandani M, Reddy DN. Per-oral cholangioscopy. J Interv Gastroenterol. 2011;1(2):70–7. PubMed Central PMCID: PMC3136857.
25. Itoi T, Neuhaus H, Chen YK. Diagnostic value of image-enhanced video cholangiopancreatoscopy. Gastrointest Endosc Clin N Am. 2009;19(4):557–66. doi:10.1016/j.giec.2009.06.002. Review.
26. Chen YK. Preclinical characterization of the Spyglass peroral cholangiopancreatoscopy system for direct access, visualization, and biopsy. Gastrointest Endosc. 2007;65(2):303–11.
27. Chen YK, Pleskow DK. SpyGlass single-operator peroral cholangiopancreatoscopy system for the diagnosis and therapy of bile-duct disorders: a clinical feasibility study (with video). Gastrointest Endosc. 2007;65(6):832–4.
28. Leung JW, Chung SS. Electrohydraulic lithotripsy with peroral choledochoscopy. BMJ. 1989;299(6699):595–8. PubMed Central PMCID: PMC1837426.
29. Binmoeller KF, Brückner M, Thonke F, Soehendra N. Treatment of difficult bile duct stones using mechanical, electrohydraulic and extracorporeal shock wave lithotripsy. Endoscopy. 1993;25(3):201–6.
30. Arya N, Nelles SE, Haber GB, Kim YI, Kortan PK. Electrohydraulic lithotripsy in 111 patients: a safe and effective therapy for difficult bile duct stones. Am J Gastroenterol. 2004;99(12):2330–4.
31. Hui CK, Lai KC, Ng M, Wong WM, Yuen MF, Lam SK, Lai CL, Wong BC. Retained common bile duct stones: a comparison

between biliary stenting and complete clearance of stones by electrohydraulic lithotripsy. Aliment Pharmacol Ther. 2003; 17(2):289–96.

32. Adamek HE, Maier M, Jakobs R, Wessbecher FR, Neuhauser T, Riemann JF. Management of retained bile duct stones: a prospective open trial comparing extracorporeal and intracorporeal lithotripsy. Gastrointest Endosc. 1996;44(1):40–7.

33. Aljebreen AM, Alharbi OR, Azzam N, Almadi MA. Efficacy of spyglass-guided electrohydraulic lithotripsy in difficult bile duct stones. Saudi J Gastroenterol. 2014;20(6):366–70. doi:10.4103/1319-3767.145329. PubMed Central PMCID: PMC4271012.

34. Lux G, Ell C, Hochberger J, Müller D, Demling L. The first successful endoscopic retrograde laser lithotripsy of common bile duct stones in man using a pulsed neodymium-YAG laser. Endoscopy. 1986;18(4):144–5.

35. Patel SN, Rosenkranz L, Hooks B, Tarnasky PR, Raijman I, Fishman DS, Sauer BG, Kahaleh M. Holmium-yttrium aluminum garnet laser lithotripsy in the treatment of biliary calculi using single-operator cholangioscopy: a multicenter experience(with video). Gastrointest Endosc. 2014;79(2):344–8. doi:10.1016/j. gie.2013.07.054. Epub 2013 Nov 22.

36. Das AK, Chiura A, Conlin MJ, Eschelman D, Bagley DH. Treatment of biliary calculi using holmium: yttrium aluminum garnet laser. Gastrointest Endosc. 1998;48(2):207–9.

37. Strunge C, Brinkmann R, Flemming G, Engelhardt R. Interspersion of fragmented fiber's splinters into tissue during pulsed alexandrite laser lithotripsy. Lasers Surg Med. 1991;11(2):183–7.

38. Kozarek RA, Low DE, Ball TJ. Tunable dye laser lithotripsy: in vitro studies and in vivo treatment of choledocholithiasis. Gastrointest Endosc. 1988;34(5):418–21.

39. Ell C, Hochberger J, May A, Fleig WE, Bauer R, Mendez L, Hahn EG. Laser lithotripsy of difficult bile duct stones by means of a rhodamine-6G laser and an integrated automatic stone-tissue detection system. Gastrointest Endosc. 1993;39(6):755–62.

40. Cho YD, Cheon YK, Moon JH, Jeong SW, Jang JY, Lee JS, Shim CS. Clinical role of frequency-doubled double-pulsed yttrium aluminum garnet laser technology for removing difficult bile duct stones (with videos). Gastrointest Endosc. 2009;70(4):684–9. doi:10.1016/j.gie.2009.03.1170. Epub 2009 Jul 1.

41. Ell C, Hochberger J, Müller D, Zirngibl H, Giedl J, Lux G, Demling L. Laser lithotripsy of gallstone by means of a pulsed neodymium-YAG laser—in vitro and animal experiments. Endoscopy. 1986;18(3):92–4. PubMed.

42. Hochberger J, Tex S, Maiss J, Hahn EG. Management of difficult common bile duct stones. Gastrointest Endosc Clin N Am. 2003;13(4):623–34. Review. PubMedPMID: 14986790.

43. Weickert U, Mühlen E, Janssen J, Johanns W, Greiner L. The holmium-YAG laser: a suitable instrument for stone fragmentation in choledocholithiasis. The assessment of the results of its use under babyscopic control]. Dtsch Med Wochenschr. 1999;124(17):514–8. German.

44. Larghi A, Waxman I. Endoscopic direct cholangioscopy by using an ultra-slim upper endoscope: a feasibility study. Gastrointest Endosc. 2006;63(6):853–7. PubMed.

45. Moon JH, Ko BM, Choi HJ, Hong SJ, Cheon YK, Cho YD, Lee JS, Lee MS, Shim CS. Intraductal balloon-guided direct peroral cholangioscopy with an ultraslim upper endoscope (with videos). Gastrointest Endosc. 2009;70(2):297–302. doi:10.1016/j. gie.2008.11.019. Epub 2009 Apr 25.

46. Moon JH, Terheggen G, Choi HJ, Neuhaus H. Peroral cholangioscopy: diagnostic and therapeutic applications. Gastroenterology. 2013;144(2):276–82. doi:10.1053/j.gastro.2012.10.045. Epub 2012 Nov 2. Review.

47. Choi HJ, Moon JH, Ko BM, Hong SJ, Koo HC, Cheon YK, Cho YD, Lee JS, Lee MS, Shim CS. Overtube-balloon-assisted

direct peroral cholangioscopy by using an ultra-slim upper endoscope (with videos). Gastrointest Endosc. 2009;69(4):935–40. doi:10.1016/j.gie.2008.08.043.

48. Moon JH, Ko BM, Choi HJ, Koo HC, Hong SJ, Cheon YK, Cho YD, Lee MS, Shim CS. Direct peroral cholangioscopy using an ultra-slim upper endoscope for the treatment of retained bile duct stones. Am J Gastroenterol. 2009;104(11):2729–33. doi:10.1038/ajg.2009.435. Epub 2009 Jul 21.

49. Moon JH, Choi HJ. The role of direct peroral cholangioscopy using an ultraslim endoscope for biliary lesions: indications, limitations, and complications. Clin Endosc. 2013;46(5):537–9. doi:10.5946/ce.2013.46.5.537. PubMed PMID: 24143317, PubMed Central PMCID: PMC3797940, Epub 2013 Sep 30. Review.

50. Sethi A, Chen YK, Austin GL, Brown WR, Brauer BC, Fukami NN, Khan AH, Shah RJ. ERCP with cholangiopancreatoscopy may be associated with higher rates of complications than ERCP alone: a single-center experience. Gastrointest Endosc. 2011;73(2):251–6. doi:10.1016/j.gie.2010.08.058. Epub 2010 Nov 24.

51. Efthymiou M, Raftopoulos S, Antonio Chirinos J, May GR. Air embolism complicated by left hemiparesis after direct cholangioscopy with an intraductal balloon anchoring system. Gastrointest Endosc. 2012;75(1):221–3. doi:10.1016/j.gie.2011.01.038. Epub 2011 Apr 5.

52. Neuhaus H, Zillinger C, Born P, Ott R, Allescher H, Rösch T, Classen M. Randomized study of intracorporeal laser lithotripsy versus extracorporeal shock-wave lithotripsy for difficult bile duct stones. Gastrointest Endosc. 1998;47(5):327–34.

53. Jakobs R, Adamek HE, Maier M, Krömer M, Benz C, Martin WR, Riemann JF. Fluoroscopically guided laser lithotripsy versus extracorporeal shock wave lithotripsy for retained bile duct stones: a prospective randomised study. Gut. 1997;40(5):678–82. PubMed PMID: 9203950, PubMed Central PMCID: PMC1027174.

54. Bland KI, Jones RS, Maher JW, Cotton PB, Pennell TC, Amerson JR, Munson JL, Berci G, Fuchs GJ, Way LW, et al. Extracorporeal shock-wave lithotripsy of bile duct calculi. An interim report of the Dornier U.S. Bile Duct Lithotripsy Prospective Study. Ann Surg. 1989;209(6):743–53. PubMed PMID: 2658883, PubMed Central PMCID: PMC1494134, discussion 753–5.

55. Meyenberger C, Meierhofer U, Michel-Harder C, Knuchel J, Wirth HP, Bühler H, Münch R, Altorfer J. Long-term follow-up after treatment of common bile duct stones by extracorporeal shock-wave lithotripsy. Endoscopy. 1996;28(5):411–7.

56. Ellis RD, Jenkins AP, Thompson RP, Ede RJ. Clearance of refractory bile duct stones with extracorporeal shockwave lithotripsy. Gut. 2000;47(5):728–31. PubMed PMID: 11034593, PubMed Central PMCID: PMC1728118.

57. Nicholson DA, Martin DF, Tweedle DE, Rao PN. Management of common bile duct stones using a second-generation extracorporeal shockwave lithotriptor. Br J Surg. 1992;79(8):811–4.

58. Muratori R, Azzaroli F, Buonfiglioli F, Alessandrelli F, Cecinato P, Mazzella G, Roda E. ESWL for difficult bile duct stones: a 15-year single centre experience. World J Gastroenterol. 2010;16(33):4159–63. PubMed PMID: 20806432, PubMed Central PMCID: PMC2932919.

59. Tandan M, Reddy DN, Santosh D, Reddy V, Koppuju V, Lakhtakia S, Gupta R, Ramchandani M, Rao GV. Extracorporeal shock wave lithotripsy of large difficult common bile duct stones: efficacy and analysis of factors that favor stone fragmentation. J Gastroenterol Hepatol. 2009;24(8):1370–4. doi:10.1111/j.1440-1746.2009.05919.x.

60. Ersoz G, Tekesin O, Ozutemiz AO, Gunsar F. Biliary sphincterotomy plus dilation with a large balloon for bile duct stones that are difficult to extract. Gastrointest Endosc. 2003;57(2):156–9.

61. Lee DK, Han JW. Endoscopic papillary large balloon dilation: guidelines for pursuing zero mortality. Clin Endosc.

2012;45(3):299–304. doi:10.5946/ce.2012.45.3.299. PubMed PMID: 22977823, PubMed Central PMCID: PMC3429757, Epub 2012 Aug 22.

62. Attam R, Freeman ML. Endoscopic papillary large balloon dilation for large common bile duct stones. J Hepatobiliary Pancreat Surg. 2009;16(5):618–23. doi:10.1007/s00534-009-0134-2. Epub 2009 Jun 24. Review.

63. Donatelli G, Vergeau B, Dhumane P, Cereatti F, Fiocca F, Tuszynski T, Meduri B. Endoscopic partial sphincterotomy coupled with large balloon papilla dilation – Single stage approach for management of extra-hepatic bile ducts macro-lithiasis. Video J Encycl GI Endosc. 2013;1(3):636–9. Retrieved March 14, 2015, from http://www.sciencedirect.com/science/article/pii/S2212097113000423.

64. Minami A, Hirose S, Nomoto T, Hayakawa S. Small sphincterotomy combined with papillary dilation with large balloon permits retrieval of large stones without mechanical lithotripsy. World J Gastroenterol. 2007;13(15):2179–82. PubMed PMID: 17465497, PubMed Central PMCID: PMC4146840.

65. Maydeo A, Bhandari S. Balloon sphincteroplasty for removing difficult bile duct stones. Endoscopy. 2007;39(11):958–61. Epub 2007 Aug 15.

66. Stefanidis G, Viazis N, Pleskow D, Manolakopoulos S, Theocharis L, Christodoulou C, Kotsikoros N, Giannousis J, Sgouros S, Rodias M, Katsikani A, Chuttani R. Large balloon dilation vs. mechanical lithotripsy for the management of large bile duct stones: a prospective randomized study. Am J Gastroenterol. 2011;106(2):278–85. doi:10.1038/ajg.2010.421. Epub 2010 Nov 2.

67. Rebelo A, Ribeiro PM, Correia AP, Cotter J. Endoscopic papillary large balloon dilation after limited sphincterotomy for difficult biliary stones. World J Gastrointest Endosc. 2012;4(5):180–4. doi:10.4253/wjge.v4.i5.180. PubMed Central PMCID: PMC3355240.

68. Heo JH, Kang DH, Jung HJ, Kwon DS, An JK, Kim BS, Suh KD, Lee SY, Lee JH, Kim GH, Kim TO, Heo J, Song GA, Cho M. Endoscopic sphincterotomy plus large-balloon dilation versus endoscopic sphincterotomy for removal of bile-duct stones. Gastrointest Endosc. 2007;66(4):720–6. quiz 768, 771.

69. Itoi T, Itokawa F, Sofuni A, Kurihara T, Tsuchiya T, Ishii K, Tsuji S, Ikeuchi N, Moriyasu F. Endoscopic sphincterotomy combined with large balloon dilation can reduce the procedure time and fluoroscopy time for removal of large bile duct stones. Am J Gastroenterol. 2009;104(3):560–5. doi:10.1038/ajg.2008.67. Epub 2009 Jan 27.

70. Kim TH, Oh HJ, Lee JY, Sohn YW. Can a small endoscopic sphincterotomy plus a large-balloon dilation reduce the use of mechanical lithotripsy in patients with large bile duct stones? Surg Endosc. 2011;25(10):3330–7. doi:10.1007/s00464-011-1720-3. Epub 2011 Apr 30.

71. Draganov PV, Evans W, Fazel A, Forsmark CE. Large size balloon dilation of the ampulla after biliary sphincterotomy can facilitate endoscopic extraction of difficult bile duct stones. J Clin Gastroenterol. 2009;43(8):782–6. doi:10.1097/MCG.0b013e31818f50a2.

72. Kim HG, Cheon YK, Cho YD, Moon JH, Park DH, Lee TH, Choi HJ, Park SH, Lee JS, Lee MS. Small sphincterotomy combined with endoscopic papillary large balloon dilation versus sphincterotomy. World J Gastroenterol. 2009;15(34):4298–304. PubMed PMID: 19750573, PubMed Central PMCID: PMC2744186.

73. Attasaranya S, Cheon YK, Vittal H, Howell DA, Wakelin DE, Cunningham JT, Ajmere N, Ste Marie Jr RW, Bhattacharya K, Gupta K, Freeman ML, Sherman S, McHenry L, Watkins JL, Fogel EL, Schmidt S, Lehman GA. Large-diameter biliary orifice balloon dilation to aid in endoscopic bile duct stone removal: a multicenter series. Gastrointest Endosc.

2008;67(7):1046–52. doi:10.1016/j.gie.2007.08.047. Epub 2008 Feb 21.

74. Misra SP, Dwivedi M. Large-diameter balloon dilation after endoscopic sphincterotomy for removal of difficult bile duct stones. Endoscopy. 2008;40(3):209–13. doi:10.1055/s-2007-967040. Epub 2008 Feb 11.

75. Witte CL. Choledochal obstruction by cystic duct stone. Mirizzi's syndrome. Am Surg. 1984;50(5):241–3.

76. Mithani R, Schwesinger WH, Bingener J, Sirinek KR, Gross GW. The Mirizzi syndrome: multidisciplinary management promotes optimal outcomes. J Gastrointest Surg. 2008;12(6):1022–8. Epub 2007 Sep 14.

77. Schäfer M, Schneiter R, Krähenbühl L. Incidence and management of Mirizzi syndrome during laparoscopic cholecystectomy. Surg Endosc. 2003;17(8):1186–90. discussion 1191–2. Epub 2003 May 13.

78. McSherry CK, Ferstenberg H, Virshup H. The Mirizzi syndrome: suggested classification and surgical therapy. Surg Gastroenterol. 1982;1:219–25.

79. England RE, Martin DF. Endoscopic management of Mirizzi's syndrome. Gut. 1997;40(2):272–6. PubMed Central PMCID: PMC1027061.

80. Benninger J, Rabenstein T, Farnbacher M, Keppler J, Hahn EG, Schneider HT. Extracorporeal shockwave lithotripsy of gallstones in cystic duct remnants and Mirizzi syndrome. Gastrointest Endosc. 2004;60(3):454–9.

81. Tsuyuguchi T, Sakai Y, Sugiyama H, Ishihara T, Yokosuka O. Long-term follow-up after peroral cholangioscopy-directed lithotripsy in patients with difficult bile duct stones, including Mirizzi syndrome: an analysis of risk factors predicting stone recurrence. Surg Endosc. 2011;25(7):2179–85. doi:10.1007/s00464-010-1520-1. Epub 2010 Dec 24.

82. Huang MH, Chen CH, Yang JC, Yang CC, Yeh YH, Chou DA, Mo LR, Yueh SK, Nien CK. Long-term outcome of percutaneous transhepatic cholangioscopic lithotomy for hepatolithiasis. Am J Gastroenterol. 2003;98(12):2655–62.

83. Pitt HA, Venbrux AC, Coleman J, Prescott CA, Johnson MS, Osterman Jr FA, Cameron JL. Intrahepatic stones. The transhepatic team approach. Ann Surg. 1994;219(5):527–35. PubMed Central PMCID: PMC1243184, discussion 535–7.

84. Yoshimoto H, Ikeda S, Tanaka M, Matsumoto S, Kuroda Y. Choledochoscopic electrohydraulic lithotripsy and lithotomy for stones in the common bile duct, intrahepatic ducts, and gallbladder. Ann Surg. 1989;210(5):576–82. PubMed Central PMCID: PMC1357789.

85. Liu CL, Fan ST, Wong J. Primary biliary stones: diagnosis and management. World J Surg. 1998;22(11):1162–6.

86. Mori T, Sugiyama M, Atomi Y. Gallstone disease: management of intrahepatic stones. Best Pract Res Clin Gastroenterol. 2006;20(6):1117–37. Review.

87. Cheon YK, Cho YD, Moon JH, Lee JS, Shim CS. Evaluation of long-term results and recurrent factors after operative and nonoperative treatment for hepatolithiasis. Surgery. 2009;146(5):843–53. doi:10.1016/j.surg.2009.04.009. Epub 2009 Jun 28.

88. Jan YY, Chen MF. Percutaneous trans-hepatic cholangioscopic lithotomy for hepatolithiasis: long-term results. Gastrointest Endosc. 1995;42(1):1–5.

89. Lee SK, Seo DW, Myung SJ, Park ET, Lim BC, Kim HJ, Yoo KS, Park HJ, Joo YH, Kim MH, Min YI. Percutaneous transhepatic cholangioscopic treatment for hepatolithiasis: an evaluation of long-term results and risk factors for recurrence. Gastrointest Endosc. 2001;53(3):318–23.

90. Chen C, Huang M, Yang J, Yang C, Yeh Y, Wu H, Chou D, Yueh S, Nien C. Reappraisal of percutaneous transhepatic cholangioscopic lithotomy for primary hepatolithiasis. Surg Endosc. 2005;19(4):505–9. Epub 2005 Feb 3.

91. Neuhaus H. Endoscopic and percutaneous treatment of difficult bile duct stones. Endoscopy. 2003;35(8):S31–4. Review.

92. Kennedy RH, Thompson MH. Are duodenal diverticula associated with choledocholithiasis? Gut. 1988;29(7):1003–6. PubMed Central PMCID: PMC1433758.

93. Lee A, Shah JN. Endoscopic approach to the bile duct in the patient with surgically altered anatomy. Gastrointest Endosc Clin N Am. 2013;23(2):483–504. doi:10.1016/j.giec.2012.12.005. Epub 2013 Jan 12. Review.

94. García-Cano J. A simple technique to aid intubation of the duodenoscope in the afferent limb of Billroth II gastrectomies for endoscopic retrograde cholangiopancreatography. Endoscopy. 2008;40 Suppl 2:E21–2. doi:10.1055/s-2007-966950. Epub 2008 Feb 19.

95. Park CH, Lee WS, Joo YE, Kim HS, Choi SK, Rew JS. Cap-assisted ERCP in patients with a Billroth II gastrectomy. Gastrointest Endosc. 2007;66(3):612–5.

96. Osnes M, Rosseland AR, Aabakken L. Endoscopic retrograde cholangiography and endoscopic papillotomy in patients with a previous Billroth-II resection. Gut. 1986;27(10):1193–8. PubMed Central PMCID: PMC1433853.

97. Tyagi P, Sharma P, Sharma BC, Puri AS. Periampullary diverticula and technical success of endoscopic retrograde cholangiopancreatography. Surg Endosc. 2009;23(6):1342–5. doi:10.1007/s00464-008-0167-7. Epub 2008 Sep 26.

98. Bergman JJ, van Berkel AM, Bruno MJ, Fockens P, Rauws EA, Tijssen JG, Tytgat GN, Huibregtse K. A randomized trial of endoscopic balloon dilation and endoscopic sphincterotomy for removal of bile duct stones in patients with a prior Billroth II gastrectomy. Gastrointest Endosc. 2001;53(1):19–26.

99. Hintze RE, Adler A, Veltzke W, Abou-Rebyeh H. Endoscopic access to the papilla of Vater for endoscopic retrograde cholangiopancreatography in patients with Billroth II or Roux-en-Y gastrojejunostomy. Endoscopy. 1997;29(2):69–73.

100. Faylona JM, Qadir A, Chan AC, Lau JY, Chung SC. Small-bowel perforations related to endoscopic retrograde cholangiopancreatography (ERCP) in patients with Billroth II gastrectomy. Endoscopy. 1999;31(7):546–9.

101. Neumann H, Fry LC, Meyer F, Malfertheiner P, Monkemuller K. Endoscopic retrograde cholangiopancreatography using the single balloon enteroscope technique in patients with Roux-en-Y anastomosis. Digestion. 2009;80(1):52–7. doi:10.1159/000216351.

102. Gostout CJ, Bender CE. Cholangiopancreatography, sphincterotomy, and common duct stone removal via Roux-en-Y limb enteroscopy. Gastroenterology. 1988;95(1):156–63.

103. Elton E, Hanson BL, Qaseem T, Howell DA. Diagnostic and therapeutic ERCP using an enteroscope and a pediatric colonoscope in long-limb surgical bypass patients. Gastrointest Endosc. 1998;47(1):62–7.

104. Shimatani M, Matsushita M, Takaoka M, Koyabu M, Ikeura T, Kato K, Fukui T, Uchida K, Okazaki K. Effective "short" double-balloon enteroscope for diagnostic and therapeutic ERCP in patients with altered gastrointestinal anatomy: a large case series. Endoscopy. 2009;41(10):849–54. doi:10.1055/s-0029-1215108. Epub 2009 Sep 11.

105. Itoi T, Ishii K, Sofuni A, Itokawa F, Tsuchiya T, Kurihara T, Tsuji S, Ikeuchi N, Umeda J, Moriyasu F. Single-balloon enteroscopy-assisted ERCP in patients with Billroth II gastrectomy or Roux-en-Y anastomosis (with video). Am J Gastroenterol. 2010;105(1):93–9. doi:10.1038/ajg.2009.559. Epub 2009 Oct 6.

106. Emmett DS, Mallat DB. Double-balloon ERCP in patients who have undergone Roux-en-Y surgery: a case series. Gastrointest Endosc. 2007;66(5):1038–41.

107. Wright BE, Cass OW, Freeman ML. ERCP in patients with long-limb Roux-en-Y gastrojejunostomy and intact papilla. Gastrointest Endosc. 2002;56(2):225–32.

108. Saleem A, Baron TH, Gostout CJ, Topazian MD, Levy MJ, Petersen BT, Petersen BT, Wong Kee Song LM. Endoscopic retrograde cholangiopancreatography using a single-balloon enteroscope in patients with altered Roux-en-Y anatomy. Endoscopy. 2010;42(8):656–60. doi:10.1055/s-0030-1255557. Epub 2010 Jun 29.

109. Aabakken L, Bretthauer M, Line PD. Double-balloon enteroscopy for endoscopic retrograde cholangiography in patients with a Roux-en-Y anastomosis. Endoscopy. 2007;39(12):1068–71.

110. Wagh MS, Draganov PV. Prospective evaluation of spiral overtube-assisted ERCP in patients with surgically altered anatomy. Gastrointest Endosc. 2012;76(2):439–43. doi:10.1016/j.gie.2012.04.444.

111. Shah RJ, Smolkin M, Yen R, Ross A, Kozarek RA, Howell DA, Bakis G, Jonnalagadda SS, Al-Lehibi AA, Hardy A, Morgan DR, Sethi A, Stevens PD, Akerman PA, Thakkar SJ, Brauer BC. A multicenter, U.S. experience of single-balloon, double-balloon, and rotational overtube-assisted enteroscopy ERCP in patients with surgically altered pancreaticobiliary anatomy (with video). Gastrointest Endosc. 2013;77(4):593–600. doi:10.1016/j.gie.2012.10.015. Epub 2013 Jan 3.

112. Rimon U, Kleinmann N, Bensaid P, Golan G, Garniek A, Khaitovich B, Winkler H. Percutaneous transhepatic endoscopic holmium laser lithotripsy for intrahepatic and choledochal biliary stones. Cardiovasc Intervent Radiol. 2011;34(6):1262–6. doi:10.1007/s00270-010-0058-x. Epub 2010 Dec 16.

113. van der Velden JJ, Berger MY, Bonjer HJ, Brakel K, Laméris JS. Percutaneous treatment of bile duct stones in patients treated unsuccessfully with endoscopic retrograde procedures. Gastrointest Endosc. 2000;51(4 Pt 1):418–22.

114. Stage JG, Moesgaard F, Grønvall S, Stage P, Kehlet H. Percutaneous transhepatic cholelithotripsy for difficult common bile duct stones. Endoscopy. 1998;30(3):289–92.

115. Jeong EJ, Kang DH, Kim DU, Choi CW, Eum JS, Jung WJ, Kim PJ, Kim YW, Jung KS, Bae YM, Cho M. Percutaneous transhepatic choledochoscopic lithotomy as a rescue therapy for removal of bile duct stones in Billroth II gastrectomy patients who are difficult to perform ERCP. Eur J Gastroenterol Hepatol. 2009;21(12):1358–62. doi:10.1097/MEG.0b013e328326caa1.

116. Martinez J, Guerrero L, Byers P, Lopez P, Scagnelli T, Azuaje R, Dunkin B. Endoscopic retrograde cholangiopancreatography and gastroduodenoscopy after Roux-en-Y gastric bypass. Surg Endosc. 2006;20(10):1548–50. Epub 2006 Aug 1.

117. Baron TH, Vickers SM. Surgical gastrostomy placement as access for diagnostic and therapeutic ERCP. Gastrointest Endosc. 1998;48(6):640–1.

118. Lopes TL, Clements RH, Wilcox CM. Laparoscopy-assisted ERCP: experience of a high-volume bariatric surgery center (with video). Gastrointest Endosc. 2009;70(6):1254–9. doi:10.1016/j.gie.2009.07.035. Epub 2009 Oct 28.

119. Patel JA, Patel NA, Shinde T, Uchal M, Dhawan MK, Kulkarni A, Colella JJ. Endoscopic retrograde cholangiopancreatography after laparoscopic Roux-en-Y gastric bypass: a case series and review of the literature. Am Surg. 2008;74(8):689–93. discussion 693–4. Review.

120. Gutierrez JM, Lederer H, Krook JC, Kinney TP, Freeman ML, Jensen EH. Surgical gastrostomy for pancreatobiliary and duodenal access following Roux en Y gastric bypass. J Gastrointest Surg. 2009;13(12):2170–5. doi:10.1007/s11605-009-0991-7. Epub 2009 Sep 24.

121. Tsuyuguchi T, Saisho H, Ishihara T, Yamaguchi T, Onuma EK. Long-term follow-up after treatment of Mirizzi syndrome by peroral cholangioscopy. Gastrointest Endosc. 2000;52(5):639–44.

122. Maranki J, Hernandez AJ, Arslan B, Jaffan AA, Angle JF, Shami VM, Kahaleh M. Interventional endoscopic ultrasound-guided cholangiography: long-term experience of an emerging alterna-

tive to percutaneous transhepatic cholangiography. Endoscopy. 2009;41(6):532–8. doi:10.1055/s-0029-1214712. Epub 2009 Jun 16.

123. Dhir V, Bhandari S, Bapat M, Maydeo A. Comparison of EUS-guided rendezvous and precut papillotomy techniques for biliary access (with videos). Gastrointest Endosc. 2012;75(2):354–9. doi:10.1016/j.gie.2011.07.075.

124. Iwashita T, Lee JG, Shinoura S, Nakai Y, Park DH, Muthusamy VR, Chang KJ. Endoscopic ultrasound-guided rendezvous for biliary access after failed cannulation. Endoscopy. 2012;44(1): 60–5. doi:10.1055/s-0030-1256871. Epub 2011 Nov 29.

125. Iwashita T, Yasuda I, Doi S, Yamauchi T, Uemura S, Okuno M, Moriwaki H. Endoscopic ultrasound-guided antegrade papillary balloon dilation for treating a common bile duct stone. Dig Endosc. 2013;25(1):89–90. doi:10.1111/j.1443-1661.2012.01381.x.

126. Weilert F, Binmoeller KF, Marson F, Bhat Y, Shah JN. Endoscopic ultrasound-guided anterograde treatment of biliary stones following gastric bypass. Endoscopy. 2011;43(12):1105–8. doi:10.1055/s-0030-1256961. Epub 2011 Nov 4.

127. Di Giorgio P, Manes G, Grimaldi E, Schettino M, D'Alessandro A, Di Giorgio A, Giannattasio F. Endoscopic plastic stenting for bile duct stones: stent changing on demand or every 3 months. A prospective comparison study. Endoscopy. 2013;45(12):1014–7. doi:10.1055/s-0033-1344556. Epub 2013 Nov 28.

128. Lee TH, Han JH, Kim HJ, Park SM, Park SH, Kim SJ. Is the addition of choleretic agents in multiple double-pigtail biliary stents effective for difficult common bile duct stones in elderly patients? A prospective, multicenter study. Gastrointest Endosc. 2011;74(1):96–102. doi:10.1016/j.gie.2011.03.005. Epub 2011 Apr 30.

ERCP in Patients with Chronic Pancreatitis

Virendra Joshi and Laura Alder

Etiology

Chronic pancreatitis (CP) is a disease of varied etiology characterized by progressive and irreversible damage to the pancreas with resultant loss of both endocrine and exocrine function. Alcohol, smoking, genetic factors, autoimmune, congenital, and metabolic disorders are common etiological causes. One elegant attempt at classification of chronic pancreatitis based on pathophysiology is worth mentioning—TIGAR-O (Toxic, Idiopathic, Genetic, Autoimmune, Recurrent acute pancreatitis, Obstructive) [1].

Evaluation and Diagnosis

Computed Tomography (CT) scanning is the most sensitive and accurate noninvasive method to identify pancreatic calcifications, which often signifies the presence of scarring within the pancreas (Fig. 3.1). Magnetic resonance with cholangiopancreatography (MRCP) is the best noninvasive

Electronic supplementary material: The online version of this chapter (doi:10.1007/978-3-319-26854-5_3) contains supplementary material, which is available to authorized users. Videos can also be accessed at http://link.springer.com/chapter/10.1007/978-3-319-26854-5_3.

V. Joshi, M.D., A.G.A.F. (✉)
Tulane School of Medicine, New Orleans, LA USA

University of Queensland School of Medicine, Brisbane, QLD, Australia

Department of Gastroenterology, Advanced Endoscopy, Ochsner Medical Center, Ochsner Cancer Institute, 1514, Jefferson Hwy, New Orleans, LA 70121, USA
e-mail: vjoshi@ochsner.org

L. Alder
Department of Gastroenterology, Advanced Endoscopy, Ochsner Medical Center, Ochsner Cancer Institute, 1514, Jefferson Hwy, New Orleans, LA 70121, USA

Mayne Medical School, University of Queensland School of Medicine, Brisbane, QLD, Australia

technique to assess the anatomy of the biliary tree, of the pancreatic ducts, and of inflammatory pancreatic fluid collections including pseudocysts and necrosis. CT scans are often obtained to assist in planning treatments for patients with chronic pancreatitis. A combination of other imaging modalities (e.g., MRCP or endoscopic ultrasonography [EUS] plus CT scanning or abdominal X-ray) may be preferable in specific circumstances (e.g., suspected anatomical variants of the pancreatic ducts, CBD strictures, or drainage of post-necrotic pancreatic fluid collections).

Chronic pancreatitis is associated with an increased risk of pancreatic cancer. It can sometimes be difficult to distinguish chronic pancreatitis from pancreatic cancer, and the two can also occur simultaneously. In patients with a pancreatic mass or a main pancreatic duct (MPD) or common bile duct (CBD) stricture in the context of chronic pancreatitis, an adequate workup should be performed to reasonably rule out a pancreatic cancer, cystic neoplasms of pancreas or autoimmune pancreatitis (although chronic pancreatitis can cause all of these ductal abnormalities and can often mimic malignancy).

In the past, ERCP was frequently used both for diagnosis and management of patients with CP (Fig. 3.2). ERCP has a sensitivity of 73–94 % and specificity of 90–100 % in visualizing duct related changes in CP [2]. The emergence of magnetic resonance cholangiopancreatography (MRCP) with secretin stimulation, as well as EUS, has minimized the role of ERCP in diagnosing CP. EUS is a better diagnostic modality, especially in early and less advanced CP, as it identifies both ductal and parenchymal changes, and poses minimal risk to patients [3]. EUS has a diagnostic sensitivity of close to 100 % as compared to 80 % with ERCP in patients with early CP [3]. MRCP is completely noninvasive and provides a "roadmap" prior to ERCP for evaluating ductal changes.

ERCP, a once purely diagnostic procedure, is now mainly a therapeutic tool in managing the complications arising from chronic pancreatitis. ERCP provides direct access to the pancreatic duct for evaluation and treatment of symptomatic stones, strictures, leaks and pseudocysts, which can occur alone or in combination. ERCP is not entirely benign and

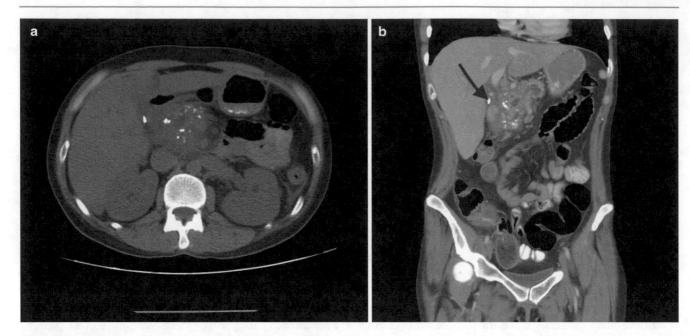

Fig. 3.1 (**a** and **b**) Axial and coronal CT scan images of chronic pancreatitis showing dense calcifications (*arrow*) and pancreatic ductal dilation

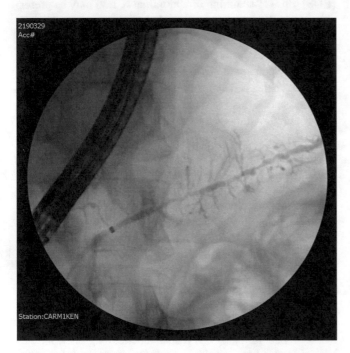

Fig. 3.2 Pancreatogram obtained during ERCP showing dilated main pancreatic duct and dilated side branches consistent with chronic pancreatitis

even in expert hands it carries a risk of acute pancreatitis, hemorrhage, perforation, and in very rare cases, death [4].

Minimal Change Chronic Pancreatitis

Painful CP can occasionally present with minimal or no ductal dilation and in the absence of ductal strictures or stones. This is classified as mild CP as per the Cambridge classification [5]. Endoscopic pancreatic sphincterotomy (EPS) is a documented mode of therapy and offers symptomatic relief in some of these patients. Both the standard pull type and the needle knife sphincterotomy over a stent can be performed. A 64 % relief in pain on follow-up of 6.5 years has been reported following EPS in patients with minimal change chronic pancreatitis [6]. High success rates of 98 % and low complication rates of around 4 % have been reported in one retrospective analysis [7]. Randomized studies have shown a higher incidence of pancreatitis in high risk patients following pull type sphincterotomy as compared to the needle knife technique, although the former is most commonly performed due to its speed and technical ease [8]. Approximately 12 % of patients with CP undergoing EPS will develop post-ERCP pancreatitis (PEP) [9–11]. Placement of a pancreatic stent can reduce this incidence significantly [12]. Recent data showing a reduced risk of PEP with rectal NSAIDs such as indomethacin apply to this patient population as well [13, 14]. Re-stenosis of the pancreatic sphincter orifice is reported in up to 14 % of patients on long-term follow-up [15]. It is believed that re-stenosis is less common following the longer incision often created with pull type sphincterotomes as compared to those created via the needle knife technique [16]. The presence of periductal fibrosis seen in patients with CP may lower the incidence of post procedure pancreatitis. An additional biliary sphincterotomy may also indicated in the following conditions [17]: (1) presence of cholangitis, (2) CBD >12 mm diameter, (3) serum alkaline phosphatase >2 times upper limit of normal, (4) difficult access to MPD, and (5) need for other biliary intervention.

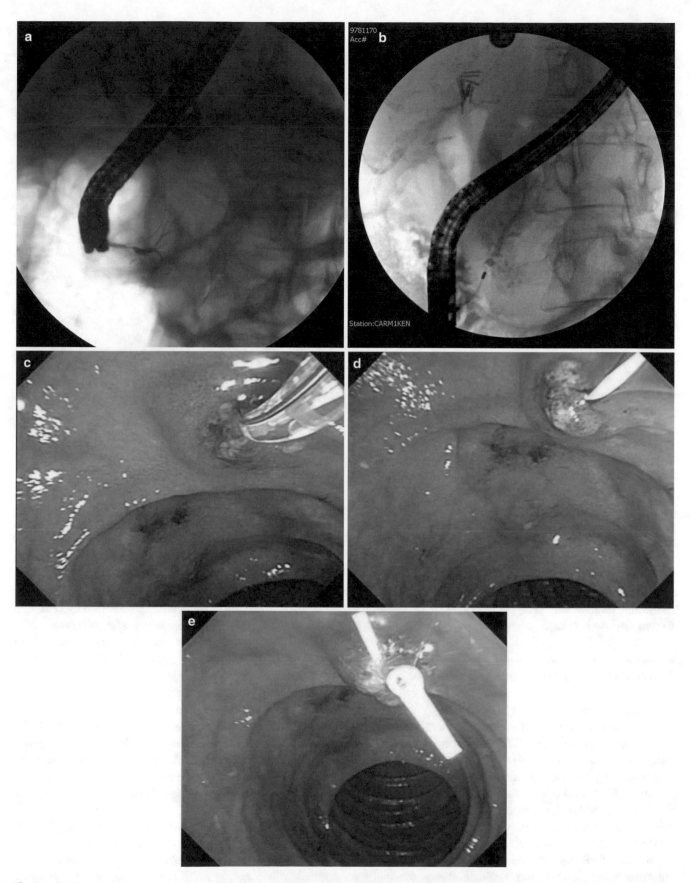

Fig. 3.3 (**a**) Pancreas Divisum. Cannulation of the pancreatic duct at the major papilla only visualized the ventral duct that does not communicate with the main duct. A separate wire is in the biliary tree. (Image courtesy of Douglas G. Adler MD). (**b**) Pancreas divisum in a different patient than (**a**). Cannulation of the minor papilla results in opacification of the dorsal pancreatic duct to the tail. Note that the pancreatic duct is dilated with dilated side branches. (**c**) Cannulation of the minor papilla with a pull-type sphinc-terotome in a patient with chronic pancreatitis and pancreas divisum. (Image courtesy of Douglas G. Adler MD). (**d**) Image of minor papilla following minor papillotomy. Note that the actual length of the cut in this patient is quite short when compared to a typical biliary sphincterotomy. (Image courtesy of Douglas G. Adler MD). (**e**) Pancreatic duct stent place-ment was performed at the minor papilla following papillotomy. (Image courtesy of Douglas G. Adler MD)

Minor Papilla Endoscopic Sphincterotomy in Chronic Pancreatitis

Minor papilla endoscopic sphincterotomy (MiES) was first performed by Cotton [18]. It is indicated in those patients with CP with minimal ductal changes who have a pancreas divisum or a dominant dorsal duct. Both the pull type and needle knife technique can be used.

If a pull type sphincterotome is used, deep access to the dorsal duct is obtained with a guidewire and the sphincterotomy is done in a standard fashion, recognizing that the cut itself may be very short as compared to, say, a biliary sphincterotomy (Fig. 3.3). The needle-knife technique used for minor papillotomy is similar to that of EPS of the major papilla. Following wire-guided cannulation, a small diameter 3- or 5-F pancreatic stent is first placed over the wire and through the minor papillary orifice into the proximal dorsal duct. Once the stent is in position and the guidewire is removed, a needle-knife is used to cut the portion of the minor papillary mound above the stent. The needle-knife cutting wire is generally directed in the 11 o'clock position along the course of the dorsal duct as the minor papilla is 'unroofed'. Again, either blended current or pure cutting current may be used. The evidence of any definite benefit from MiES is debatable as studies include small numbers of heterogeneous patients and are not conclusive. Significant pain relief on a 2-year follow-up has been reported following MiES and stenting of patients with CP [19]. Relief of pain is also seen in 41 % of patients with CP following MiES as compared to 77 % with acute recurrent pancreatitis or 33 % of patients with CP with no pain [20]. Post ERCP pancreatitis has been reported in up to 15 % of patients [21] and re-stenosis of the minor papilla was seen in 20–24 % of patients on a 6-year follow-up [22].

Pancreatic Sphincterotomy Techniques

Endoscopic pancreatic sphincterotomy (EPS) at the major papilla is the cornerstone of endoscopic therapy in patients with chronic pancreatitis [23–25]. Once pancreatic duct access is obtained, EPS may be used as a single therapeutic maneuver (e.g., to treat pancreatic-type sphincter of Oddi dysfunction), or in combination with other endoscopic therapeutic techniques such as stone extraction, stricture dilation, and stent placement [23–25].

Once a clear indication for sphincterotomy has been established, EPS is most often performed with a pull-type sphincterotome. Like biliary sphincterotomy, the incision should be created in a careful and controlled manner [26]. The direction of the sphincterotomy itself should be towards the 1–2 o'clock position [27, 28] (Fig. 3.4). Only a small

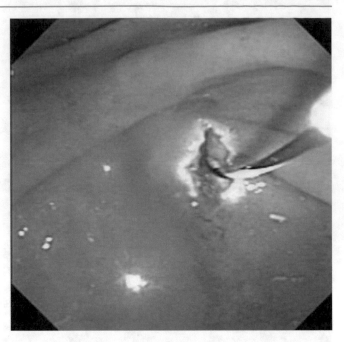

Fig. 3.4 Pancreatic sphincterotomy in a patient with chronic pancreatitis. Note the 1 o'clock orientation of the sphincterotomy. (Image courtesy of Douglas G. Adler MD)

amount of cutting wire should be used to make the actual cut to maximize current density and to minimize tissue trauma. In other words, most of the cutting wire should be visible outside the papillary orifice during the actual creation of the sphincterotomy. Note that the direction of the cut in a pancreatic sphincterotomy is very different from that of a biliary sphincterotomy (where the cutting direction is usually towards the 11 o'clock position) [27].

Another approach to pancreatic sphincterotomy is using a needle-knife at the pancreatic orifice after placement of a pancreatic duct stent. The stent provides ductal drainage and a guide for the direction of the pancreatic duct and the pancreatic sphincter complex during the actual sphincterotomy. The incision can be made from the ampullary orifice in an upwards direction or from a more superior position in a downwards direction. The overall length of the incision with any type of sphincterotomy has to be individualized. Some have postulated that a prior biliary sphincterotomy can be of assistance when performing a pancreatic sphincterotomy, as it often helps expose the pancreatobiliary septum during pancreatic sphincterotomy [15].

The so-called "pre-cut pancreatic sphincterotomy" refers to pancreatic sphincterotomy being performed prior to achieving deep pancreatic ductal access. This can be performed with a needle knife sphincterotome or a standard pull-type sphincterotome inserted into the ampullary orifice. This maneuver is usually undertaken when access to the pancreatic duct is blocked in some manner (e.g., an impacted stone) [29–31]. Once the pancreatic duct is accessed and a guidewire has been advanced into the pancreatic duct, the sphincterotomy can be completed with either device.

Management of Pancreatic Stones

Chronic pancreatitis can cause both pancreatic-duct dilatation and obstruction. Obstructing pancreatic stones may contribute to abdominal pain or flares of pancreatitis in patients with chronic pancreatitis (Fig. 3.5). Approximately one third of patients with chronic pancreatitis will have pancreatic stones. Approximately half of those people with stones will have the majority of their stone burden within the main duct in the pancreatic head or body. Such patients typically have a pancreatic duct stricture downstream from the stones which presumably contribute to stone formation.

The sensitivity and the specificity of ERCP for detecting main duct pancreatic stones is over 95 %; small stones are missed occasionally. Removing pancreatic stones endoscopically is less invasive compared to surgery but is more likely to be successful when the stone burden is small and stones are located only in the main duct [32–34].

Endoscopic management of pancreatic duct stones is a significant undertaking. It is relatively high risk, may involve multiple procedures, and offers no guarantee of relief from pain even in patients whose ducts are cleared of all stones. Patients should be willing to undergo repeat procedures as needed before undergoing endoscopic pancreatic duct removal as it is unusual to completely clear the duct in a single procedure.

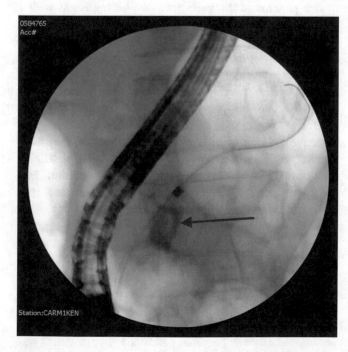

Fig. 3.5 Large pancreatic duct stone in the ventral duct (*arrow*)

From a technical point of view, pancreatic duct stone removal often involves a combination of many techniques including pancreatic sphincterotomy, stricture dilation, lithotripsy, stone removal, and pancreatic duct stenting. Endoscopists should undertake pancreatic stone removal recognizing that some or all of these techniques may be required for a given patient.

If pancreatic duct stones are non-obstructing and the patient does not have appreciable pancreatic duct strictures, removal is often straightforward and accomplished with baskets and balloons (Fig. 3.6).

If pancreatic duct stones are located above a stricture, the stricture must be crossed and dilated before endoscopic therapy for the stones can be initiated. In theory, this sounds simple but in practice this can be tremendously difficult and, in some patients, impossible. Often, multiple attempts with different guidewires and catheters are required to successfully traverse a tight pancreatic duct stricture. If a pancreatic stricture cannot be crossed by endoscopic means the patient may warrant surgical evaluation for pancreatic duct decompression and stone removal.

Pancreatic duct stones may also obstruct the pancreatic duct in the absence of a pancreatic stricture. This obstruction is often, at least in part, a cause of the patient's pancreatic-type pain. If a guidewire can be advanced past the stone then the stone can typically be reached by endoscopic accessories to facilitate removal. Techniques such as mechanical lithotripsy, laser lithotripsy, or electrohydraulic shockwave lithotripsy may be used to fragment the stone or stones prior to removal with baskets or balloons (Fig. 3.7).

Impacted stones that obstruct the pancreatic duct may require extracorporeal shockwave lithotripsy (ESWL) to fragment before endoscopic removal can be attempted. ESWL, often performed by urologists or interventional radiologists, uses focused sound waves to try to fracture pancreatic duct stones. ESWL for pancreatic stones is a difficult procedure even in experienced hands, has significant risks, and patients may require protracted therapy (>10 sessions) to obtain successful fracture of stones and eventual clearance of the pancreatic duct. While some investigators have reported high success rates with this technique (with or without pancreatic stents), others have had much less impressive results, with improvement in pain seen in less than 35 % of patients, whereas other large series have reported that, despite successful ESWL, most patients experience no improvement in pain [33, 34].

Some encouraging short-term (77–100 %) and long-term (54–86 %) improvements in pain have been reported with the treatment of pancreatic duct stones. Other, larger series have been less encouraging. One large series of 1000 patients with chronic pancreatitis with long-term follow-up found that only 65 % of patients with strictures and stones could benefit from pancreatic endotherapy with

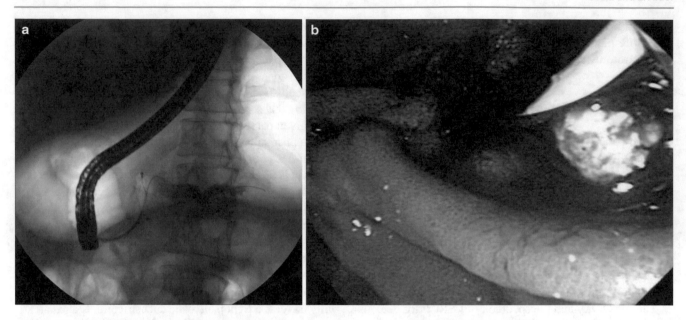

Fig. 3.6 (**a**) A 1.5 cm stone retrieval basket is used to capture stones in a dilated pancreatic duct in a patient with chronic pancreatitis. (Image courtesy of Douglas G. Adler MD). (**b**) Endoscopic image of a pancre- atic duct stone in the duodenum after removal from the pancreatic duct. (Image courtesy of Douglas G. Adler MD)

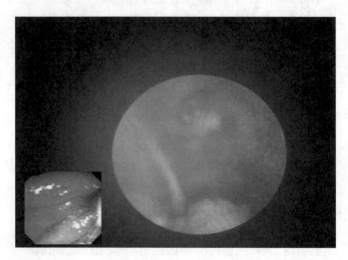

Fig. 3.7 A cluster of pancreatic duct stones seen on fiber optic pancreatoscopy. The stones were causing pancreatic duct obstruction in the absence of a pancreatic duct stricture. The stones were then cleared using balloon and basket sweeps. (Image courtesy of Douglas G. Adler MD)

regard to pain but that endotherapy did not improve pancreatic function [33, 35]. Also, this same study found that 24 % of patients ultimately underwent some form of surgery to treat their chronic pancreatitis.

Pancreatic Duct Strictures

Strictures of the main pancreatic duct (MPD) are seen in about half of patients of chronic pancreatitis. Most strictures are inflammatory and fibrotic and difficult to cannulate

(Video 3.1) (Fig. 3.8). A Soehendra stent retriever can be used to attempt to simultaneously traverse and dilate a pancreatic duct stricture. Once a stricture has been dilated (Video 3.2), placement of a pancreatic stent (Video 3.3) across the stricture helps promote stricture patency and facilitates future procedures wherein the stricture can be dilated further as needed. Patients who undergo successful stenting of pancreatic duct strictures may often be able to avoid pancreatic decompressive surgery [36–39].

If a pancreatic duct stricture can be traversed with a guidewire, dilation can be performed with a biliary dilation balloon or a tapered biliary dilation catheter a.k.a a passage dilator [40, 41] (Fig. 3.9) (Video 3.2). In patients with pancreatic-type pain and pancreatic structures, if the stricture can be traversed with a wire, dilated and stented, the MPD can be functionally decompressed and the patient's pain can then be reevaluated. Some patients will have marked improvement in pain while others may have no change in symptoms. This latter outcome highlights the fact that pain in chronic pancreatitis is often multifactorial in nature and that endoscopic success does not always translate into clinical success.

In one randomized trial of endoscopic and surgical therapy for patients with strictures and painful chronic pancreatitis, surgery was superior for durability in patients with painful obstructive chronic pancreatitis, although endotherapy is typically the first line of treatment given its less invasive nature [38].

In a single center experience of 1000 patients who underwent ESWL, the incidence of pancreatic duct strictures was 18 % [39]. MPD strictures are defined as a high grade narrowing of MPD with one of the following: (1) MPD dilatation

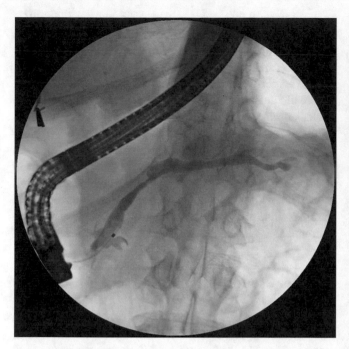

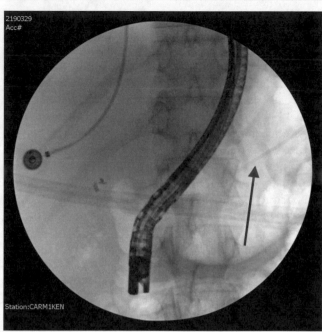

Fig. 3.8 Fluoroscopic image of a pancreatic duct stricture in the genu in a patient with painful chronic pancreatitis. (Image courtesy of Douglas G. Adler MD)

Fig. 3.10 Fluoroscopic image of a proximally migrated pancreatic duct stent (*arrow*)

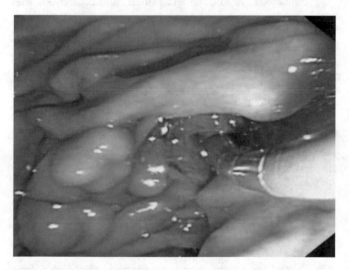

Fig. 3.9 Endoscopic image of a passage dilator being advanced into the pancreatic duct to treat a pancreatic duct stricture

>6 mm beyond the stricture; (2) failure of contrast to flow through the stricture [40, 41]. Endotherapy is ideal for single strictures in the head while isolated strictures in the tail or multiple strictures with a chain of lake appearance are often not amenable to endotherapy [40].

Large bore stents 7–10 Fr should be used, if possible, when treating pancreatic duct strictures as they have longer patency [41]. Delhaye et al. [41] proposed a protocol where a single stent was placed across a stricture and exchanged every 6 months or when the patient developed recurrent

symptoms. Stents were placed for 24 months. Patients were restented if symptoms recurred. Surgery can be considered if patients responded to stent placement but needed frequent or repeated stenting.

Cumulative data from several investigators revealed pain relief between 70 and 94 % for a single pancreatic stent on follow-up of 14–69 months [40]. Recurrence of strictures was reported in 38 % of patients after 2 years follow-up [42]. The concept of multiple plastic stenting for MPD strictures not responding to a single stent placement was advocated by Costamagna et al. [43]. These authors proposed that after a round of treatment with a single pancreatic duct stent the stricture was dilated and multiple plastic stents 8.5–11.5 Fr diameter were placed. A mean of three stents were used per patient. The stents were removed 12 months later. Stricture resolution was seen in 95 % of patients and pain relief in 84 % at 38 months follow-up. In patients with a normal pancreas, long-term stenting of the pancreatic duct is usually avoided to reduce the risk of pancreatic duct fibrosis [44], although this is much less of a concern in patients with chronic pancreatitis [45].

Complications with pancreatic stenting can occur, and new types of pancreatic stents are still being developed to reduce the limitations of these devices [46, 47]. Stent occlusion and/or migration will occur in up to 10 % of patients [44] (Fig. 3.10). Distal migration and impaction on the opposite duodenal wall can rarely cause perforation while proximal migration into the pancreas is a technical challenge for the endoscopist. Some proximally migrated pancreatic duct stents cannot be removed endoscopically and need to be removed via surgical means.

The use of covered metal biliary stents (CSEMS) for pancreatic strictures is also under evaluation. Standard or novel CSEMS can be used in an off label manner to treat pancreatic duct strictures in patients with chronic pancreatitis [48, 49]. Advantages to this approach include their large diameters and high radial force which can be very effective in treating even densely fibrotic strictures. Downsides to this approach include the risks of migration (especially proximal migration), higher costs, and potential obstruction of pancreatic duct side branches. CSEMS can also be associated with de novo stricture formation at their ends.

European Society of Gastrointestinal Endoscopy (ESGE) guidelines state that dominant PD strictures be treated by placing a single 10 Fr stent with stent exchanges planned for 1 year [50]. Multiple plastic stents should be deployed in a stricture which persists after 1 year of single stent placement [43]. Uncovered SEMS (self expanding metal stents) should, with rare exception, not be placed in MPD as they are very likely to become permanent implants that cannot be removed endoscopically.

Pancreatic Duct Leaks

Leaks from the MPD or side branches can occur following rupture of the ducts due to obstruction by stone or strictures (Fig. 3.11). A pancreatic duct leak is defined as extravasation of

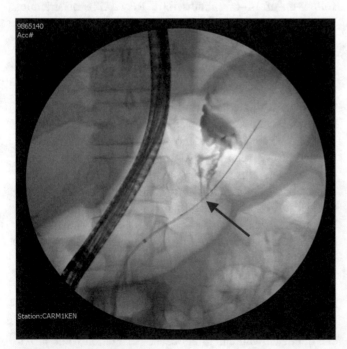

Fig. 3.11 Fluoroscopic image of a pancreatic duct leak in a patient with chronic pancreatitis

contrast material from the ductal system confirmed via ERCP [51–54]. Disruption may be partial or complete and can lead to fluid collection, pseudocyst formation, pancreatic ascites, pleural effusion and external or internal fistulas [41, 45, 52].

The cornerstone of treatment for pancreatic duct leaks is pancreatic duct stenting. If possible, the stent should bridge the leak itself to promote resolution of the leak and duct continuity. Resolution of pancreatic duct leaks was seen in 92 % of patients when a stent bridged the disruption, in 50 % when the stent was placed near to the level of disruption and in 44 % when a short transpapillary stent was placed [51–53]. In patients with complete transection of the pancreatic duct stenting alone may not be adequate and surgery may be warranted.

ERCP for Pseudocyst Management in Chronic Pancreatitis

Management of pancreatic fluid collections are covered in detail in Chap. 14. This section will briefly cover the role of endoscopy in pseudocysts (Videos 3.4 and 3.5) in patients with chronic pancreatitis.

Pseudocysts are nonepithelial lined fluid collections that result from transient or persistent pancreatic duct disruption. Pancreatic pseudocysts may occur in the setting of acute or chronic pancreatitis. In the setting of chronic pancreatitis, symptomatic pseudocysts are commonly seen in a setting of coexistent stones or strictures that also need to be addressed. Pseudocysts can be treated via transampullary drainage, transmural drainage, or a combination thereof 80–90 % of endoscopically treated pseudocysts resolve within 1–2 months at which time stents are removed. A 15 % recurrence rate has been reported [54].

Pseudocyst formation in patients with chronic pancreatitis is usually the result of disruption of the MPD or one of its side branches and occurs in 20–40 % of patients [55]. Disruption generally follows obstruction by stones or strictures but can be purely due to inflammation. Treatment is indicated for symptomatic pseudocysts-size alone does not dictate the need for intervention [56]. Symptoms most commonly result due to compression of adjacent structures, bleeding, and/or infection. There is generally a low rate of spontaneous resolution of pseudocysts in patients with chronic pancreatitis regardless of the presence or absence of symptoms [57].

Transpapillary drainage of pseudocysts is usually performed if EUS or cross sectional imaging suggests communication between the main pancreatic duct and the cyst itself. In transpapillary drainage, the stent can promote primary drainage of the cyst through the main pancreatic duct and can also promote healing of any disruption of the pancreatic duct itself. The latter effect also minimizes ongoing backfilling of the

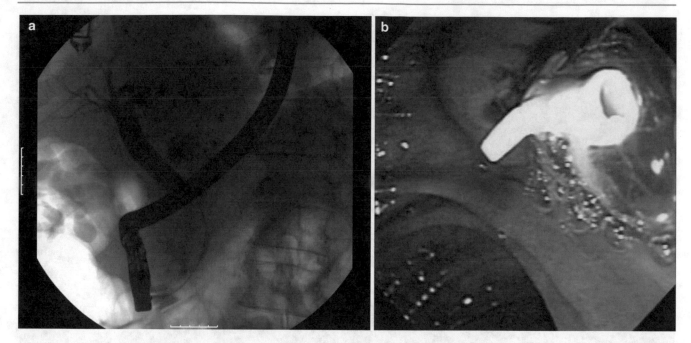

Fig. 3.12 (**a**) Fluoroscopic image of a pseudocyst that communicates with the main pancreatic duct in a patient with chronic pancreatitis. (Image courtesy of Douglas G. Adler MD). (**b**) Endoscopic image of pseudocyst-type fluid draining through a transampullary stent. (Image courtesy of Douglas G. Adler MD)

cyst. In patients who undergo transpapillary drainage of pancreatic pseudocysts, follow-up cross sectional imaging usually dictates the stent indwell time. Stent removal can be accomplished at the time of cyst collapse or resolution (Fig. 3.12).

Transmural drainage is often selected for symptomatic cysts that extrinsically compress the stomach, duodenum, and or bile duct. Some have suggested that transduodenal (as opposed to transgastric) drainage offers the best chance for long-term success because the drainage tracts created by transduodenal approaches tend to remain patent longer than those created by transgastric approaches, although in practice transgastric approaches are much more common [58]. Transmural drainage of simple pseudocyst (those without significant solid debris) can be performed under ERCP or EUS guidance, and usually involves the placement of two or more double pigtail plastic stents or a metal stent across the cystenterostomy [23, 59]. The ideal amount of time stents should be left in place is unknown but as a general rule 6–8 weeks is a typical timeframe to assess a patient for stent removal, usually by a combination of endoscopic and radiologic means [52].

Pseudoaneurysm can complicate management of pancreatic pseudocysts because of the associated risk of hemorrhage and its associated morbidity and mortaliy [60]. Delhaye et al. [41] recommend prophylactic embolization of pseudoaneurysms prior to drainage of an adjacent PPC.

The endoscopic drainage of nonbulging pseudocysts is usually accomplished using EUS-based approaches. Comparison of EUS guided drainage with surgical therapy for pseudocysts in one randomized clinical trial demonstrated that endoscopic drainage was superior to surgery in terms of cost and length of stay over a 3 month follow-up [61]. Complications include bleed, infection and leak of around 4 % each with a mortality of 0.5 % [62].

Of note, routine antibiotic administration is recommended for patients undergoing endoscopic drainage of pancreatic pseudocysts [63]. With a success rate of 80–95 % at most centers, a recurrence rate of 10–20 %, and results comparable to or better than those obtained via, endoscopy is the preferred first line of management for patients with PPC in the background of CP [41, 52].

ERCP for Chronic Pancreatitis-Associated Benign Biliary Strictures

Extrahepatic biliary strictures are common in patients with chronic pancreatitis. Distal common bile duct strictures will develop in approximately 3–46 % of patients with chronic pancreatitis [31, 53, 64, 65]. The stenosis arises most commonly as a consequence of fibrosis in the head of the pancreas with compression of the distal common bile duct, but adjacent pseudocysts can also compress the bile duct (Videos 3.4 and 3.5) The consequences of the obstruction include jaundice which may be associated with cholangitis. Secondary biliary cirrhosis can develop from chronic untreated obstruction.

The earliest manifestation of biliary obstruction may be an asymptomatic increase of the serum alkaline phosphatase level.

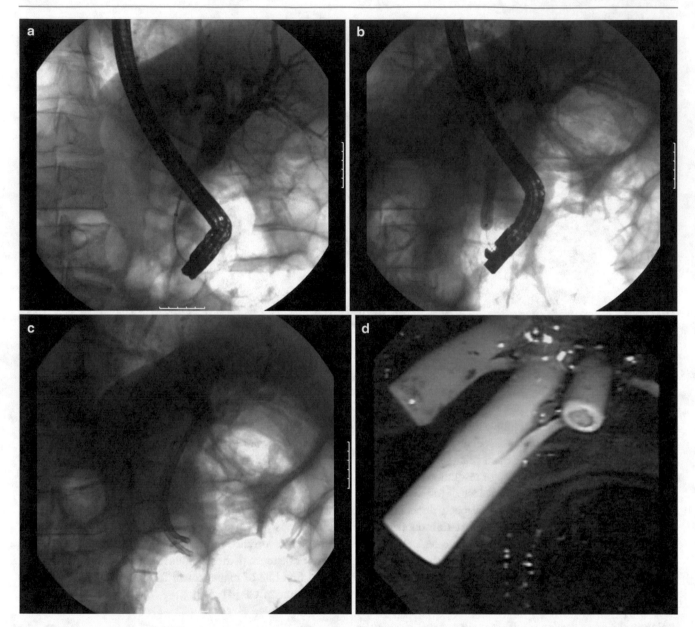

Fig. 3.13 Multiple plastic stents to treat a biliary stricture in a patient with chronic pancreatitis. (**a**) Fluoroscopic view of a distal CBD stricture with proximal intra- and extrahepatic ductal dilation. (Image courtesy of Douglas G. Adler MD). (**b**) Fluoroscopic view as the stricture is dilated with a biliary dilating balloon. (Image courtesy of Douglas G. Adler MD). (**c**) Fluoroscopic view of three plastic biliary stents placed across the stricture. (Image courtesy of Douglas G. Adler MD). (**d**) Endoscopic view of three plastic biliary stents in side-by-side configuration. (Image courtesy of Douglas G. Adler MD)

Biliary strictures can be encountered at the time of diagnosis of chronic pancreatitis, during the course of disease in association `tis in the setting of otherwise quiescent disease.

Endoscopic biliary stenting has a high technical success rate and provides short-term resolution of jaundice and cholangitis and can provide long-term relief of biliary obstruction in some patients. ERCP with the placement of one or more biliary stents is considered first-line therapy. The presence of periductal calcifications also portends a high endoscopic failure rate as it suggests that the surrounding pancreatic tissue is densely fibrotic and scarred [64]. Patients with recalcitrant strictures or patients who cannot undergo repeated endoscopic procedures are often better treated via surgical biliary bypass [66–68].

Placement of a single plastic stent in the CBD is associated with poor long-term success rates, although if the stricture is very tight the placement of a single plastic stent may be all that is achievable on the initial ERCP. Long-term results with a single plastic stent have been disappointing and sustained benefit is seen in around 25 % of patients on follow-up of

46 months [53, 65]. Single plastic stent use is also associated with poor stricture resolution and a higher relapse rate.

The placement of multiple, side by side, plastic stents in patients with biliary strictures due to chronic pancreatitis is widely performed. Multiple stents allow for more aggressive stricture dilation and allow for biliary drainage both through and between the stents. Between two and five plastic stents are commonly employed at one time with this method [66] (Fig. 3.13). Complete therapy requires approxi-

mately four ERCP procedures and stent exchanges performed every 3 months for 1 year. In one study, single stents provided relief in 31 % of 350 patients as compared to 62 % in 50 patients who received multiple stents [52]. In a nonrandomized study comparing single and multiple plastic stents in patients with chronic pancreatitis and biliary strictures long-term success was reported in 92 % of patients treated with multiple stents as compared to 24 % treated with single stents [65].

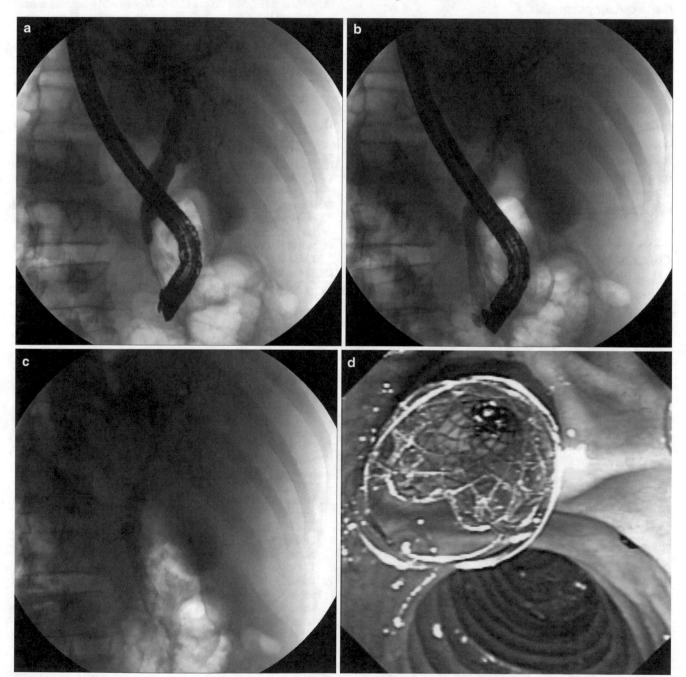

Fig. 3.14 Fully covered metal biliary stent placement for a biliary stricture in a patient with chronic pancreatitis. (**a**) Fluoroscopic view of a distal CBD stricture in a patient with chronic pancreatitis. (Image courtesy of Douglas G. Adler MD). (**b**) A 10×40 mm fully covered self expanding metal stent is deployed across the stricture. (Image courtesy of Douglas G. Adler MD). (**c**) Final fluoroscopic position of stent after endoscope removal. The stent was left in place for 3 months at which time the stricture had resolved. (Image courtesy of Douglas G. Adler MD). (**d**) Endoscopic view of fully covered metal stent after deployment. (Image courtesy of Douglas G. Adler MD)

While uncovered SEMS for biliary strictures related to chronic pancreatitis are not recommended, partially or fully covered SEMS have been used with a success rate of 50–80 % on follow-up of 22–28 months (Fig. 3.14) [67, 69, 70]. Covered stents may be easier to place than multiple plastic stents and, despite their increased costs and risk of migration, are now widely used in this context. To date there are no studies comparing single or multiple plastic stents and metal stents and surgery in patients with biliary strictures due to chronic pancreatitis.

It should be emphasized that some patients with biliary and pancreatic strictures due to chronic pancreatitis will fail even the most aggressive endoscopic therapy. Surgical drainage is always an option for these patients [71–73]. Surgical options include a biliary bypass (i.e., hepaticojejunostomy or choledochoduodenostomy) or more complex operations in patients with pain due to concomitant pancreatic duct obstruction (pancreaticoduodenectomy or duodenal preserving pancreatectomy, as is seen the Frey or the Beger procedure). However, due to its morbidity and mortality, surgery should be carefully balanced in patients with potentially reversible strictures.

Conclusion

Chronic pancreatitis remains a commonly encountered clinical entity. ERCP plays a vital role in the diagnosis and management of patients with symptomatic chronic pancreatitis. Endoscopic therapy of pancreatic duct stones, strictures, and leaks is considered a first line therapy. Pancreatic fluid collections are often amenable to endoscopic approaches as well. Biliary strictures associated with chronic pancreatitis are also common, and both plastic and metal stents are established treatment modalities for this problem. Surgery to treat the biliary and pancreatic complications of chronic pancreatitis is often reserved for poor candidates for repeat endoscopic procedures or in those who have failed prior endoscopic therapy.

Video Legend
Video 3.1 Demonstrating key procedures in management of chronic pancreatitis. Pancreatic and biliary cannulation, sphincterotomy, stenting and dilation, drainage of pancreatic fluid collections.

References

1. Whitcomb DC. Chronic pancreatitis: diagnosis, classification, and new genetic developments. Gastroenterology. 2001;120(3):682–707.
2. Enríquez WK. Diagnostic and therapeutic endoscopy of pancreas and biliary tract. Rev Gastroenterol Mex. 2006;71 Suppl 1:36–8.
3. Kahl S, Glasbrenner B, Leodolter A, Pross M, Schulz HU, Malfertheiner P. EUS in the diagnosis of early chronic pancreatitis: a prospective follow-up study. Gastrointest Endosc. 2002;55:507–11.
4. Freeman ML. Adverse outcomes of ERCP. Gastrointest Endosc. 2002;56(6 Suppl):S273–82.
5. Sarner M, Cotton PB. Classification of pancreatitis. Gut. 1984;25(7):756–9.
6. Gabbrielli A, Mutigani M, Pondolfi M, Perri V, Costamagna G. Endotherapy of early onset idiopathic chronic pancreatitis: results with long-term follow-up. Gastrointestinal Endosc. 2002;55(4):488–93.
7. Ell C, Rabinstein T, Bulling D. Safety and efficacy of pancreatic sphincterotomy in chronic pancreatitis. Gastrointestinal Endosc. 1998;48(3):244–9.
8. Varadarajulu S, Mel Wilcox C. Randomized trial comparing needle-knife and pull-sphincterotome techniques for pancreatic sphincterotomy in high-risk patients. Gastrointest Endosc. 2006;64(5):716–22.
9. Freeman ML, DiSario JA, Nelson DB, Fennerty MB, Lee JG, Bjorkman DJ, et al. Risk factors for post-ERCP pancreatitis: a prospective, multicenter study. Gastrointest Endosc. 2001;54(4):425–34.
10. Vandervoort J, Soetikno RM, Tham TCK, Wong RCK, Ferrari Jr AP, Montes H, et al. Risk factors for complications after performance of ERCP. Gastrointest Endosc. 2002;56(5):652–6.
11. Gottlieb K, Sherman S. ERCP and endoscopic biliary sphincterotomy-induced pancreatitis. Gastrointest Endosc Clin N Am. 1998;8:87–114.
12. Hookey L, Tinto R, Delhaye M, Baize M, Le Moine O, Devière J. Risk factors for pancreatitis after pancreatic sphincterotomy: a review of 572 cases. Endoscopy. 2006;38(7):670–6.
13. Klibansky DA, Gordon SR, Gardner TB. Rectal indomethacin for the prevention of post-ERCP pancreatitis: a valuable tool to keep in your back pocket. Gastroenterology. 2012;143(5):1387–8.
14. Rectal indomethacin to prevent post-ERCP pancreatitis. N Engl J Med 2012;367(3):277–9.
15. Kozarek RA, Ball TJ, Patterson DJ, Brandabur JJ, William Traverso L, Raltz S. Endoscopic pancreatic duct sphincterotomy: indications, technique, and analysis of results. Gastrointest Endosc. 1994;40(5):592–8.
16. Siegel JH, Cohen SA. Pull or push pancreatic sphincterotomy for sphincter of Oddi dysfunction? A conundrum for experts only. Gastrointestinal Endosc. 2006;64(5):723–5.
17. Kim MH, Myung SJ, Kim YS, Kim HJ, Seo DW, Nam SW, Ahn JH, Lee SK, Min YI. Routine biliary sphincterotomy may not be indispensable for endoscopic pancreatic sphincterotomy. Endoscopy. 1998;30:697–701.
18. Cotton PB. Duodenoscopic papillotomy at the minor papilla for recurrent dorsal pancreatitis. Endosc Digest. 1978;3:27–8.
19. Vitale GC, Vitale M, Vitale DS, Binford JC, Hill B. Long-term follow-up of endoscopic stenting in patients with chronic pancreatitis secondary to pancreas divisum. Surg Endosc. 2007;21:2199–202.
20. Watkins JL, Lehman GA. Minor papilla endoscopic sphincterotomy. In: Kozareck R, Carr-Lock DL, Baron TH, editors. ERCP. Amsterdam: Elsevier; 2008. p. 143–57.
21. Lehman GA, Sherman S, Nisi R, Hawes RH. Pancreas divisum: results of minor papilla sphincterotomy. Gastrointest Endosc. 1993;39:1–8.
22. Attwell A, Borak G, Hawes R, Cotton P, Romagnuolo J. Endoscopic pancreatic sphincterotomy for pancreas divisum by using a needle-knife or standard pull-type technique: safety and reintervention rates. Gastrointest Endosc. 2006;64:705–11.
23. Howell DA, Holbrook RF, Bosco JJ, Muggia RA, Biber BP. Endoscopic needle localization of pancreatic pseudocysts before transmural drainage. Gastrointest Endosc. 1993;39:693–8.
24. Elton E, Howell DA, Parsons WG, Qaseem T, Hanson BL. Endoscopic pancreatic sphincterotomy: indications, outcome, and a safe stentless technique. Gastrointest Endosc. 1998;47:240–9.
25. Cremer M, Deviere J. Chronic pancreatitis. In: Testoni PA, Tittobello A, editors. Endoscopy in pancreatic disease: diagnosis and therapy. Chicago: Mosby-Wolfe; 1997. p. 99–112.

26. Shields SJ, Carr-Locke DL. Sphincterotomy techniques and risks. Gastrointest Endosc Clin N Am. 1996;6:17–42.
27. Cotton PB, Williams CB. Practical gastrointestinal endoscopy. 3rd ed. London: Blackwell; 1990. p. 118–56.
28. Delhaye M, Matos C, Devière J. Endoscopic management of chronic pancreatitis. Gastrointest Endosc Clin N Am. 2003;13:717–42.
29. Maydeo A, Borkar D. Techniques of selective cannulation and sphincterotomy. Endoscopy. 2003;35:S19–23.
30. Freeman ML, Guda NM. ERCP cannulation: a review of reported techniques. Gastrointest Endosc. 2005;61:112–25.
31. Novack DJ, Al-Kawas F. Endoscopic management of bile duct obstruction and sphincter of Oddi dysfunction. In: Bayless TM, Diehl AM, editors. Advanced therapy in gastroenterology and liver disease. Hamilton: B.C. Decker; 2005. p. 766–73.
32. Sherman S, Lehman GA, Hawes RH, et al. Pancreatic ductal stones: frequency of successful endoscopic removal and improvement in symptoms. Gastrointest Endosc. 1991;37:511–7.
33. Adamek HE, Jakobs R, Buttmann A, Adamek MU, Schneider AR, Riemann JF. Long term follow up of patients with chronic pancreatitis and pancreatic stones treated with extracorporeal shock wave lithotripsy. Gut. 1999;45:402–5.
34. Delhaye M, Arvanitakis M, Verset G, Cremer M, Deviere J. Long-term clinical outcome after endoscopic pancreatic ductal drainage for patients with painful chronic pancreatitis. Clin Gastroenterol Hepatol. 2004;2:1096–106.
35. Guda NM, Freeman ML, Smith C. Role of extracorporeal shock wave lithotripsy in the treatment of pancreatic stones. Rev Gastroenterol Disord. 2005;5:73–81.
36. Morgan DE, Smith JK, Hawkins K, et al. Endoscopic stent therapy in advanced chronic pancreatitis: relationships between ductal changes, clinical response, and stent patency. Am J Gastroenterol. 2003;98:821–6.
37. Binmoeller KF, Jue P, Seifert H, et al. Endoscopic pancreatic stent drainage in chronic pancreatitis and a dominant stricture: long-term results. Endoscopy. 1995;27:638–44.
38. Cahen DL, Gouma DJ, Huibregtse K, Bruno MJ. Endoscopic versus surgical drainage of the pancreatic duct in chronic pancreatitis. N Engl J Med. 2007;356(7):676–84.
39. Tandan M, Reddy DN, Santosh D, Vinod K, Ramchandani M, Rajesh G, Rama K, Lakhtakia S, Banerjee R, Pratap N, et al. Extracorporeal shock wave lithotripsy and endotherapy for pancreatic calculi-a large single center experience. Indian J Gastroenterol. 2010;29:143–8.
40. Adler DG, Lichtenstein D, Baron TH, Davila R, Egan JV, Gan SL, Qureshi WA, Rajan E, Shen B, Zuckerman MJ, et al. The role of endoscopy in patients with chronic pancreatitis. Gastrointest Endosc. 2006;63:933–7.
41. Delhaye M, Matos C, Devière J. Endoscopic technique for the management of pancreatitis and its complications. Best Pract Res Clin Gastroenterol. 2004;18:155–81.
42. Eleftheriadis N, Dinu F, Delhaye M, Le Moine O, Baize M, Vandermeeren A, Hookey L, Devière J. Long-term outcome after pancreatic stenting in severe chronic pancreatitis. Endoscopy. 2005;37:223–30.
43. Costamagna G, Bulajic M, Tringali A, Pandolfi M, Gabbrielli A, Spada C, Petruzziello L, Familiari P, Mutignani M. Multiple stenting of refractory pancreatic duct strictures in severe chronic pancreatitis: long-term results. Endoscopy. 2006;38:254–9.
44. Kozarek RA. Pancreatic stents can induce ductal changes consistent with chronic pancreatitis. Gastrointest Endosc. 1990;36:93–5.
45. Tringali A, Boskoski I, Costamagna G. The role of endoscopy in the therapy of chronic pancreatitis. Best Pract Res Clin Gastroenterol. 2008;22:145–65.
46. Raju GS, Gomez G, Xiao SY, Ahmed I, Brining D, Bhutani MS, Kalloo AN, Pasricha PJ. Effect of a novel pancreatic stent design on short-term pancreatic injury in a canine model. Endoscopy. 2006;38:260–5.
47. Ishihara T, Yamaguchi T, Seza K, Tadenuma H, Saisho H. Efficacy of s-type stents for the treatment of the main pancreatic duct stricture in patients with chronic pancreatitis. Scand J Gastroenterol. 2006;41:744–50.
48. Park do H, Kim MH, Moon SH, Lee SS, Seo DW, Lee SK. Feasibility and safety of placement of a newly designed, fully covered self-expandable metal stent for refractory benign pancreatic ductal strictures: a pilot study (with video). Gastrointest Endosc. 2008;68:1182–9.
49. Moon SH, Kim MH, Park do H, Song TJ, Eum J, Lee SS, Seo DW, Lee SK. Modified fully covered self-expandable metal stents with antimigration features for benign pancreatic-duct strictures in advanced chronic pancreatitis, with a focus on the safety profile and reducing migration. Gastrointest Endosc. 2010;72:86–91.
50. Dumonceau JM, Delhaye M, Tringali A, Dominguez-Munoz JE, Poley JW, Arvanitaki M, Costamagna G, Costea F, Devière J, Eisendrath P, et al. Endoscopic treatment of chronic pancreatitis: European Society of Gastrointestinal Endoscopy (ESGE) Clinical Guideline. Endoscopy. 2012;44:784–800.
51. Telford JJ, Farrell JJ, Saltzman JR, Shields SJ, Banks PA, Lichtenstein DR, Johannes RS, Kelsey PB, Carr-Locke DL. Pancreatic stent placement for duct disruption. Gastrointest Endosc. 2002;56:18–24.
52. Adler DG, Baron TH, Davila RE, Egan J, Hirota WK, Leighton JA, et al. ASGE guideline: the role of ERCP in diseases of the biliary tract and the pancreas. Gastrointest Endosc. 2005;62(1):1–8.
53. Seicean A, Vultur S. Endoscopic therapy in chronic pancreatitis: current perspectives. Clin Exp Gastroenterol. 2015;8:1–11. doi:10.2147/CEG.S43096.
54. Lehman GA. Role of ERCP and other endoscopic modalities in chronic pancreatitis. Gastrointest Endosc. 2002;56(6 Suppl):S237–40.
55. Andrén-Sandberg A, Dervenis C. Pancreatic pseudocysts in the 21st century. Part I: classification, pathophysiology, anatomic considerations and treatment. JOP. 2004;5:8–24.
56. Lerch MM, Stier A, Wahnschaffe U, Mayerle J. Pancreatic pseudocysts: observation, endoscopic drainage, or resection? Dtsch Arztebl Int. 2009;106:614–21.
57. Andrén-Sandberg A, Dervenis C. Pancreatic pseudocysts in the 21st century. Part II: natural history. JOP. 2004;5:64–70.
58. Beckingham IJ, Krige JE, Bornman PC, Terblanche J. Endoscopic management of pancreatic pseudocysts. Br J Surg. 1997;84:1638–45.
59. Cahen D, Rauws E, Fockens P, Weverling G, Huibregtse K, Bruno M. Endoscopic drainage of pancreatic pseudocysts: long-term outcome and procedural factors associated with safe and successful treatment. Endoscopy. 2005;37:977–83.
60. Balachandra S, Siriwardena AK. Systematic appraisal of the management of the major vascular complications of pancreatitis. Am J Surg. 2005;190:489–95.
61. Varadarajulu S, Trevino J, Wilcox CM, Sutton B, Christein JD. Randomized trial comparing EUS and surgery for pancreatic pseudocyst drainage. Gastrointest Endosc. 2010;71:AB116.
62. Hookey LC, Debroux S, Delhaye M, Arvanitakis M, Le Moine O, Devière J. Endoscopic drainage of pancreatic-fluid collections in 116 patients: a comparison of etiologies, drainage techniques, and outcomes. Gastrointest Endosc. 2006;63:635–43.
63. Banerjee S, Shen B, Baron TH, Nelson DB, Anderson MA, Cash BD, Dominitz JA, Gan SI, Harrison ME, Ikenberry SO, et al. Antibiotic prophylaxis for GI endoscopy. Gastrointest Endosc. 2008;67:791–8.
64. Barthet M, Bernard JP, Duval JL, Affriat C, Sahel J. Biliary stenting in benign biliary stenosis complicating chronic calcifying pancreatitis. Endoscopy. 1994;26:569–72.
65. Kahl S, Zimmermann S, Genz I, Glasbrenner B, Pross M, Schulz HU, Mc Namara D, Schmidt U, Malfertheiner P. Risk factors for failure of endoscopic stenting of biliary strictures in chronic pancreatitis: a prospective follow-up study. Am J Gastroenterol. 2003;98:2448–53.
66. Catalano MF, Linder JD, George S, Alcocer E, Geenen JE. Treatment of symptomatic distal common bile duct stenosis

secondary to chronic pancreatitis: comparison of single vs. multiple simultaneous stents. Gastrointest Endosc. 2004;60: 945–52.

67. Cahen DL, Rauws EA, Gouma DJ, Fockens P, Bruno MJ. Removable fully covered self-expandable metal stents in the treatment of common bile duct strictures due to chronic pancreatitis: a case series. Endoscopy. 2008;40:697–700.

68. Behm B, Brock A, Clarke BW, Ellen K, Northup PG, Dumonceau JM, Kahaleh M. Partially covered self-expandable metallic stents for benign biliary strictures due to chronic pancreatitis. Endoscopy. 2009;41:547–51.

69. Deviere JM, Reddy DN, Puspok A, Ponchon T, Bruno MJ, Bourke MJ, Neuhaus H, Roy A, González-Huix F, Barkun AN, et al. 147 Preliminary results from a 187 patient multicenter prospective trial using metal stents for treatment of benign biliary strictures. Gastrointest Endosc. 2012;75:AB123.

70. Familiari P, Boškoski I, Bove V, Costamagna G. ERCP for biliary strictures associated with chronic pancreatitis. Gastrointest Endosc Clin N Am. 2013;23(4):833–45.

71. Smits ME, Badiga SM, Rauws EAJ, et al. Long-term results of pancreatic stents in chronic pancreatitis. Gastrointest Endosc. 1995;42:461–7.

72. Topazian M, Aslanian H, Andersen D. Outcome following endoscopic stenting of pancreatic duct strictures in chronic pancreatitis. J Clin Gastroenterol. 2005;39:908–11.

73. Dite P, Ruzicka M, Zboril V, et al. A prospective, randomized trial comparing endoscopic and surgical therapy for chronic pancreatitis. Endoscopy. 2003;35:553–8.

Cholangioscopy and Pancreatoscopy: Their Role in Benign and Malignant Disease

Mansour A. Parsi

Cholangioscopy and Pancreatoscopy Equipment

Performance of cholangioscopy and pancreatoscopy requires use of highly specialized equipment. Currently, peroral cholangiopancreatoscopy can be performed by two different methods: (1) by using a dedicated cholangiopancreatoscope and (2) by direct insertion of a small-diameter upper endoscope into the bile duct or the pancreatic duct (the direct method) [1].

Dedicated Cholangiopancreatoscopes

Two types of cholangiopancreatoscopy systems are manufactured solely for the purpose of pancreatic and biliary ductal visualization and include "single operator" and "dual operator" systems (Figs. 4.1 and 4.2). The terms "single operator" and "dual operator" refer to the number of endoscopists required to perform the procedure. As a general rule, dual operator cholangiopancreatoscopy systems require two endoscopists (or one endoscopist with a highly trained assistant), while single operator systems require only one endoscopist for performance [2]. Dual operator systems, however, can be maneuvered by a single operator by using appropriate accessory equipment [3].

The only single operator cholangiopancreatoscopy system currently available is the Spyglass system (Boston Scientific, Natick, MA, USA). The Spyglass Direct Visualization System,

Electronic supplementary material: The online version of this chapter (doi:10.1007/978-3-319-26854-5_4) contains supplementary material, which is available to authorized users. Videos can also be accessed at http://link.springer.com/chapter/10.1007/978-3-319-26854-5_4.

M.A. Parsi, M.D., M.P.H. (✉)
Center for Endoscopy and Pancreatobiliary Disorders, Department of Gastroenterology and Hepatology, Digestive Disease Institute, Cleveland Clinic, 9500 Euclid Ave, Cleveland, OH 44195, USA
e-mail: parsim@ccf.org

released in 2006, was fiber-optic-based and had single and multi-use components [4]. A new generation of this system, called Spyglass Digital System, using digital video imaging technology has been developed and released into the market. In addition to a better digital image quality, the new system has slightly larger accessory channel, suction capability and a "plug and play" platform requiring very little setup time.

Dual operator cholangioscopes of varying length, diameter and image quality are available [5]. There is limited commercial availability of dual operator systems with enhanced video image quality. At present, all dual operator systems with high definition image quality and narrow band imaging (NBI) capability are prototypes and are not commercially available [6]. Older, fiber optic dual operator systems are still in use at some centers.

Direct Cholangiopancreatoscopy

In direct cholangiopancreatoscopy, an ultraslim upper endoscope is inserted through the mouth and advanced to the duodenum [1]. The endoscope itself is subsequently maneuvered across the biliary or pancreatic sphincters and into the bile duct or the pancreatic duct for observation of ductal mucosa and lumen, often over a wire (Fig. 4.3) [1]. Maneuvering of the endoscope across these sphincters requires presence of a sphincterotomy and in most cases performance of a balloon sphincteroplasty. Direct cholangiopancreatoscopy offers some advantages over ductoscopy using dedicated cholangiopancreatoscopes [1]. The ultraslim endoscope uses a single-operator platform, provides high-definition digital image quality, allows simultaneous irrigation and therapy, is not fragile, and has a larger working channel enabling enhanced diagnostic sampling and therapeutic interventions [7–9]. Despite its many advantages, direct cholangiopancreatoscopy is rarely performed in nonacademic settings and has not penetrated into widespread clinical use. The biggest disadvantage of direct cholangiopancreatoscopy has been the difficult and

D.G. Adler (ed.), *Advanced Pancreaticobiliary Endoscopy*, DOI 10.1007/978-3-319-26854-5_4

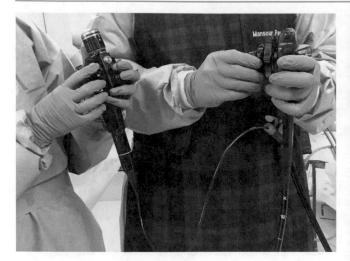

Fig. 4.1 In dual operator cholangiopancreatoscopy the duodenoscope is handled by one and the cholangiopancreatoscope by another endoscopist

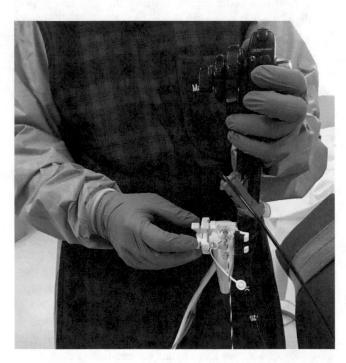

Fig. 4.2 The Spyglass Digital System is an example of a single operator cholangiopancreatoscope. The cholangiopancreatoscope is attached to the handle of the duodenoscope, allowing operation of both by one endoscopist

time-consuming task of biliary or pancreatic duct cannulation with an upper endoscope, often ending in failure even in expert hands [1]. There are several published reports with innovative suggestions on how to achieve this task. Introduction of the endoscope over a guidewire, through a regular overtube, or with the help of a double-balloon overtube are some of the suggestions [10–12]. However, despite use of these accessories, failure rate remains high [13]. Different variations of inflatable balloons used as an anchor have been introduced and shown to facilitate access [7, 8, 14, 15].

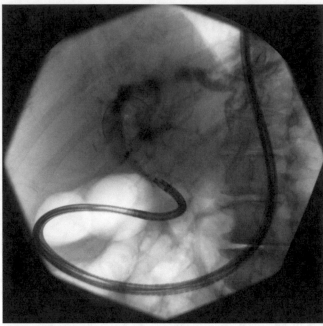

Fig. 4.3 In direct peroral cholangioscopy an ultraslim upper endoscope is directly inserted into the bile duct for examination of the biliary tree

Another disadvantage of direct cholangiopancreatoscopy is its inability to visualize the proximal segments of the pancreatic or bile ducts [7]. In the biliary tree, even with the use of anchoring balloons, direct cholangioscopy can rarely visualize the ducts proximal to the confluence of the right and left hepatic ducts [7].

Currently available ultraslim upper endoscopes have an outer diameter of 5–6 mm, which is significantly larger than the diameter of most dedicated cholangiopancreatoscopes (3–3.5 mm). Direct cholangiopancreatoscopy using the ultraslim upper endoscopes can therefore be performed only in patients with dilated pancreatic or bile ducts. In addition, the larger outer diameter requires generous sphincterotomy and sphincteroplasty for manipulation of the endoscope across the biliary or pancreatic sphincters [1]. If direct cholangiopancreatoscopy is performed, insufflation should be with carbon dioxide, if possible, to reduce the risk of air embolism.

Cholangioscopy

Technique

Peroral cholangioscopy is often performed after a biliary sphincterotomy, although this step is not mandatory, especially if the patient has previously had a biliary stent in place. The cholangioscope is advanced through the accessory channel of the duodenoscope and directed into the bile duct. Although biliary cannulation can be achieved directly with the tip of the cholangioscope, some endoscopists prefer cannulation over a guidewire. Stricture dilatation is performed as needed to facilitate passage of the cholangioscope across a lesion. The bile duct can be irrigated with sterile saline solution through the accessory channel of the cholangioscope for adequate visualization, followed by slow withdrawal of the cholangioscope, allowing systematic inspection of the biliary mucosa [16]. Sterile saline irrigation can be substituted with carbon dioxide (CO_2) insufflation (Figs. 4.4 and 4.5). In a study involving 19 patients with suspected biliary disease, Ueki et al. reported superior image quality using CO_2 insufflation compared to saline irrigation [17]. Another study involving 36 patients, however, reported that although the median time required to obtain a clear endoscopic image using CO_2 insufflation was significantly shorter than that required for saline irrigation, the quality of the endoscopic images obtained was similar in the majority of cases [18]. Air insufflation during direct cholangioscopy has been associated with serious adverse events, notably air embolus as mentioned above, and its use has been discouraged [7, 19]. If available, narrow band imaging (NBI) can be used in the evaluation of biliary strictures to assess the presence or absence of neovascularization [6].

Common Indications

Peroral cholangioscopy has been used for multiple indications. Currently the most common indications for cholangioscopy are evaluation of indeterminate biliary strictures and removal of bile duct stones that cannot be removed by traditional means [2]. Multiple less common indications

have also been described and will be discussed in this chapter as well.

Evaluation of Indeterminate Biliary Strictures

Visual Impression

Biliary strictures can be benign or malignant. Distinguishing between the two is essential for treatment planning and the correct choice of therapy, such as surgical resection or endoscopic stenting. In clinical practice, indeterminate biliary strictures are common. Classification of biliary strictures as benign or malignant often involves a stepwise investigation that starts with patient history, laboratory tests, and noninvasive cross-sectional imaging followed by invasive tests such as endoscopic retrograde cholangiopancreatography (ERCP) and endoscopic ultrasound (EUS). Often the nature of a stricture becomes clear after a limited initial investigation. However, in some patients with indeterminate biliary strictures differentiation of malignant from benign ductal lesions may pose a significant challenge. While there is no consensus definition for "indeterminate strictures," the term usually refers to biliary strictures where initial investigation including cross-sectional imaging and laboratory testing has been unrevealing. For many years, ERCP with retrograde biliary brushing has been the initial mode of investigation for diagnosis of indeterminate biliary strictures. In such patients, ERCP is often needed for biliary drainage and relief of symptoms. Since endoscopic retrograde brush cytology is safe, does not require special expertise and adds little to the cost of ERCP, it is routinely performed during therapeutic ERCP and

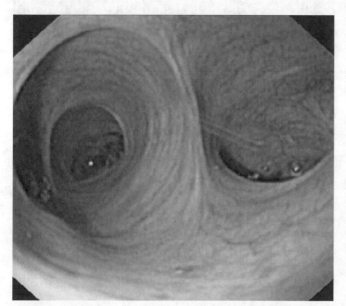

Fig. 4.4 High-definition video cholangioscopy image of the biliary confluence (bifurcation) using saline for irrigation

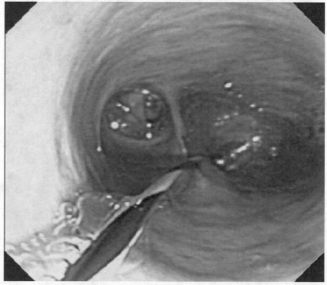

Fig. 4.5 High-definition video cholangioscopy image of the cystic duct insertion to the common bile duct using CO_2 for insufflation. Note the guidewire in the bile duct which was used to steer the cholangioscope into appropriate position

has become the preferred initial method of pursuing a diagnosis in many patients with pancreatobiliary strictures. Brush cytology performed during ERCP has a very high specificity, approaching 100 % in most large institutions. Its sensitivity, however, is often disappointing [20, 21]. In our institution, brush cytology obtained during ERCP has a sensitivity of 40 % and a specificity of 100 % [21]. In other words when positive, brush cytology is very reliable but when negative, it cannot be reliably felt to exclude malignancy.

The low sensitivity of brush cytology has encouraged investigation of other modalities to improve diagnosis. One of those modalities has been cholangioscopy. Peroral cholangioscopy as an adjunct to ERCP allows direct visualization of the stricture and performance of targeted biopsies. Direct endoscopic visualization of the strictures has been shown to be of value in determining the nature of indeterminate biliary strictures as there are certain clues suggestive of malignancy [2]. One such clue is the visualization of abnormally tortuous and dilated capillaries at the site of strictures (Fig. 4.6) [22, 23]. These abnormal vessels are best known as "tumor vessels" and are often indicative of ongoing neovascularization process. It has long been known that malignant tumors promote formation of new blood vessels to meet their blood supply needs [24]. This process is driven by secretion of various substances such as vascular endothelial growth factor (VEGF) from the cancer cells [24]. Neovascularization is the result of angiogenesis, a vital process in the progression of cancer [25]. To grow beyond 1 mm in diameter, a tumor needs an independent blood supply, which is acquired by expressing growth factors that recruit new vasculature from existing

blood vessels [25]. Visualization of tumor vessels on cholangioscopy is therefore a fairly reliable sign of malignancy. In a study of 63 patients, 41 with malignant and 22 patients with benign biliary strictures, tumor vessels were seen in 25 of 41 patients with malignancy (sensitivity 61 %) and none of those with benign strictures (specificity 100 %) [22].

It has been suggested that newer cholangioscopes with high definition image and NBI can diagnose neovascularization at an earlier stage and thus increase the sensitivity of this finding for diagnosis of malignant strictures (Fig. 4.7) [6]. Indeed, in a study of 18 patients with indeterminate biliary strictures, high-definition cholangioscopy identified all cholangiocarcinomas but labeled as malignant only one of four strictures caused by pancreatic cancer (sensitivity 73 %). All benign strictures were correctly labeled (specificity 100 %) [26]. In another study, using high definition cholangioscopy for evaluation of indeterminate biliary strictures, neovascularization was seen in all patients with biliary malignancy and none of those with benign stricture [16].

Another visual clue suggestive of malignancy is presence of raised nodules at the site of strictures [27]. Such nodules usually have an irregular surface mucosa which at times can contain tumor vessels (Figs. 4.8 and 4.9) [27]. Papillary mucosal projections are yet another characteristic finding in certain types of malignant biliary strictures [27]. Such projections can mimic biliary papillomatosis, another type of papillary tumor [28]. Although biliary papillomatosis is basically a collection of benign papillary adenomas, these lesions can transform into papillary adenocarcinoma and sometimes require surgery in suitable candidates (Fig. 4.10) [28]. Biliary

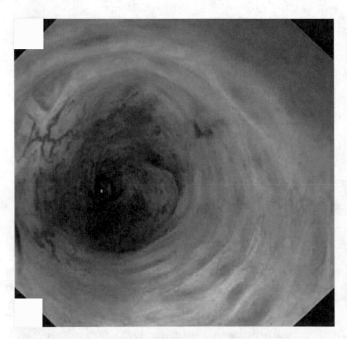

Fig. 4.6 Neovascularization at the site of a biliary stricture seen during direct peroral cholangioscopy using white light

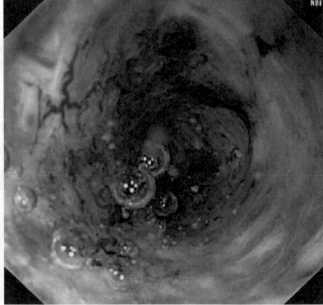

Fig. 4.7 Neovascularization at the site of a biliary stricture seen during direct peroral cholangioscopy with narrow band imaging (NBI). Use of NBI accentuates the abnormal vessels

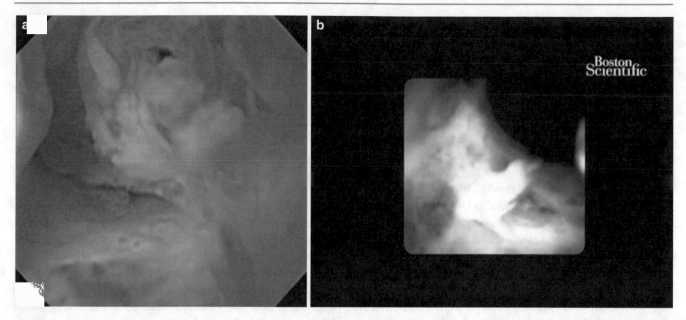

Fig. 4.8 Different appearances of nodules in patients with cholangiocarcinoma. (**a**) Biliary nodule in the common bile duct seen during cholangioscopy in a patient with biliary stricture. Biopsies confirmed diagnosis of cholangiocarcinoma. (**b**) Subtle biliary nodules along *left* *side* of image seen during cholangioscopy in a patient with elevated serum CA 19-9. Biopsies and brushings in this case confirmed cholangiocarcinoma (Image courtesy of Douglas G. Adler MD).

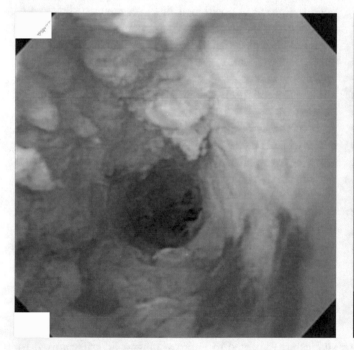

Fig. 4.9 High definition cholangioscopic image of several small nodules along the ductal wall in a patient with cholangiocarcinoma

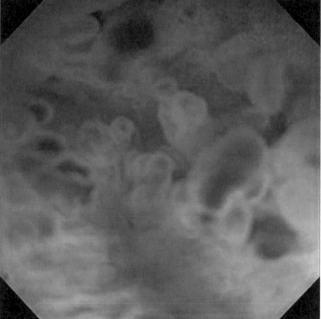

Fig. 4.10 Cholangioscopic views of biliary papillomatosis

papillomatosis can sometimes be found incidentally in elderly patients, not all of whom may be candidates for aggressive biliary surgery.

Other visual clues such as irregularity of mucosa at the site of strictures have been suggested as clues to malignancy, but such clues do not have a high specificity, leading to false positive results [29]. Studies evaluating the sensitivity and specificity of visual evaluation of the stricture sites for diagnosis of malignancy have shown wide variation, likely due to use of different criteria for diagnosis of malignancy. The image quality of the cholangioscope used for this purpose may also affect the sensitivity of the test for diagnosis of malignant lesions as high definition cholangioscopes are able to detect vascular and mucosal abnormalities such as tumor vessels and raised nodules at an earlier stage [6].

In one of the largest cholangioscopic studies to date, diagnostic fiber-optic cholangioscopy using the first generation Spyglass system was performed in 226 patients with various biliary disorders. In patients with biliary stricture, the sensitivity for the diagnosis of malignancy was 51 % for ERCP impression, 78 % for cholangioscopic impression, and 49 % for targeted biopsy [30]. Other studies using high definition cholangioscopes have reported higher sensitivity [26, 31]. The specificity of visual impression at cholangioscopy for diagnosis of malignant strictures also varies likely as a result of using differing criteria for labeling a stricture as malignant. Tumor vessels and raised nodule seem to be more specific than irregularity of the mucosa. Studies that have used mucosal irregularity at the site of a stricture as a criterion for malignancy seem to have lower specificity [29] and thus higher false positive results than those using more strict criteria [16, 26, 31]. Although, undoubtedly, direct visualization of indeterminate biliary strictures can aid in the diagnosis of indeterminate biliary strictures, the sensitivity and specificity of various cholangioscopic clues for distinguishing benign from malignant strictures has not been vigorously studied.

Cholangioscopy-Guided Targeted Biopsy

In addition to visual impression, cholangioscopy allows targeted biopsy of the strictures. Targeted biopsy is defined as obtaining tissue from sites that are clearly affected by disease [2]. Although it is logical to assume that biopsy of areas that are clearly affected should improve sensitivity of tissue acquisition, in practice targeted biopsy under cholangioscopic guidance has not been shown to significantly increase the sensitivity of the specimens for diagnosis of malignant pancreatobiliary strictures.

In a large international multicenter study, the sensitivity of fiber-optic cholangioscopy-guided targeted biopsy for diagnosis of indeterminate biliary strictures was only 49 %, far below the sensitivity of cholangioscopic visualization (78 %) [30]. In that study, however, the specificity of targeted biopsy was higher than cholangioscopic visualization alone (98 % vs. 82 %) [30]. Another study compared the diagnostic accuracy of peroral video cholangioscopic visual findings with that of video cholangioscopy-guided forceps biopsy for diagnosis of indeterminate biliary lesions. The sensitivity and specificity for visual findings were 100 and 91.7 % and for biopsy were 38.1 and 100 %, respectively [32]. In another study involving 89 patients, the diagnostic performance of fluoroscopy-guided and cholangioscopy-guided biopsies for diagnosis of indeterminate biliary strictures were compared [33]. While 100 % specificity was achieved with both methods, fluoroscopy-guided biopsy had a higher sensitivity (76 %) than cholangioscopy-guided biopsy (57 %). According to the authors, the most likely reason for this finding was the larger cup size of the fluoroscopic-guided biopsy

forceps along with the greater ease of passing a biopsy forceps through the working channel of a duodenoscope than the smaller accessory channel of a cholangioscope [33]. A positive association between the size of biopsy specimens and their sensitivity for detection of malignancy in biliary strictures has been previously described [34]. Currently available biopsy forceps for cholangioscopy and pancreatoscopy are only able to obtain very small and superficial tissue samples, limiting their clinical value.

Confocal Laser Endomicroscopy

Confocal laser endomicroscopy (CLE) is an imaging technique that allows microscopic visualization of the epithelial and subepithelial layers of the mucosa in vivo [35]. It is performed after intravenous injection of a contrast agent, usually fluorescein [36, 37]. Fluorescein diffuses through the capillaries and stains the extracellular matrix of the surface epithelium [35, 36]. Confocal laser endomicroscopy in the bile duct is carried out by using specialized probes that can be introduced through the working channel of a cholangioscope or through the lumen of various ERCP catheters [38]. The radiopaque tip of the probe assists with localization of the probe within the bile duct by fluoroscopy. On a practical note, the probe is positioned in direct contact with and as perpendicular as possible to the mucosa at the site of the stricture. Various catheters or sphincterotomes can be used to enable this orientation [39]. Differences in contrast uptake, blood flow and contrast leakage through the capillaries may allow differentiation of normal surface mucosa from neoplastic tissue.

Several criteria have been proposed to diagnose malignancy with CLE, although none of these have replaced tissue sampling to establish a diagnosis of malignancy. Although initial studies have reported encouraging results, current technology seems to lack adequate specificity for diagnosing malignancy especially in the presence of inflammation [40]. For instance, in a recent international multicenter study, 112 patients with indeterminate biliary strictures were evaluated, 71 of whom were eventually diagnosed with malignant lesions. Tissue sampling alone was 56 % sensitive, and 100 % specific, while CLE was 89 % sensitive and only 71 % specific [41].

CLE hardware is expensive and has found only limited use in clinical practice at most large ERCP centers. Ongoing studies are expected to improve diagnostic criteria used for diagnosing malignancy and shed more light on the role of this technology in evaluation of indeterminate biliary strictures.

Management of Biliary Stones

Difficult to Remove Biliary Stones

Cholelithiasis or gallstone disease is common in adult subjects and has been estimated to affect 15 % of the general population in the United States [42, 43]. Between 10 and

20 % of people undergoing cholecystectomy for gallstones have bile duct stones or choledocholithiasis [42]. Stones in the bile ducts are typically removed since they can cause complications such as jaundice, pain, cholangitis, and pancreatitis [43, 44]. Removal of bile duct stones is commonly done by ERCP. In approximately 90 % of cases, ERCP can successfully remove bile duct stones by using conventional methods such as sphincterotomy with or without sphincter dilatation, use of extraction balloons or retrieval baskets, mechanical lithotripsy, or a combination of these methods [2]. At times, however, stone extraction by standard methods is not possible or meets with limited success.

Multiple factors have been postulated to be associated with failure of endoscopic extraction of bile duct stones. Among the most common factors are abnormal anatomy primarily due to difficulties in accessing the bile duct (periampullary diverticulum, sigmoid shaped CBD, post-gastrectomy Billroth type II anatomy, Roux-en-Y-gastrojejunostomy), large number of stones (greater than 10), large size of stones (stones with a diameter >15 mm which cannot be grasped with a basket), unusually shaped stones (barrel-shaped), or location of the stones (intrahepatic, within the cystic duct, proximal to biliary strictures) [2, 45, 46]. In addition, endoscopic management becomes challenging in Mirizzi syndrome, in which stones in the cystic duct cause obstruction of the main bile duct [47].

Kim and colleagues prospectively evaluated the factors influencing the technical difficulty of endoscopic clearance of bile duct stones [48]. They reported that older age (>65 years), previous gastrojejunostomy, large stone size (≥15 mm), impaction of stones, shorter length of the distal common bile duct arm (≤36 mm), and more acute distal common bile duct angulation (≤135°) are all factors that can contribute to technical difficulty of endoscopic biliary stone removal [48]. In a more recent study involving 1390 patients, older age (≥85 years), presence of periampullary diverticula, multiple stones (>4), and large diameter of stones (≥15 mm) were associated with failed endoscopic stone extraction [49].

A variety of methods have been devised for endoscopic extraction of stones that cannot be removed by conventional means during ERCP. As a general rule, these methods involve using shock waves to fragment the stones inside the bile duct, with subsequent removal of the fragments. The shock waves for fragmentation of biliary stones are usually generated using electric spark (electrohydraulic lithotripsy) or laser light (laser lithotripsy) [47, 50]. For shock wave lithotripsy of biliary stones during ERCP, laser or electrohydraulic lithotripsy probes are positioned close to the stone (and away from the bile duct wall) [51]. The bile duct is then irrigated by saline while the shock waves are delivered to the stone. The aqueous medium facilitates transfer of energy produced by the shockwaves to nearby stones resulting in their fragmentation. The shock waves can cause inadvertent injury or perforation of the bile duct wall if the probe is not deployed close to the stone and away from the ductal wall. Shock wave lithotripsy can be performed under fluoroscopic guidance by using centering balloons [52, 53]. The disadvantage of using only fluoroscopic guidance is related to the two-dimensional imaging and the inability to confirm correct positioning of the probe. Both electrohydraulic and laser lithotripsy are ideally, and most commonly, performed under direct visual control using a cholangioscope [51]. Direct visualization ensures that the shock waves are aimed at the stone and not the bile duct wall. Direct visualization by cholangioscopy also allows distinction between stone fragments, air bubbles or blood clots, which can be indistinguishable on contrast cholangiography [2, 54]. Probes that pass through the accessory channels of cholangioscopes for laser or electrohydraulic lithotripsy are commercially available. Laser and electrohydraulic lithotripsy have been used for fragmentation and subsequent extraction of difficult to remove stones for many years, and both techniques have been shown to be safe and effective. Based on cumulative results of small studies, both EHL and laser lithotripsy can lead to clearance of stones in over 90 % of patients with bile-duct stones that are refractory to standard endoscopic therapy [55]. However, repeated procedures and/or combination with other forms of stone extraction may be required [55]. In an international multicenter study, cholangioscopy-guided laser or electrohydraulic lithotripsy were effective in >92 % of the cases [30]. There are currently no randomized studies comparing the effectiveness of laser and electrohydraulic lithotripsy for fragmentation and subsequent extraction of difficult-to-remove biliary stones. Laser lithotripsy has a potential advantage of relatively precise targeting of stones that reduces the risk of injury to surrounding tissue [55]. On the other hand, Laser generators are more expensive than electrohydraulic lithotripsy generators and the use of laser requires special training and protective equipment [55]. Video 4.1 shows successful laser lithotripsy of a large bile duct stone that could not be removed with conventional means during ERCP.

Detection of Missed Stones

Inability to detect certain stones in the bile ducts during ERCP is a well-known phenomenon. Small stones can be "drowned" in contrast (have contrast on both sides of them relative to the fluoroscope, thus rendering them "invisible"), especially in a dilated bile duct, and be missed [2]. Larger stones can block a duct, thus preventing passage of contrast, and evade detection during ERCP [2]. Cholangioscopy allows detection of stones that might have been missed during ERCP (Fig. 4.11). In a study of patients with primary sclerosing cholangitis, stones were not detectable on cholangiography in 7 of 23 patients (30 %) [56]. In a more recent international multicenter study of 66 patients who underwent

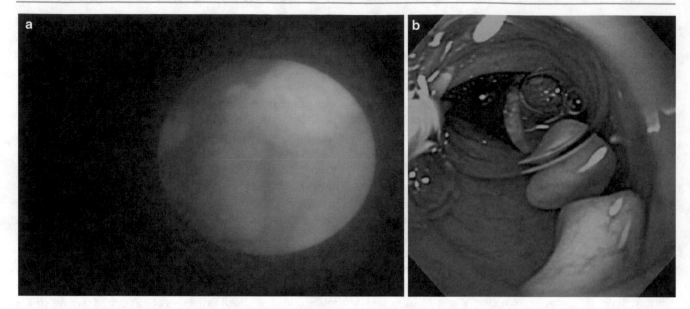

Fig. 4.11 Stones missed on fluoroscopy but detected by cholangioscopy as seen by different types of cholangioscopes. (**a**) Small residual stones seen with fiber optic cholangioscopy. (Image courtesy of Douglas

G. Adler MD). (**b**) Direct peroral cholangioscopy image of the common bile duct containing multiple small cholesterol stones

cholangioscopy-directed EHL or laser lithotripsy, 11 % had one or more stones identified only by cholangioscopy but not ERCP [30]. The ability of cholangioscopy to detect stones missed by ERCP has also been demonstrated in other studies [3, 26, 29].

Less Common Indications for Cholangioscopy

Between 10 and 20 % of peroral cholangioscopy procedures are performed for indications other than biliary stricture diagnosis or removal of biliary stones [2]. Some of these indications are mentioned below.

Assessing Post-liver-Transplantation Biliary Complications

Improvements in surgical techniques and postoperative care have reduced the incidence of complications after liver transplantation. Biliary complications, however, continue to be a significant cause of morbidity after liver transplantation [57–59]. In select cases, cholangioscopy may be of benefit in diagnosis and treatment of biliary complications after liver transplantation (Fig. 4.12). In a study of 20 liver transplant patients, cholangioscopy aided diagnosis of ischemia, ulcerations, scar tissue, intraductal clots, and retained suture material, which otherwise might have been missed by ERCP alone [60]. In another study of 21 patients, 6 of whom had undergone liver transplantation, high definition cholangioscopy revealed sloughing of the mucosa, blood clots and hyperplastic tissue causing irregularities at the anastomotic site [16]. Other studies have confirmed usefulness of cholan-

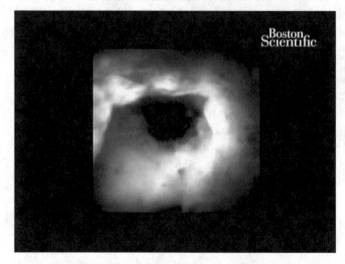

Fig. 4.12 Anastomotic stricture in a patient following liver transplantation viewed with Spyglass Digital System cholangioscope. Courtesy of Douglas G. Adler MD

gioscopy for evaluation of the bile ducts in liver transplant patients [26]. Case series have also suggested that there are differences in appearance of duct-to-duct anastomosis in liver transplant patients that may affect response to endoscopic therapy [16, 61].

Assistance with Guidewire Placement

ERCP is the procedure of choice for treatment of biliary strictures and biliary stones. Success of ERCP, however, depends on the ability to traverse the stricture or the stone with a guidewire that is subsequently used to direct accessory equipment such as balloons or baskets [62]. Traversing strictures or stones with a guidewire is accomplished with ease in an overwhelming majority of cases. In rare occasions, however, it can represent a time-consuming challenge, and in some studies, a failure rate of up to 20 % has been reported [63]. In such cases, cholangioscopy can facilitate guidewire placement and prevent more invasive procedures such as percutaneous transhepatic access or surgery. Several reports have highlighted the value of cholangioscopy in such instances [62, 64].

Assessment of Strictures in Patients with Primary Sclerosing Cholangitis

Primary sclerosing cholangitis (PSC) is a progressive disease with no specific treatment except liver transplantation. Patients with PSC are at increased risk of developing a variety of malignancies including cholangiocarcinoma. The lifetime

risk of cholangiocarcinoma in PSC patients has been estimated to be between 10 and 15 %, with an estimated annual risk of 1.5 % [65].

Cholangiocarcinoma has poor prognosis unless detected early. PSC patients often present with biliary strictures. However, diagnosis of cholangiocarcinoma is particularly difficult in PSC because fibrotic changes may decrease the yield of brush cytology and other tissue acquisition methods. In a study of 30 patients with PSC, cholangioscopy with narrow band imaging allowed visualization of tumor margins in cholangiocarcinoma but did not improve dysplasia detection [66]. This is likely due to presence of inflammation at the stricture site in patients with PSC which can be difficult to distinguish from malignancy on cholangioscopy (Fig. 4.13).

In another study involving 47 patients with PSC and a median follow-up time of 27 months, only one of three

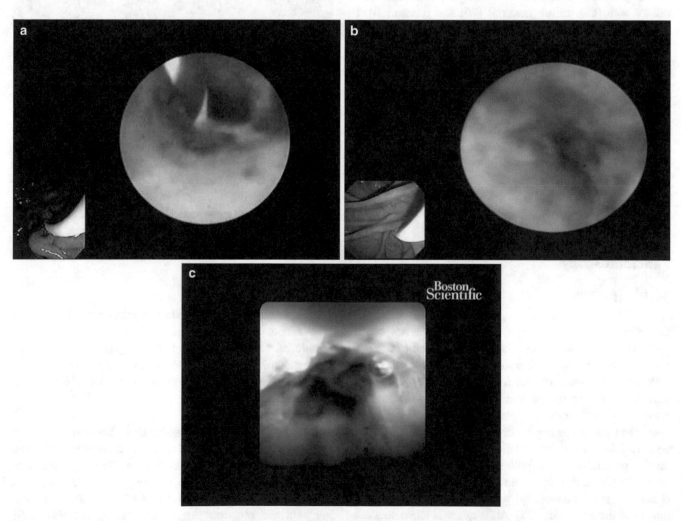

Fig. 4.13 Cholangioscopic view of strictures in patients with PSC. (a) Mild PSC stricture as seen with fiber optic Spyglass cholangioscope. Note luminal narrowing and erythematous, inflamed bile duct epithelium. (b) Moderate to severe stricture as seen with fiber optic Spyglass cholangioscope. Note more severe loss of duct lumen and "angry" appearance of bile duct epithelium with some tissue sloughing. (c) Moderate stricture as seen with digital Spyglass cholangioscope. Note increased image resolution as well as erythematous duct walls with luminal narrowing. ((a), (b), and (c) courtesy of Douglas G. Adler MD)

patients with a final diagnosis of cholangiocarcinoma was diagnosed at the time of cholangioscopy, leading to a sensitivity and specificity of 33 % and 100 % respectively [67].

Characterization of Indeterminate Intraductal Lesions or Filling Defects

Increased use of imaging studies such as CT, MRI and EUS has led to an increase in incidental findings such as intraductal biliary lesions or filling defects. Although, most often these findings are real, they can also be due to artifacts [2]. Direct visualization of the intraluminal biliary tree is the most appropriate way to investigate further the nature of these findings [2]. Cholangioscopy has been shown to be effective for this purpose [29, 68].

Determining the Cause of Unexplained Recurrent Choledocholithiasis

Cholangioscopic diagnosis of biliary papillomatosis [28], biliary web [69], suture material [70] and retained T-tube after cholecystectomy [71] in the bile duct leading to recurrent choledocholithiasis have been reported. In these case reports, standard imaging modalities such as CT, MRCP, ERCP and EUS had failed to diagnose the underlying etiology.

Other

Use of cholangioscopy for evaluation of recurrent acute pancreatitis [71], determination of sources of bleeding in hemobilia [72–75], and staging and ablation of biliary neoplasms [76] has been reported. Cholangioscopy has also been used for removal of embedded and migrated biliary stents [77].

Pancreatoscopy

Technique

Compared to cholangioscopy, the relatively narrow caliber and tortuosity of the pancreatic duct limits ability of endoscopic endoluminal examination of the pancreatic duct by an endoscope. In cases suitable for pancreatoscopy, the procedure is performed during and as an adjunct to endoscopic retrograde cholangiopancreatography (ERCP). Prior to attempt at pancreatoscopy, access to the pancreatic duct is achieved by ERCP, pancreatic sphincterotomy is almost always performed and a guidewire placed in the pancreatic duct. The pancreatoscope is advanced through the accessory channel of the duodenoscope and steered into the pancreatic duct over the guidewire [78]. Although pancreatic duct cannulation can be achieved directly with the tip of the pancreatoscope, most endoscopists prefer cannulation over a guidewire (Fig. 4.14). Stricture dilatation is performed as needed to facilitate passage of the pancreatoscope across a

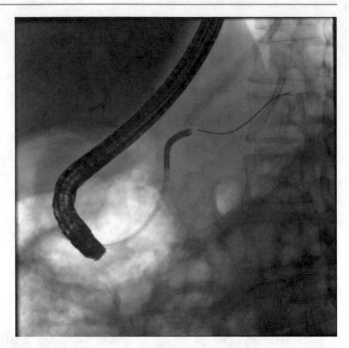

Fig. 4.14 Passage of Spyglass Digital System to the pancreatic duct over a guidewire

lesion. Once the pancreatoscope is advanced to the target location, the guidewire can be removed to enhance visualization and to permit use of the working channel of the pancreatoscope [78]. Removal of the guidewire also improves the tip deflection of the pancreatoscope. The pancreatic duct can be irrigated through the accessory channel of the pancreatoscope with sterile saline solution followed by slow withdrawal of the pancreatoscope, allowing systematic inspection of the ductal mucosa and lumen.

Indications

Pancreatoscopy can been used for management of main pancreatic duct stones, assessment of ductal involvement in intraductal pancreatic mucinous neoplasms (IPMN) and evaluation of indeterminate strictures in the pancreatic duct. With increasing use of pancreatoscopy, the list of indications is expected to grow.

Treatment of Main Pancreatic Duct Stones

Pancreatic duct calcifications are common in chronic pancreatitis. Up to 90 % of patients with chronic pancreatitis develop pancreatic duct stones at long-term follow-up [79]. Pancreatic duct calculi can lead to outflow obstruction, causing pain and recurrent attacks of acute pancreatitis [80]. Restoration of ductal flow is necessary to prevent further attacks of acute pancreatitis and alleviate the pain. Pancreatic duct calculi can be removed by surgical or endoscopic techniques or by extracorporeal shockwave lithotripsy [80].

Extracorporeal shockwave lithotripsy requires special equipment and expertise. Surgical removal is invasive and associated with significant morbidity and occasional mortality. Compared with surgery, conventional endoscopic removal by endoscopic retrograde cholangiopancreatography (ERCP) is far less invasive, but unlikely to be successful with stones >10 mm in diameter, presence of a downstream stricture, or stone impaction [81, 82]. Pancreatoscopy allows identification and shockwave lithotripsy of pancreatic stones under safety of direct vision (Fig. 4.15).

In a series of 46 patients who underwent peroral pancreatoscopy using either an endoscope or a catheter-based system, complete clearance was achieved in 70 % of the patients [83]. In another study, 28 patients underwent pancreatoscopy-guided lithotripsy for pancreatic duct stones. Complete ductal clearance was achieved in 22 patients (79 %) while partial ductal clearance occurred in 3 (11 %) [84].

Multiple case series and case reports have shown that pancreatoscopy-guided lithotripsy either by using laser or EHL is an effective and safe method for removal of main pancreatic duct stones [78, 85, 86]. Improved image quality of the new spyglass system and more widespread access to pancreatoscopes with high-definition image capability is expected to improve success rates of pancreatoscopy-guided lithotripsy for treatment of pancreatic duct stones.

Defining the Extent of Ductal Involvement in IPMN

Pancreatoscopy can be used to define the extent of ductal involvement in patients with intraductal papillary mucinous

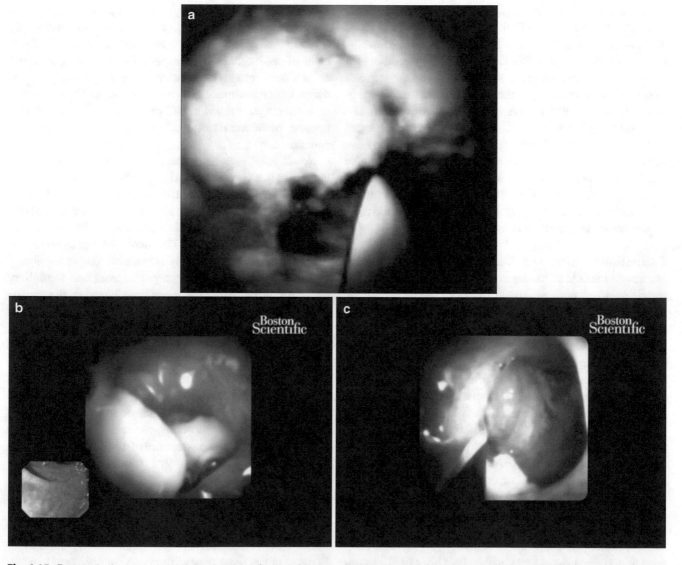

Fig. 4.15 Pancreatic duct stones. (**a**) A large pancreatic stone is seen by Spyglass Digital System. Note the guidewire in the pancreatic duct. (**b**) Multiple large pancreatic duct stones seen by Spyglass Digital System. Note in this case a guidewire is not being used. (**c**) A small pancreatic duct stone is seen in a dilated pancreatic duct by Spyglass Digital System (**b** and **c** -Courtesy of Douglas G. Adler MD)

neoplasia (IPMN). IPMN are cystic tumors of the pancreas that are diagnosed increasingly often as a result of increasing use of cross-sectional imaging modalities such as computerized tomography (CT) and magnetic resonance imaging (MRI). The entity IPMN as a neoplastic lesion was included in the World Health Organization (WHO) classification system in 1996 [87, 88]. Anatomically and prognostically, a distinction is made between main-duct IPMN and branch-duct IPMN as the risk of high-grade dysplasia and progression to malignancy is higher with involvement of the main pancreatic duct compared to side-branches alone [89]. Determining involvement of the main pancreatic duct can at times be difficult. Furthermore, although CT and MRI studies are helpful in the detection of cystic pancreatic lesions, distinguishing ductal dilation of IPMN from chronic pancreatitis can at times pose a challenge. In such instances pancreatoscopy can ascertain involvement of the main pancreatic duct with greater degree of certainty [88] and help distinguish IPMN from chronic pancreatitis [90]. Main duct IPMN is treated with surgical resection as the risk of progression to malignancy is fairly high [91]. The aim of operative resection is to remove all adenomatous or malignant ductal epithelium and to ensure that recurrence in the pancreatic remnant is minimized. However, IPMN can have a discontinuous pattern and so-called "skip lesions" have been reported in between 6 and 19 % of patients in different series [92]. Pancreatoscopy can detect the extent of pancreatic duct involvement and also skip lesions and aid in clinical decision making regarding the extent of surgical resection, potentially reducing the rate of missed lesions during surgery and subsequently the risk of recurrence in the pancreatic remnant [93–95].

Evaluation of Pancreatic Duct Strictures

Studies on the role of pancreatoscopy for evaluation of pancreatic duct strictures are small. In one of the largest series, 115 patients, 55 of whom had indeterminate pancreatic duct strictures, underwent fiber-optic pancreatoscopy [96]. Thirty-five strictures were histologically confirmed as malignant and 20 as benign. Only 22 of the malignant and 16 of the benign strictures could be observed directly with the pancreatoscope. Among the malignant strictures, pancreatoscopy findings were coarse mucosa (59 %), friability (50 %), erythema (36 %), protrusion (27 %), tumor vessels (23 %), and papillary projections (14 %). Benign strictures were noted to have a smooth stenosis (62 %), erythema (25 %), and coarse mucosa (13 %) [96]. Of all of the pancreatoscopy findings, coarse mucosa and friability had the highest sensitivities for malignancy of 59 % and 50 %, respectively, whereas protrusion, friability, tumor vessels, and papillary projections each had a specificity of 100 % for malignancy [96, 97]. The presence of erythema alone was nonspecific. Other smaller studies have also suggested that pancreatoscopy could be of value in assessing pancreatic duct strictures [97].

Adverse Events and Things to Watch for

With the exception of a retrospective study [98], cholangioscopy and pancreatoscopy studies have reported similar rates of adverse events associated with ERCP with and without cholangioscopy or pancreatoscopy [99, 100]. Addition of these procedures to ERCP does not seem to significantly increase the risk of adverse events. One reason behind this finding may be careful selection of patients for performance of these procedures. There are, however, risks associated with cholangioscopy and pancreatoscopy that need special attention. Vigorous irrigation during cholangioscopy can lead to translocation of biliary bacteria to the proximal biliary radicals and liver sinusoids and therefor lead to cholangitis, liver abscess formation, bacteremia, or even sepsis. Saline irrigation should therefore be kept to the minimum rate that provides adequate visualization. It is also important to avoid performing cholangioscopy in patients with active cholangitis. In such cases, if possible, cholangioscopy should be deferred to after completion of antibiotic treatment of cholangitis. Some experts recommend routine use of antibiotic prophylaxis prior to cholangioscopy procedures. In our institution we routinely use antibiotic prophylaxis only in patients with PSC who undergo cholangioscopy because of increased rate of cholangitis in this group of patients.

Another potential adverse event is air embolism. Air embolism is a rare complication that has been reported with various endoscopic procedures including EGD and ERCP [101]. Direct cholangioscopy with air insufflation directly into the bile duct, however, is a particularly strong risk factor for air embolism [101]. The increased risk of air embolism in direct cholangioscopy is probably due to the ability of the ultraslim upper endoscopes to insufflate the biliary tree with air, while at the same time blocking the escape rout of the insufflated air [7]. Reports of air embolization during direct cholangioscopy have been published [19, 102, 103]. In fact, it was this adverse event that prompted one of the medical manufacturers to withdraw their biliary anchoring balloon from the market [7]. The withdrawn anchoring balloon facilitated insertion of ultraslim upper endoscopes into the bile ducts for direct cholangioscopy. In both direct and dedicated cholangioscopy, air insufflation should be avoided [7, 104]. For distention of the bile ducts during cholangioscopy, CO_2 and saline irrigation seem to be safe and effective [7, 104].

When using saline irrigation, we recommend performance of cholangioscopy and pancreatoscopy under general anesthesia with endotracheal intubation since prolonged saline irrigation increases risk of pulmonary aspiration. Because of the same reason, thorough suctioning of any fluids in the duodenum and stomach prior to duodenoscope withdrawal is recommended.

Finally, in patients undergoing pancreatoscopy we advise rectal indomethacin during the procedure and placement of a prophylactic pancreatic stent at the end of the procedure to decrease the risk of post procedure pancreatitis.

Video Legend

Video 4.1 Laser lithotripsy of biliary stones using the Spyglass Digital System.

References

1. Parsi MA. Direct peroral cholangioscopy. World J Gastrointest Endosc. 2014;6:1–5.
2. Parsi MA. Peroral cholangioscopy in the new millennium. World J Gastroenterol. 2011;17:1–6.
3. Farrell JJ, Bounds BC, Al-Shalabi S, et al. Single-operator duodenoscope-assisted cholangioscopy is an effective alternative in the management of choledocholithiasis not removed by conventional methods, including mechanical lithotripsy. Endoscopy. 2005;37:542–7.
4. Chen YK, Pleskow DK. SpyGlass single-operator peroral cholangiopancreatoscopy system for the diagnosis and therapy of bile-duct disorders: a clinical feasibility study (with video). Gastrointest Endosc. 2007;65:832–41.
5. Shah RJ, Adler DG, Conway JD, et al. Cholangiopancreatoscopy. Gastrointest Endosc. 2008;68:411–21.
6. Parsi MA. High-definition endoscopy and narrow-band imaging of the bile ducts: new possibilities for diagnosis of indeterminate strictures. Gastroenterology. 2014;146:343–4.
7. Parsi MA, Stevens T, Vargo JJ. Diagnostic and therapeutic direct peroral cholangioscopy using an intraductal anchoring balloon. World J Gastroenterol. 2012;18:3992–6.
8. Waxman I, Dillon T, Chmura K, et al. Feasibility of a novel system for intraductal balloon-anchored direct peroral cholangioscopy and endotherapy with an ultraslim endoscope (with videos). Gastrointest Endosc. 2010;72:1052–6.
9. Pohl J, Meves VC, Mayer G, et al. Prospective randomized comparison of short-access mother-baby cholangioscopy versus direct cholangioscopy with ultraslim gastroscopes. Gastrointest Endosc. 2013;78:609–16.
10. Larghi A, Waxman I. Endoscopic direct cholangioscopy by using an ultra-slim upper endoscope: a feasibility study. Gastrointest Endosc. 2006;63:853–7.
11. Bohle W. A simple and rapid technique of direct cholangioscopy. Gastrointest Endosc. 2007;65:559.
12. Choi HJ, Moon JH, Ko BM, et al. Overtube-balloon-assisted direct peroral cholangioscopy by using an ultra-slim upper endoscope (with videos). Gastrointest Endosc. 2009;69:935–40.
13. Terheggen G, Neuhaus H. New options of cholangioscopy. Gastroenterol Clin North Am. 2010;39:827–44.
14. Moon JH, Ko BM, Choi HJ, et al. Intraductal balloon-guided direct peroral cholangioscopy with an ultraslim upper endoscope (with videos). Gastrointest Endosc. 2009;70:297–302.
15. Sola-Vera J, Uceda F, Cuesta R, et al. Direct peroral cholangioscopy using an ultrathin endoscope: making technique easier. Rev Esp Enferm Dig. 2014;106:30–6.
16. Parsi MA, Stevens T, Collins J, et al. Utility of a prototype peroral video cholangioscopy system with narrow-band imaging for evaluation of biliary disorders (with videos). Gastrointest Endosc. 2011;74:1148–51.
17. Ueki T, Mizuno M, Ota S, et al. Carbon dioxide insufflation is useful for obtaining clear images of the bile duct during peroral cholangioscopy (with video). Gastrointest Endosc. 2010;71:1046–51.
18. Doi S, Yasuda I, Nakashima M, et al. Carbon dioxide insufflation vs. conventional saline irrigation for peroral video cholangioscopy. Endoscopy. 2011;43:1070–5.
19. Efthymiou M, Raftopoulos S, Antonio Chirinos J, et al. Air embolism complicated by left hemiparesis after direct cholangioscopy with an intraductal balloon anchoring system. Gastrointest Endosc. 2012;75:221–3.
20. Parsi MA, Li A, Li CP, et al. DNA methylation alterations in endoscopic retrograde cholangiopancreatography brush samples of patients with suspected pancreaticobiliary disease. Clin Gastroenterol Hepatol. 2008;6:1270–8.
21. Parsi MA, Deepinder F, Lopez R, et al. Factors affecting the yield of brush cytology for the diagnosis of pancreatic and biliary cancers. Pancreas. 2011;40:52–4.
22. Kim HJ, Kim MH, Lee SK, et al. Tumor vessel: a valuable cholangioscopic clue of malignant biliary stricture. Gastrointest Endosc. 2000;52:635–8.
23. Parsi MA. Neovascularization at the site of biliary strictures: a cholangioscopic sign of malignancy. Clin Gastroenterol Hepatol. 2015;13:A17–8.
24. Nishida N, Yano H, Nishida T, et al. Angiogenesis in cancer. Vasc Health Risk Manag. 2006;2:213–9.
25. Hanahan D, Folkman J. Patterns and emerging mechanisms of the angiogenic switch during tumorigenesis. Cell. 1996;86:353–64.
26. Parsi MA, Jang S, Sanaka M, et al. Diagnostic and therapeutic cholangiopancreatoscopy: performance of a new digital cholangioscope. Gastrointest Endosc. 2014;79:936–42.
27. Seo DW, Lee SK, Yoo KS, et al. Cholangioscopic findings in bile duct tumors. Gastrointest Endosc. 2000;52:630–4.
28. Parsi MA. Biliary papillomatosis: diagnosis with direct peroral cholangioscopy. Gastrointest Endosc. 2015;81:231–2.
29. Fukuda Y, Tsuyuguchi T, Sakai Y, et al. Diagnostic utility of peroral cholangioscopy for various bile-duct lesions. Gastrointest Endosc. 2005;62:374–82.
30. Chen YK, Parsi MA, Binmoeller KF, et al. Single-operator cholangioscopy in patients requiring evaluation of bile duct disease or therapy of biliary stones (with videos). Gastrointest Endosc. 2011;74:805–14.
31. Itoi T, Osanai M, Igarashi Y, et al. Diagnostic peroral video cholangioscopy is an accurate diagnostic tool for patients with bile duct lesions. Clin Gastroenterol Hepatol. 2010;8:934–8.
32. Nishikawa T, Tsuyuguchi T, Sakai Y, et al. Comparison of the diagnostic accuracy of peroral video-cholangioscopic visual findings and cholangioscopy-guided forceps biopsy findings for indeterminate biliary lesions: a prospective study. Gastrointest Endosc. 2013;77:219–26.
33. Hartman DJ, Slivka A, Giusto DA, et al. Tissue yield and diagnostic efficacy of fluoroscopic and cholangioscopic techniques to assess indeterminate biliary strictures. Clin Gastroenterol Hepatol. 2012;10:1042–6.
34. Ikeda M, Maetani I, Terada K, et al. Usefulness of endoscopic retrograde biliary biopsy using large-capacity forceps for extrahepatic biliary strictures: a prospective randomized study. Endoscopy. 2010;42:837–41.
35. Kiesslich R, Goetz M, Neurath MF. Confocal laser endomicroscopy for gastrointestinal diseases. Gastrointest Endosc Clin N Am. 2008;18:451–66. viii.
36. Paramsothy S, Leong RW. Endoscopy: fluorescein contrast in confocal laser endomicroscopy. Nat Rev Gastroenterol Hepatol. 2010;7:366–8.
37. Wallace MB, Meining A, Canto MI, et al. The safety of intravenous fluorescein for confocal laser endomicroscopy in the gastrointestinal tract. Aliment Pharmacol Ther. 2010;31:548–52.
38. Wallace MB, Fockens P. Probe-based confocal laser endomicroscopy. Gastroenterology. 2009;136:1509–13.
39. Loeser CS, Robert ME, Mennone A, et al. Confocal endomicroscopic examination of malignant biliary strictures and histologic

correlation with lymphatics. J Clin Gastroenterol. 2011;45: 246–52.

40. Caillol F, Filoche B, Gaidhane M, et al. Refined probe-based confocal laser endomicroscopy classification for biliary strictures: the Paris Classification. Dig Dis Sci. 2013;58:1784–9.

41. Slivka A, Gan I, Jamidar P, et al. Validation of the diagnostic accuracy of probe-based confocal laser endomicroscopy for the characterization of indeterminate biliary strictures: results of a prospective multicenter international study. Gastrointest Endosc. 2015;81:282–90.

42. Dasari BV, Tan CJ, Gurusamy KS, et al. Surgical versus endoscopic treatment of bile duct stones. Cochrane Database Syst Rev. 2013;9, CD003327.

43. Williams EJ, Green J, Beckingham I, et al. Guidelines on the management of common bile duct stones (CBDS). Gut. 2008;57: 1004–21.

44. Caddy GR, Tham TC. Gallstone disease: symptoms, diagnosis and endoscopic management of common bile duct stones. Best Pract Res Clin Gastroenterol. 2006;20:1085–101.

45. Binmoeller KF, Bruckner M, Thonke F, et al. Treatment of difficult bile duct stones using mechanical, electrohydraulic and extracorporeal shock wave lithotripsy. Endoscopy. 1993;25:201–6.

46. Trikudanathan G, Navaneethan U, Parsi MA. Endoscopic management of difficult common bile duct stones. World J Gastroenterol. 2013;19:165–73.

47. McHenry L, Lehman G. Difficult bile duct stones. Curr Treat Options Gastroenterol. 2006;9:123–32.

48. Kim HJ, Choi HS, Park JH, et al. Factors influencing the technical difficulty of endoscopic clearance of bile duct stones. Gastrointest Endosc. 2007;66:1154–60.

49. Christoforidis E, Vasiliadis K, Tsalis K, et al. Factors significantly contributing to a failed conventional endoscopic stone clearance in patients with "difficult" choledecholithiasis: a single-center experience. Diagn Ther Endosc. 2014;2014:861689.

50. Seitz U, Bapaye A, Bohnacker S, et al. Advances in therapeutic endoscopic treatment of common bile duct stones. World J Surg. 1998;22:1133–44.

51. Yoo KS, Lehman GA. Endoscopic management of biliary ductal stones. Gastroenterol Clin North Am. 2010;39:209–27. viii.

52. Cho YD, Cheon YK, Moon JH, et al. Clinical role of frequency-doubled double-pulsed yttrium aluminum garnet laser technology for removing difficult bile duct stones (with videos). Gastrointest Endosc. 2009;70:684–9.

53. Moon JH, Cha SW, Ryu CB, et al. Endoscopic treatment of retained bile-duct stones by using a balloon catheter for electrohydraulic lithotripsy without cholangioscopy. Gastrointest Endosc. 2004;60:562–6.

54. Darcy M, Picus D. Cholangioscopy. Tech Vasc Interv Radiol. 2008;11:133–42.

55. DiSario J, Chuttani R, Croffie J, et al. Biliary and pancreatic lithotripsy devices. Gastrointest Endosc. 2007;65:750–6.

56. Awadallah NS, Chen YK, Piraka C, et al. Is there a role for cholangioscopy in patients with primary sclerosing cholangitis? Am J Gastroenterol. 2006;101:284–91.

57. Kochhar G, Parungao JM, Hanouneh IA, et al. Biliary complications following liver transplantation. World J Gastroenterol. 2013;19:2841–6.

58. Shah SA, Grant DR, McGilvray ID, et al. Biliary strictures in 130 consecutive right lobe living donor liver transplant recipients: results of a Western center. Am J Transplant. 2007;7:161–7.

59. Tashiro H, Itamoto T, Sasaki T, et al. Biliary complications after duct-to-duct biliary reconstruction in living-donor liver transplantation: causes and treatment. World J Surg. 2007;31:2222–9.

60. Siddique I, Galati J, Ankoma-Sey V, et al. The role of choledochoscopy in the diagnosis and management of biliary tract diseases. Gastrointest Endosc. 1999;50:67–73.

61. Balderramo D, Sendino O, Miquel R, et al. Prospective evaluation of single-operator peroral cholangioscopy in liver transplant recipients requiring an evaluation of the biliary tract. Liver Transpl. 2013;19:199–206.

62. Parsi MA, Guardino J, Vargo JJ. Peroral cholangioscopy-guided stricture therapy in living donor liver transplantation. Liver Transpl. 2009;15:263–5.

63. Hisatsune H, Yazumi S, Egawa H, et al. Endoscopic management of biliary strictures after duct-to-duct biliary reconstruction in right-lobe living-donor liver transplantation. Transplantation. 2003;76:810–5.

64. Parsi MA. Peroral cholangioscopy-assisted guidewire placement for removal of impacted stones in the cystic duct remnant. World J Gastrointest Surg. 2009;1:59–61.

65. Bergquist A, Ekbom A, Olsson R, et al. Hepatic and extrahepatic malignancies in primary sclerosing cholangitis. J Hepatol. 2002;36:321–7.

66. Azeem N, Gostout CJ, Knipschield M, et al. Cholangioscopy with narrow-band imaging in patients with primary sclerosing cholangitis undergoing ERCP. Gastrointest Endosc. 2014;79: 773–9. e2.

67. Arnelo U, von Seth E, Bergquist A. Prospective evaluation of the clinical utility of single-operator peroral cholangioscopy in patients with primary sclerosing cholangitis. Endoscopy. 2015; 47(8):696–702.

68. Abdel Aziz AM, Sherman S, Binmoeller KF, Deviere J, Hawes RH, Haluszka O, Neuhaus H, Pleskow D, Raijman I. SpyGlass cholangioscopy—impact on patients with bile duct filling defect(s) of uncertain etiology. Gastrointest Endosc. 2008;67: AB325.

69. Parsi MA. Biliary web: diagnosis with high-definition videocholangioscopy. Clin Gastroenterol Hepatol. 2014;12:A29.

70. Parsi MA, Bhatt A, Stevens T, et al. Cholangioscopic diagnosis of iatrogenic recurrent choledocholithiasis. Gastrointest Endosc. 2015;81(5):1263–4.

71. Parsi MA, Sanaka MR, Dumot JA. Iatrogenic recurrent pancreatitis. Pancreatology. 2007;7:539.

72. Hayashi S, Baba Y, Ueno K, et al. Small arteriovenous malformation of the common bile duct causing hemobilia in a patient with hereditary hemorrhagic telangiectasia. Cardiovasc Intervent Radiol. 2008;31 Suppl 2:S131–4.

73. Prasad GA, Abraham SC, Baron TH, et al. Hemobilia caused by cytomegalovirus cholangiopathy. Am J Gastroenterol. 2005; 100:2592–5.

74. Parsi MA. Hemobilia: endoscopic, fluoroscopic, and cholangioscopic diagnosis. Hepatology. 2010;52:2237–8.

75. Komaki Y, Kanmura S, Funakawa K, et al. A case of hereditary hemorrhagic telangiectasia with repeated hemobilia arrested by argon plasma coagulation under direct peroral cholangioscopy. Gastrointest Endosc. 2014;80:528–9.

76. Lu XL, Itoi T, Kubota K. Cholangioscopy by using narrow-band imaging and transpapillary radiotherapy for mucin-producing bile duct tumor. Clin Gastroenterol Hepatol. 2009;7:e34–5.

77. Sejpal DV, Vamadevan AS, Trindade AJ. Removal of an embedded, migrated plastic biliary stent with the use of cholangioscopy. Gastrointest Endosc. 2015.

78. Parsi MA, Bakhru M, Vargo JJ. Therapeutic peroral pancreatoscopy: shockwave lithotripsy of pancreatic duct stones under direct vision. Gastroenterology. 2013;145:1203–4.

79. Ammann RW, Muench R, Otto R, et al. Evolution and regression of pancreatic calcification in chronic pancreatitis. A prospective long-term study of 107 patients. Gastroenterology. 1988;95: 1018–28.

80. Parsi MA, Stevens T, Lopez R, et al. Extracorporeal shock wave lithotripsy for prevention of recurrent pancreatitis caused by obstructive pancreatic stones. Pancreas. 2010;39:153–5.

81. Sherman S, Lehman GA, Hawes RH, et al. Pancreatic ductal stones: frequency of successful endoscopic removal and improvement in symptoms. Gastrointest Endosc. 1991;37:511–7.

82. Kozarek RA, Ball TJ, Patterson DJ. Endoscopic approach to pancreatic duct calculi and obstructive pancreatitis. Am J Gastroenterol. 1992;87:600–3.

83. Attwell AR, Brauer BC, Chen YK, et al. Endoscopic retrograde cholangiopancreatography with per oral pancreatoscopy for calcific chronic pancreatitis using endoscope and catheter-based pancreatoscopes: a 10-year single-center experience. Pancreas. 2014;43:268–74.

84. Attwell AR, Patel S, Kahaleh M, et al. ERCP with per-oral pancreatoscopy-guided laser lithotripsy for calcific chronic pancreatitis: a multicenter U.S. experience. Gastrointest Endosc. 2015;82:311–8.

85. Adler DG. Pancreatoscopy for pancreatic duct stones. Gastrointest Endosc. 2014;79:208.

86. Alatawi A, Leblanc S, Vienne A, et al. Pancreatoscopy-guided intracorporeal laser lithotripsy for difficult pancreatic duct stones: a case series with prospective follow-up (with video). Gastrointest Endosc. 2013;78:179–83.

87. Hruban RH, Takaori K, Klimstra DS, et al. An illustrated consensus on the classification of pancreatic intraepithelial neoplasia and intraductal papillary mucinous neoplasms. Am J Surg Pathol. 2004;28:977–87.

88. Tanaka M, Chari S, Adsay V, et al. International consensus guidelines for management of intraductal papillary mucinous neoplasms and mucinous cystic neoplasms of the pancreas. Pancreatology. 2006;6:17–32.

89. Tanaka M, Fernandez-del Castillo C, Adsay V, et al. International consensus guidelines 2012 for the management of IPMN and MCN of the pancreas. Pancreatology. 2012;12:183–97.

90. Kachaamy T, Salah W, Dzeletovic I, et al. Intraoperative laparoscopic-assisted pancreatoscopy and its role in differentiating main duct intraductal papillary mucinous neoplasm from chronic pancreatitis. Gastrointest Endosc. 2015;81:459–60.

91. Levy P, Jouannaud V, O'Toole D, et al. Natural history of intraductal papillary mucinous tumors of the pancreas: actuarial risk of malignancy. Clin Gastroenterol Hepatol. 2006;4:460–8.

92. Sauvanet A, Couvelard A, Belghiti J. Role of frozen section assessment for intraductal papillary and mucinous tumor of the pancreas. World J Gastrointest Surg. 2010;2:352–8.

93. Pucci MJ, Johnson CM, Punja VP, et al. Intraoperative pancreatoscopy: a valuable tool for pancreatic surgeons? J Gastrointest Surg. 2014;18:1100–7.

94. Nagayoshi Y, Aso T, Ohtsuka T, et al. Peroral pancreatoscopy using the SpyGlass system for the assessment of intraductal papillary mucinous neoplasm of the pancreas. J Hepatobiliary Pancreat Sci. 2014;21:410–7.

95. Arnelo U, Siiki A, Swahn F, et al. Single-operator pancreatoscopy is helpful in the evaluation of suspected intraductal papillary mucinous neoplasms (IPMN). Pancreatology. 2014;14:510–4.

96. Yamao K, Ohashi K, Nakamura T, et al. Efficacy of peroral pancreatoscopy in the diagnosis of pancreatic diseases. Gastrointest Endosc. 2003;57:205–9.

97. Ringold DA, Shah RJ. Peroral pancreatoscopy in the diagnosis and management of intraductal papillary mucinous neoplasia and indeterminate pancreatic duct pathology. Gastrointest Endosc Clin N Am. 2009;19:601–13.

98. Sethi A, Chen YK, Austin GL, et al. ERCP with cholangiopancreatoscopy may be associated with higher rates of complications than ERCP alone: a single-center experience. Gastrointest Endosc. 2011;73:251–6.

99. Hammerle CW, Haider S, Chung M, et al. Endoscopic retrograde cholangiopancreatography complications in the era of cholangioscopy: is there an increased risk? Dig Liver Dis. 2012;44:754–8.

100. Draganov PV, Lin T, Chauhan S, et al. Prospective evaluation of the clinical utility of ERCP-guided cholangiopancreatoscopy with a new direct visualization system. Gastrointest Endosc. 2011;73:971–9.

101. Donepudi S, Chavalitdhamrong D, Pu L, et al. Air embolism complicating gastrointestinal endoscopy: a systematic review. World J Gastrointest Endosc. 2013;5:359–65.

102. Albert JG, Friedrich-Rust M, Elhendawy M, et al. Peroral cholangioscopy for diagnosis and therapy of biliary tract disease using an ultra-slim gastroscope. Endoscopy. 2011;43:1004–9.

103. Farnik H, Weigt J, Malfertheiner P, et al. A multicenter study on the role of direct retrograde cholangioscopy in patients with inconclusive endoscopic retrograde cholangiography. Endoscopy. 2014;46:16–21.

104. Moon JH, Choi HJ. The role of direct peroral cholangioscopy using an ultraslim endoscope for biliary lesions: indications, limitations, and complications. Clin Endosc. 2013;46:537–9.

The Endoscopic Management of Biliary and Pancreatic Injury

Matthew J. Hudson, Raymond G. Kim, and Eric Goldberg

Pancreaticobiliary injuries are frequently encountered by interventional endoscopists and are a common cause of morbidity and even mortality. They are seen postoperatively after cholecystectomy, liver transplantation, pancreatectomy, and splenectomy. They may also result from blunt and penetrating trauma, and may even be related to gastrointestinal interventions like ERCP or liver biopsy. Early recognition and a multidisciplinary approach to treatment are crucial to limit systemic effects of the injury and prevent associated morbidity. Principles of therapy are often similar whether the injury is iatrogenic or traumatic. This chapter focuses on the endoscopic management of these biliary and pancreatic injuries rather than stone disease or neoplastic processes.

Bile Leak

Bile leaks (BL) can occur after any procedure in which the hepatobiliary system is manipulated, and may also result from blunt or penetrating trauma. The typical signs and symptoms include abdominal pain and the accumulation of bile rich fluid in the peritoneal cavity or external drains. It is important to note that liver function tests may be normal with BL because bile flow is typically not obstructed. If a leak is identified during surgery, surgical repair is warranted at that time. Bile leaks identified postoperatively are optimally

managed with percutaneous drainage and/or ERCP. Repeat surgical intervention is generally deferred unless mandated by a deteriorating patient condition or presence of a completely disconnected duct. This section addresses the utility of ERCP in diagnosing and managing BL.

Historically, the definition of a bile leak has lacked standardization. Past definitions have been based on the volume (20–50 mL) of fluid accumulating postoperatively, the bilirubin concentration (5–20 mg/dL) of the fluid, and timing of the leak. More recently, the International Study Group of Liver Surgery proposed a consensus definition [1] in which bile leakage was defined as:

- Increased bilirubin concentration in the abdominal drain or in the intra-abdominal fluid (define as three times greater than the serum bilirubin concentration).
- Leak occurrence on or after postoperative day 3.
- Leak requiring radiologic intervention (i.e., interventional drainage) or re-laparotomy resulting from bile peritonitis.

Because up to 24 % of patients have some degree of fluid collection in the gallbladder fossa after resection, these criteria help to delineate a clinically significant bile leak from clinically inconsequential fluid accumulation [2]. A grading system for bile leaks has also been proposed to determine the severity of leaks:

- *Bile leakage grade A*: BL characterized by clinical stability in the patient and adequate leakage control by an intra-abdominal drain. Leakage should decrease and resolve by 7 days.
- *Bile leakage grade B*: Clinical deterioration of the patient is seen due to the leak (sepsis, abscess formation, pain,

Electronic supplementary material: The online version of this chapter (doi:10.1007/978-3-319-26854-5_5) contains supplementary material, which is available to authorized users. Videos can also be accessed at http://link.springer.com/chapter/10.1007/978-3-319-26854-5_5.

M.J. Hudson, M.D.
Gastroenterology and Hepatology, Buffalo General Medical Center, Buffalo, NY, USA

R.G. Kim, M.D.
Gastroenterology and Hepatology, University of Maryland Medical Center, Baltimore, MD, USA

E. Goldberg, M.D. (✉)
Gastroenterology and Hepatology, University of Maryland, School of Medicine, 22 S. Greene St N3W62, Baltimore, MD 21201, USA
e-mail: egoldber@medicine.umaryland.edu

© Springer International Publishing Switzerland 2016
D.G. Adler (ed.), *Advanced Pancreaticobiliary Endoscopy*, DOI 10.1007/978-3-319-26854-5_5

etc.). Grade A leaks that persist for greater than 7 days are included as well. Intra-abdominal drainage alone is inadequate, and these require additional radiologic or endoscopic intervention. Surgery may be avoidable.

- *Bile leakage grade C*: Require repeat surgical intervention to control the complication. The postoperative course of the patients is prolonged, and secondary postoperative complications (e.g., abdominal wound infection) may result.

Technique

The goal of endoscopic management of BL is to reduce the transpapillary pressure gradient between the bile duct and duodenum via sphincterotomy and/or endoprosthesis placement. This results in a preferential flow of bile into the duodenum rather than through the leak site. The placement of a stent can also bridge the lesion, further protecting the leak site.

It is worthwhile to understand certain endoscopic principles when managing patients with BL. Guidewire cannulation is preferential, with recognition that cannulation may be more difficult in patients with BL due to the upstream decompression of the ducts that results from the leak. After cannulation, a complete cholangiogram should be performed to identify the leak and determine its size. A *large bile leak* is one in which the leak is identified prior to filling the intrahepatic branches (Fig. 5.1a, b). A *small bile leak*, conversely, is a BL that is seen after filling of the intrahepatic biliary tree (Fig. 5.2a, b). The cholangiogram can also be utilized to identify retained intraductal stones or areas of stenosis that may be contributing to the BL. These are then treated as indicated.

While sphincterotomy alone may be considered for small leaks, data suggests a greater likelihood of leak resolution with the use of stents, with or without sphincterotomy, than biliary sphincterotomy alone [3]. Sphincterotomy can be deferred in patients with coagulopathies or other adverse risk for bleeding. After sphincterotomy, a stent is deployed into the biliary tree (Fig. 5.3a, b). In general, 10 F plastic biliary stents are preferred over 7 or 8.5 F stents as they have a more durable patency profile and improve downstream flow. While bridging the lesion is not essential, it should be considered if technically feasible. For hepatic, intrahepatic, and subvesical bile duct (duct of Luschka) leaks, placement of the proximal aspect of the stent into the affected system involved should be attempted as possible.

Ninety-five percent of BL resolve within 2 weeks utilizing stent therapy as described [4–6]. Therefore, stents should be maintained for at least 14 days and up to 6 weeks, at which time they should be removed. Many endoscopists perform cholangiography at the time of stent removal to document leak resolution, although this is not mandated if the BL is felt to have resolved at the time of stent removal (Fig. 5.3c). If contrast dye is injected, it is important not to overfill the biliary tree, as too much pressure can reopen the leak. Occlusion cholangiography is thus discouraged. For persistent leaks, a stent may need to be replaced and exchanged until resolution is confirmed. For persistent large bile leaks, a covered self-expanding metal stent (SEMS) may be considered to provide a greater decrease in pressure gradient across the ampulla and better facilitate "bridging" over the injury. While upfront costs may be more, early use of covered SEMS for BL may decrease the need for reintervention and thus may make this a cost-effective approach.

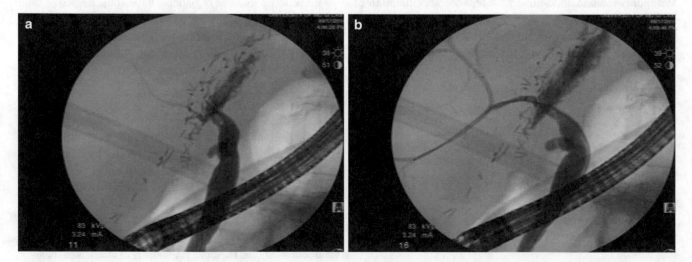

Fig. 5.1 Large anastomotic bile leak after living donor liver transplantation (**a**). The leak is seen prior to complete filling of the intrahepatic ducts (**b**)

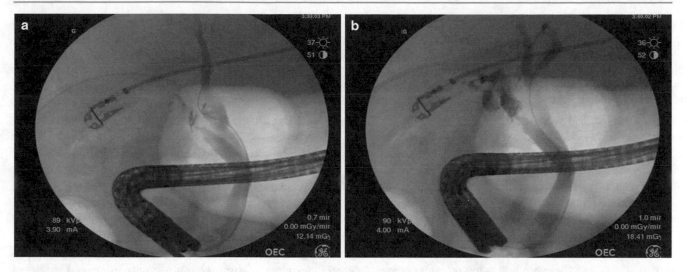

Fig. 5.2 No bile leak is seen initially in a patient after cholecystectomy (**a**). A small bile leak at the cystic duct remnant is seen only after filling of the intrahepatic ducts (**b**)

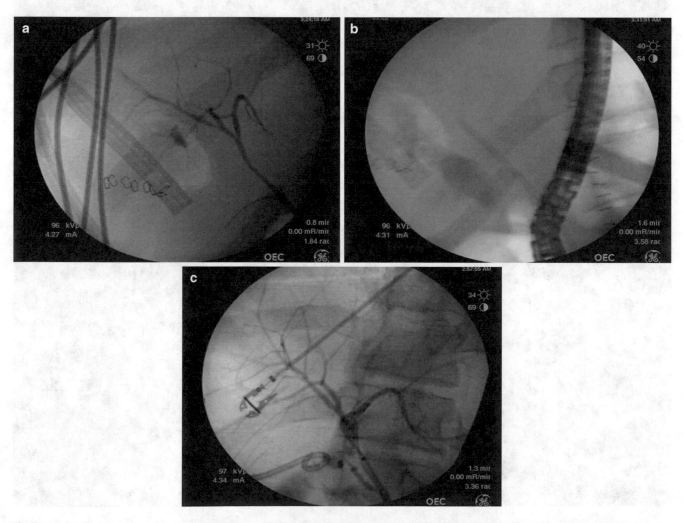

Fig. 5.3 A bile leak is seen at the resected gallbladder bed (**a**). A plastic biliary stent is places after sphincterotomy (**b**). The leak is resolved after 4 weeks of stent dwell time (**c**)

Bile Leak After Cholecystectomy

Significant post-cholecystectomy (post-CCY) bile leaks occur in 0.2–2 % of cases, with rates being higher when laparoscopic approaches are utilized over open cholecystectomy [6, 7]. ERCP serves as a good diagnostic value for evaluating BL after CCY, with sensitivities ranging between 83 and 98 % and technical success rates higher than 95 % [5, 6, 8]. After cholecystectomy, leaks typically occur at the cystic duct or the subvesicular bile ducts (ducts of Luschka), with these sites representing 54–78 % and 13–24 % of post-cholecystectomy leaks, respectively [3, 6, 8] (Fig. 5.4a). In cases of complicated cholecystitis, limited visibility may result in incomplete gallbladder resection and subsequent large bile leaks (Fig. 5.4b). Leaks can also be seen from the common bile duct, common hepatic duct, or branching hepatic ducts, but these are less common after cholecystec-

tomy than they are after liver resection. Complete disruption of the main bile duct, including inadvertent bile duct ligation, is rare, but can be identified readily with ERCP [9]. In up to a third of cases, retained bile duct stones of strictures may be contributing to post-cholecystectomy leaks and are identified on initial cholangiogram.

ERCP with sphincterotomy and stent placement have historically shown leak resolution rates of 70–100 % for post-cholecystectomy BL [4–6] (Fig. 5.5a, b). Sandha et al. showed a resolution rate of 91 % and 100 % amongst 207 patients with high-grade and low-grade bile leaks, respectively, while Kaffes and colleagues showed a resolution rate of 92 % in 100 patients with leaks after gallbladder resection [3, 6]. In another study of 127 patients, a single ERCP led to a 91 % resolution that improved to 95 % when additional endoscopic interventions were

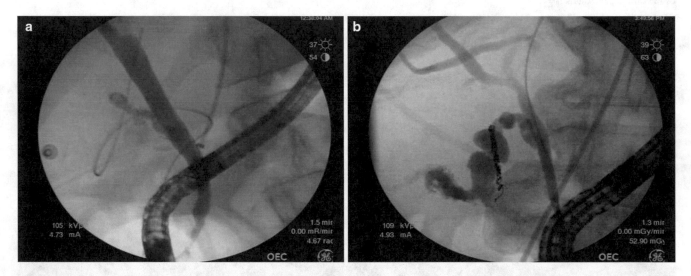

Fig. 5.4 Cystic duct stump leak (**a**). Leak from retained gallbladder remnant (**b**)

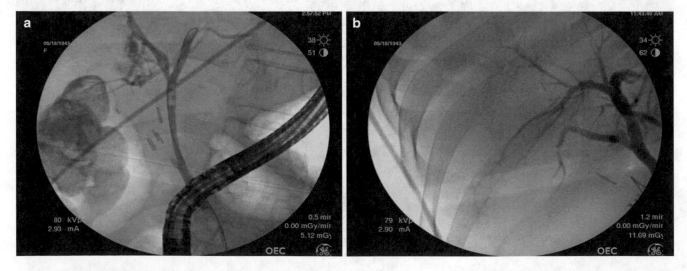

Fig. 5.5 A leak is seen within a segmental branch of the right hepatic ductal system (**a**). The leak is resolved after endoscopic sphincterotomy and a period of transpapillary stenting (**b**)

permitted [8]. While two studies suggest that biliary sphincterotomy alone may be adequate for low-grade leaks (leak resolution rates of 87–91 %), several other studies have shown sphincterotomy alone is significantly associated with treatment failure when compared to biliary stent placement alone or endoscopic sphincterotomy and stent placement as combined therapy [3, 8]. Stent placement is thus generally recommended for managing leaks after cholecystectomy where technically feasible.

Resolution of leak after cholecystectomy is typically reported within 7–14 days after stent placement [3, 10]. Median time to stent removal has been variable, but stents are generally removed at 4–6 weeks. A longer duration of stent placement is required if BL are associated with strictures. Performance of ERCP for post-CCY bile leaks has a complication rate if 1–4 %, a rate similar to other non-high risk ERCPS [6].

Bile Leak After Liver Resection

Liver resection (LR) is a well-established means of treating both benign and malignant liver diseases. While technical expertise has been improving as utilization increases, LR continues to be complicated by bile leak in approximately 15 % of cases [11–13]. Given the morbidity and mortality associated with such leaks, early recognition and management becomes imperative.

Postoperative BL following LR can be categorized as central bile leaks from the hilum or common hepatic duct, or peripheral bile leaks from the resection surface (Fig. 5.6a). Risk factors for bile leak after LR are generally related to technical aspects of the surgery, including longer operative time, left hemi-hepatectomy, and segment IV resection [12–14]. Central bile leaks after LR tend to manifest as larger volumes of bile spillage into the peritoneum, and have been associated with a worse prognosis than peripheral leaks. Options for managing post-LR leaks include surgical repair, percutaneous drainage, and endoscopic therapy. While timing is not well-defined, current literature suggests that it may be safe to wait up to 2 weeks after surgery for spontaneous resolution as long as percutaneous drainage is established and output is closely monitored [15]. Careful attention should be made toward the patient's PO intake to prevent dehydration from fluid losses in the bile in the case of large leaks, with IV hydration when needed.

All patients with LR leaks should have an endoprosthesis placed via ERCP. As a general rule, spanning the area of leak is preferential for central leaks. For peripheral leaks after LR bridging the leak is often difficult. Generally 7 or 10 F stents are utilized, with 10 F being preferred. After 2–6 weeks, endoscopic cholangiography is repeated and the stents replaced if the leak persists (Fig. 5.6b).

Success rates of ERCP for post-LR bile leaks have been reported to be between 59 and 100 % [15]. In one study, use of a bile duct endoprosthesis was associated with a better response rate than sphincterotomy alone. Central leaks have been shown to be less responsive than peripheral leaks in this context, but success rates of 59–72 % have been reported for central BL after LR [15]. The number of interventions are variable, but one study showed more ERCPs were required for leaks after hepatobiliary surgery than for those following cholecystectomy (1.4 versus 1.1) [8].

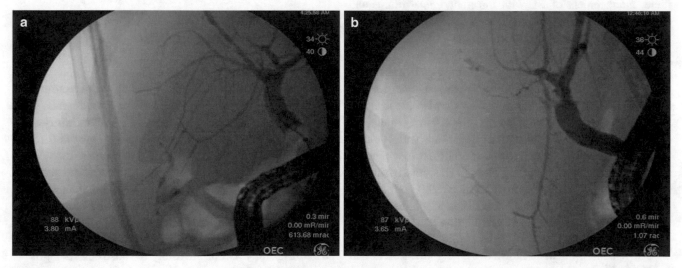

Fig. 5.6 A bile leak is seen at a subvesical duct along the resected gallbladder bed (**a**). This leak is resolved after a month of transpapillary biliary stent placement (**b**)

Traumatic Bile Leak

A prolonged bile leak as a consequence of hepatic trauma has been reported to occur in as few as 0.5 % and as many as 20 % of patients after their presenting injury [16]. When they do occur, patients with post-traumatic BL require more therapeutic procedures, have longer hospital courses, and require higher hospital charges than those without BL [17–19]. Given that up to 97 % of traumatic bile duct injuries occur in the context of trauma to other intra-abdominal organs or vascular structures, most are managed surgically if identified during initial injury screening or during initial laparotomy. When identification is delayed, endoscopic therapy has been shown to be successful in cases where repeat surgery is not appropriate or deemed too high risk for the patient.

There are limited reports about the endoscopic management and outcomes of biliary injury after blunt or penetrating abdominal trauma. This is in part due to a low frequency of presentation, with traumatic bile duct injuries representing only 0.1–2 % of all trauma admissions [20–22]. Intrahepatic duct injuries typically occur in the small sub-segmental ducts following blunt hepatic trauma, and generally are self-limiting. When they do not resolve, percutaneous drainage, endoscopic therapy, or surgery are required. Simple drainage remains the most common management option for a biliary leak from the intrahepatic biliary tree, and the majority will close without further intervention. Extra-hepatic bile duct injury generally occurs in the context of injury to other intra-abdominal organs, typically following blunt trauma. Concomitant duodenal, pancreatic, or vascular injuries are typically seen. While repair can be attempted during peritoneal exploration, this is not always possible, or biliary injury may be overlooked at initial laparotomy. In circumstances such as these, or when control of posttraumatic BL is incomplete, management of BL with intra-abdominal drains and concomitant ERCP should be considered.

Several small retrospective studies have shown that ERCP yields a treatment success of 89–100 % for traumatic bile duct injuries manifesting as BL. Bridges and colleagues achieved a resolution in nine of ten patients with penetrating or blunt liver injury after endoprosthesis placement alone, including eight patients with severe (grade 4 or 5) injury. An Israeli study noted resolution in all 11 patients with BL after hepatic trauma when treated with both endoscopic sphincterotomy and stent placement [23]. Bajaj et al. similarly showed BL resolution after ERCP in eight of nine (89 %) of patients, seven of whom received stents in addition to sphincterotomy [24]. Earlier studies also showed resolution rates of 100 % in studies including five to eight patients [25–28].

One special clinical situation deserving attention is that in which duodenal or small intestinal injury mimics a traumatic bile duct injury. In this circumstance, an ERCP is requested on account of bile-rich fluid accumulation in the peritoneum or external drain. If the cholangiogram is negative for a leak, a bowel perforation should be considered. Oral contrast-enhanced imaging should be performed when the diagnosis remains in doubt.

Endoscopic treatment protocols for traumatic biliary injuries are similar to those for iatrogenic bile duct injuries (Video 5.1). In general, a 7 to 10 F stent is placed, with the latter favored if a dilated ductal system is seen. While bridging the ductal system is not mandated, attempts should be made to place a stent within the left or right ductal system that suffered the injury. For peripheral leaks, a smaller stent may be preferred to approximate the leak more easily within the segmental branches of the intrahepatic biliary systems [19]. Anecdotal experience at the University of Maryland's Shock Trauma Center suggests traumatic bile duct injuries may take longer to resolve and often require multiple stent exchanges. Larger stents (10 F) are favored to facilitate leak resolution.

Postoperative Biliary Strictures

Benign biliary strictures result from a number of processes, including chronic pancreatitis, PSC, and postoperative biliary strictures (POBS). POBS will be the focus of this section.

POBS are most often associated with cholecystectomy or liver transplantation, although any surgery in which trauma or ischemia to the biliary tree result may be implicated in stricture formation. Biliary decompression is required in instances in which clinically significant obstruction occurs (i.e., jaundice, cholangitis, secondary biliary cirrhosis, hepatic graft dysfunction). ERCP with endoprosthesis placement is the primary treatment modality for POBS where technically possible. For refractory strictures surgical diversion via hepatico- or choledochoenterostomy may be required.

Laparoscopic Cholecystectomy

Introduction and Pathogenesis

While the evolution of laparoscopic cholecystectomy has led to shorter hospital stays and other improvements, these have come at a cost of higher rates of bile duct injury compared with open cholecystectomy (1–2 % versus 0.15 %) [6, 7]. This is in part due to the fact that laparoscopic cholecystectomy allows less complete traction of the gallbladder and cystic duct than open surgery, leading to incomplete isolation of anatomical structures and the potential for traction, thermal or penetrating injury to the bile ducts. When the degree of injury is substantial enough, biliary stricturing may occur, leading to obstructive signs or symptoms in the postoperative period. Incorrect placed clips or ligatures are less common but do occur, and typically manifest much earlier than strictures developing from healing tissue injuries along the biliary tract.

Diagnosis

Clinically significant biliary strictures after cholecystectomy typically demonstrate signs of obstruction. These include jaundice, pain, and signs of sepsis. Elevated alkaline phosphatase or bilirubin may also be seen and should raise suspicion of a bile duct injury in someone with a prior biliary surgery. Cross-sectional imaging usually demonstrates ductal dilation proximal to the stricture unless there is associated leak. MRCP has been shown to have particularly good accuracy for postoperative biliary strictures, which appear as a smooth tapering of the luminal signal. Multislice technique can help to avoid overestimation of stricture length so that proper endoscopic or surgical planning can be made [29].

Management

Technical success rates for the endoscopic treatment of benign post-cholecystectomy strictures with ERCP are greater than 90 %. While balloon dilation alone achieves suboptimal stricture resolution rates of only 25–38 %, endoscopic therapy utilizing stents with or without dilation yields clinical success rates of 80–95 % [30–37]. It is thus recommended that stents be utilized when possible for postoperative strictures. Complications have been reported in 22–33 % of patients and are usually related to stent migration or stent obstruction.

Endoscopic Technique

Standard wire-guided cannulation is performed and identification of the area of stenosis is made with cholangiography (Fig. 5.7a). While a sphincterotomy is not mandatory, it facilitates placement of multiple stents when required. Cytologic brushings should be obtained at least one time, as malignancy is sometimes misdiagnosed as a post-cholecystectomy stricture. Balloon dilation (4–10 mm) is then employed to open up the stricture. The use of contrast to inflate the dilation balloon permits visualization of the

balloon fluoroscopically, and the waist of the balloon can be visualized to ensure obliteration of the stenotic area. For tight strictures, a Soehendra biliary dilation device (4–7 F) may be employed, followed by balloon dilation of the stenosis. For very tight strictures, an angioplasty balloon may be required to permit the initial dilation. After dilation, a single plastic stent (7 F, 8.5 F, 10 F) or multiple plastic biliary stents are then placed across the stricture (Fig. 5.7b). Treatment generally consists of sequential ERCP and stent exchange every 3 months, with increasing stent numbers sequentially placed during a 12-month treatment period until stricture resolution [36].

When utilizing a multiple stent strategy, stricture resolution is achieved in 80–95 % of patients with postsurgical strictures [33, 35, 38, 39]. Use of multiple, side-by-side plastic stents may lead to improved success rates when compared to single plastic stents alone. A review of 47 studies in which extrahepatic POBS of varying etiologies were treated, clinical success rates were achieved in 94 % with multiple plastic stents versus 59 % with single stent use. For benign POBS other than OLT, clinical success rates with multiple plastic stents were reported in 81 % [40]. Complication rates were also lower when multiple stents are placed compared to single stent use.

Several small series have demonstrated the successful use of covered self-expanding metal stents (SEMS) for benign POBS of varying etiologies (Fig. 5.8a, b). Technical success rates have exceeded 98 %. When fully or partially covered 10-mm SEMS were used for benign POBS after cholecystectomy, clinical success rates of 62.3 % were reported in a 2009 systematic review. This was lower than that seen with multiple plastic stents (81.3 %) and may support the former as the first line option for POBS management [40]. However, formal comparisons between multiple plastic stents and SEMS are lacking at present. A more recent prospective study has shown stricture resolution rates of 72 % for post-

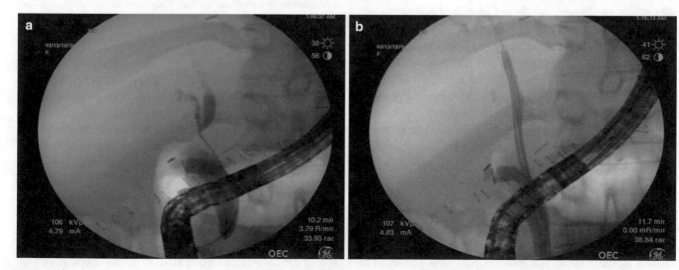

Fig. 5.7 A guide wire traverses a post-cholecystectomy biliary stricture (**a**). A stent is placed across the biliary stricture after dilation (**b**)

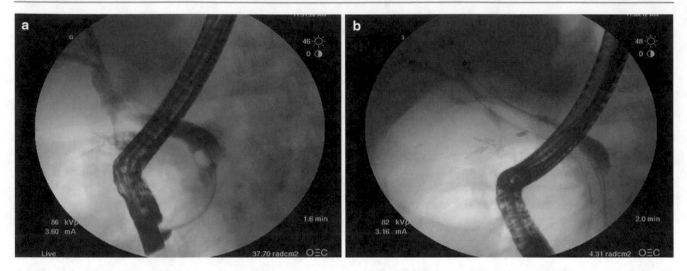

Fig. 5.8 A benign biliary stricture and bile leak are seen post-cholecystectomy and prior self-expanding metal stent (SEMS) placement (**a**). Both the leak and stricture are treated with another SEMS (**b**)

cholecystectomy strictures when SEMSs are used with a dwell of 10–12 months [41]. Stent migration remains a concern with covered SEMS, however, and appears to increase with stent indwell duration. Migration rates of 16.7, 22.2, and 66.7 % reported at 3-, 6- and 12 months have been reported [41]. Generally, SEMSs should not be used for longer than 12 month, and a change after 3–6 months should be considered. Because of the difficulty in removing uncovered SEMSs, their use for benign POBS is not recommended [36].

Exceptional Circumstances After Cholecystectomy

Complete transection of the bile duct is a rare complication of laparoscopic cholecystectomy in which traction applied to the gallbladder gulf leads to distortion and inadvertent ligation of the choledochus (Fig. 5.9). If discovered intraoperatively, an end-to-end choledochocholedochostomy or a hepaticojejunostomy is performed. When not identified during surgery, ductal transection is usually identified by ERCP carried out for the presence of a bile collection by imaging or drain output.

When identified postoperatively, a minimally invasive treatment utilizing a rendezvous between ERCP and percutaneous transhepatic cholangiography has become a preferred management option. A multidisciplinary team consisting of an endoscopist and an interventional radiologist is needed [42]. A guidewire is advanced across the papilla, into the bile duct, and into the subhepatic space. At the same time, the radiologist performs a percutaneous transhepatic cholangiography of the hepatic ducts, typically dilating them to 10 F in order to introduce a snare loop. The snare is advanced to the subhepatic space to catch the guidewire, which is externally advanced across the percutaneous entry point. Balloon dilation of the transected region is performed from both the

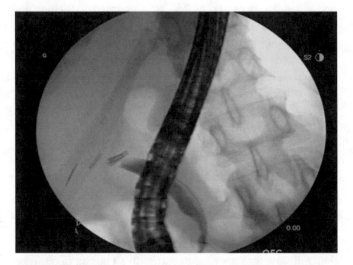

Fig. 5.9 Inadvertent placement of clips is noted across the common bile duct. The duct disruption was treated with endoscopic balloon dilation followed by transpapillary stent placement. In some circumstances, a rendezvous procedure utilizing percutaneous transhepatic cholangiography may also be required

percutaneous and transpapillary approaches in order to open the clips and permit the percutaneous insertion of an internal–external biliary drain. This drain is left in placed to avoid bile spillage into the abdomen. A percutaneous abdominal drainage may also be placed if necessary based on imaging or suspicion on ongoing leak despite ductal drainage. After 2–4 weeks, multiple 10 F plastic stents are placed, and are left in for at least 3 months, with stent changes as required. In their series, Fiocca et al. utilized and initial right hepatic approach followed by an additional left hepatic approach at 2–3 weeks to ultimately place four 10 F stents across the transected region (two in the left hepatic system and two in the right). With this method, 16 patients of the 22 patients who had completed treatment were asymptomatic 4 years after first endoscopic intervention [43].

Liver Transplantation

Introduction

There are several potential causes of cholestatic liver injury after liver transplantation, including reperfusion injury, delayed graft function, vascular complications, bile leaks, functional ampullary obstruction, and biliary stricture. Biliary stenosis can be difficult to distinguish clinically from the other causes, and radiographic tools like HIDA scan or MRCP may have a limited ability to effectively rule out an obstruction in the immediate and long-term postoperative period. Cholangiography remains the gold standard for diagnosing both anastomotic and non-anastomotic strictures after liver transplantation. While ERCP is the first line therapy for anastomotic strictures, its role for non-anastomotic strictures is more limited.

Considerations Before Cholangiography

Biliary strictures occur between 4 and 13 % of patients after orthotopic liver transplant (OLT) and in up to 19–32 % of living-donor liver transplant (LDLT) recipients [44–50]. Retrospective studies show that most strictures will present within 6 months of transplantation [51]. Strictures may come to clinical attention in a variety of ways: elevated conjugated bilirubin and alkaline phosphatase, abnormal imaging, jaundice, or evidence of cholangitis or other biliary complications. It is important to note that due to the denervation of the donor liver, the typical symptoms of biliary obstruction may be lacking. As such, serologies testing, and imaging should be performed prior to considering ERCP. Supplementary information from liver biopsy may be necessary to exclude non-stricturing causes of the laboratory abnormalities, including rejection, recurrent hepatitis, or infectious (viral) etiologies.

Radiography has a limited role for evaluating for biliary strictures after both OLT and LDLT. Less than 40–50 % of transplant recipients with anastomotic strictures show upstream biliary dilation, a limitation attributed to the denervation of the transplanted liver and fibrosis of the donor biliary system that occurs after transplantation [52–55]. HIDA scans are of limited benefit because of post-transplant graft dysfunction, medication effects, postoperative edema at the anastomosis and other confounding factors affecting the sensitivity. While one study showed HIDA scan had a negative predictive value of greater than 90 % in patients in the immediate postoperative period, other studies have shown a limited role for HIDA scan for the workup of post-transplantation strictures [56–58]. Similarly, while MRCP has been shown to have a sensitivity and sensitivity as high as 94–97 % for detecting biliary stenosis after transplant, this pooled data comes from small studies which have variable radiographic standards and which lack correlation with cholangiographic and clinical endpoints. As a whole, radiographic modalities are still considered less reliable for detecting biliary obstruction in the post-transplant population than they are for benign strictures from other etiologies.

Thus, when the suspicion for a biliary stenosis is high enough, ERCP remains the preferred diagnostic and therapeutic modality.

Classification of Biliary Strictures After Liver Transplantation

Most classification systems for post-liver transplantation strictures take into account the location of the stricture in relation to the surgical anastomosis. Most biliary strictures after transplant are anastomotic strictures (AS) and involve the choledochocholedochostomy. This is compared to those at site other than the anastomosis, or non-anastomotic strictures (NAS) (Fig. 5.10a–d). The clinical outcomes for AS versus NAS are significantly different, as are their respective responses to endoscopic therapy [59].

Pathogenesis

Technical problems remain the main cause of up to 80 % of post-OLT anastomotic strictures. These include fibrosis and ischemia resulting from donor-to-recipient duct mismatch, small-sized bile ducts, tension at the anastomosis, electrocautery or suture effect, or local infection [60–62]. Preceding bile leak is associated with late-onset AS, as is ischemic injury at the terminus of the donor duct over time [30, 59]. Studies have shown that AS tend to occur more often in LDLT than after OLT, in hepaticojejunostomy rather than duct-to-duct anastomosis, and that the use of T-tube in duct-to-duct anastomoses is generally protective when compared to those made without T-tubes [30, 63–65]. Other risk factors for AS include a BMI > 25 and recurrent HCV in the donor graft, the latter of which tends to lead to later onset AS.

Non-anastomotic strictures are typically due to ischemic complications inherent to OLT, including those related to hepatic artery thrombosis and prolonged cold ischemia time of the graft. NAS are also attributed to recurrent liver disease, chronic rejection, blood-type mismatch incompatibility, older age of donors (>60) and CMV infection [59, 66, 67]. Ischemia-associated NAS tends to present within 1 year of transplant, while immunogenic causes are more delayed in onset [30, 61]. NAS have been shown to occur earlier than AS, with a occurrences generally seen in the 3–6 month range [68, 69].

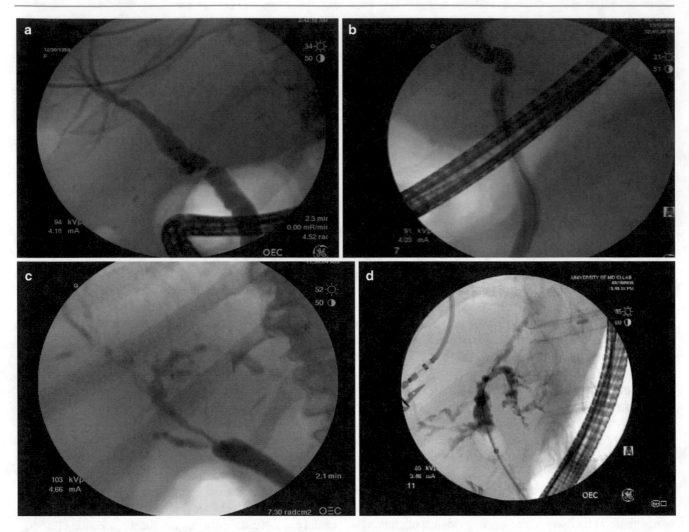

Fig. 5.10 An anastomotic stricture is identified after orthotopic liver transplantation (**a**). This stricture is patent after 6 weeks of therapy with a plastic biliary stent (**b**). Non-anastomotic strictures are seen in the secondary and tertiary branches of the donor intrahepatic system after orthotopic liver transplantation (**c** and **d**)

Management

Early reports from the transplant literature favored surgery and PTC as treatment modalities for post-liver transplantation biliary strictures. Percutaneous trans-hepatic management had been considered the preferred nonoperative treatment modality, with success rates of greater than 85 %. Both modalities are limited in terms of desirability, however, as they are invasive, and each carries its own significant morbidities. Recent advances in endoscopic techniques have been such that ERCP has now supplanted both surgery and percutaneous cholangiography as the preferred diagnostic and therapeutic modality.

Anastomotic Strictures (OLT)

The first challenge of AS is gaining wire access across the stricture. Anastomoses may be tortuous or kinked with multiple cystic duct remnants (both recipient and donor) across which to navigate. Care should be taken with wire passage,

especially in the early postoperative period (within 30 days). Once access is obtained, a combination of dilation and stenting should be attempted (Fig. 5.11a–c). (NOTE: dilation should be avoided in early anastomoses due to a concern for dehiscence at this site). While balloon dilation with a 4-, 6-, or 10-mm balloon alone can be considered, success rates of only 25–38 % have been reported with this technique [70, 71]. The use of endoprosthesis after dilation appears to offer a more durable stricture response rate, with stricture resolution reported in 64–100 % of post-OLT patients when a strategy of increasing plastic stents or SEMS is utilized [72–82].

For a strategy using multiple plastic stents, one to two 7 or 10 F stents are initially placed (Video 5.2). Subsequent ERCP with balloon dilation and stent insertion occurs every 8–12 weeks with increasing numbers of stents placed as possible until the stricture resolves. While some studies utilized time intervals as short as 2-week intervals between ERCP, intervals of 8–12 weeks are typically performed in clinical

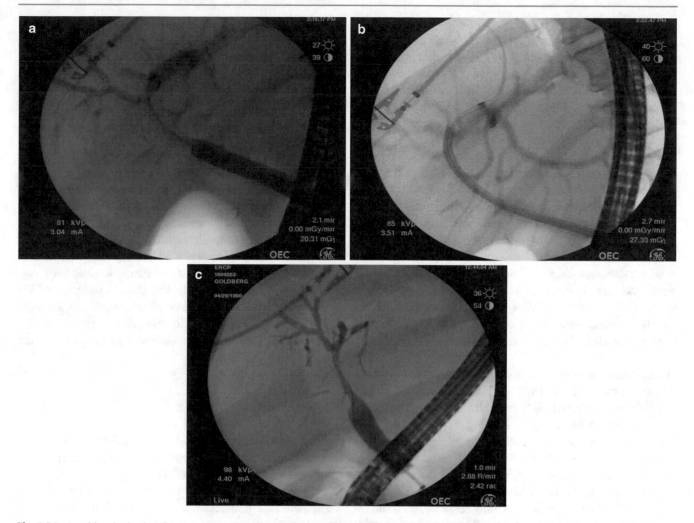

Fig. 5.11 A guide wire is placed across an anastomotic stricture and balloon dilation is performed (**a**). This is followed by a period of stent placement across the anastomosis (**b**). The stenosed area is improved after stent removal (**c**)

settings [72, 74, 83, 84]. In a review of eight studies and 440 patients, an average of two to three stents were placed per ERCP, with stent duration of 3.6–15 months. Using such a strategy, clinical success rates of 84 % and 86 % were reported for early- and late-onset AS, respectively [51]. Stent duration for greater than 12 months was associated with higher stricture resolution rates and lower stricture recurrence rates than stents placed for less than a year (97 % versus 78.3 % and 1.5 % versus 14.2 %, respectively) [51].

When plastic stents fail to yield adequate stricture resolution, the use of partially or fully covered biliary SEMS can be considered. Some small studies have also used SEMS as the primary therapy for AS when feasible. Most studies using SEMS exchanged or removed the stents at intervals of 2–3 months [76–81]. In a review of ten studies and 200 patients, a stricture resolution rate of 78–82 % was reported. Stent duration of greater than 3 months was associated with higher stricture resolution rates and lower stricture recurrence rates

than stents placed for less than 3 months (89.5 % versus 71.8 % and 8 % versus 15.3 %, respectively) [51].

There are no trials directly comparing using multiple plastic stents and SEMS, and the former are generally the preferred initial strategy in most institutions. A stent migration rate of 16 % SEMS further supports the use of plastic stents initially where possible [51]. Anecdotal reports of anastomotic dehiscence with SEMS are also available.

Non-anastomotic Strictures

NAS are more difficult to treat and are generally less responsive to endoscopic therapies than AS. Success rates in the vicinity of 60 % have been reported after OLT, but rates are lower in the context of LDLT (25–33 %) [48]. Furthermore, stent patency is limited by biliary sludge accumulation. Therefore, patients with complex NAS often require retransplantation, and the role of ERCP becomes one of a bridge to surgery rather than a definitive treatment modality in itself [48].

Endoscopic therapy of NAS typically consists of balloon dilation of all accessible strictures and extraction of biliary sludge and casts proximal to the lesions. This may be followed by the placement of plastic stents with replacement every 3 months until strictures are deemed adequately patent. Given their refractory character, NAS typically require multiple treatments. In one study, a median of six treatments were done every 8–10 weeks [85]. In cases in which obstruction does not improve or does so for only a short duration, multidisciplinary discussions with the surgeon are thus warranted, as early retransplantation may be indicated to prevent cholangitis, abscess formation, and progressive graft loss.

Endoscopic success as defined by improvement of cholestatic parameters and cholangiographic patency occur in 6–91 %, although the proximal location of NAS may permit stent placement in a few as 31 % of patients [68, 85]. In a study of 72 patients with NAS, of whom 85 % were treated, 68 (94.4 %) had persistent strictures and 22 (31 %) required retransplantation. Only 25 % received stents [68].

Living-Donor Related Transplantation (LDLT)

Biliary complications, including stricture formation and leak, occur in approximately one-third of living donor liver transplantation recipients [48, 86] (Fig. 5.12). Furthermore, studies show these complications are more refractory to treatment than those after orthotopic liver transplantation. For anastomotic strictures arising after LDLT, the treatment success rates of 31–100 % have been reported [30, 48, 86, 87]. Multiple treatments are generally required, with studies showing an average of 2.7–4 procedures required to meet success endpoints [51].

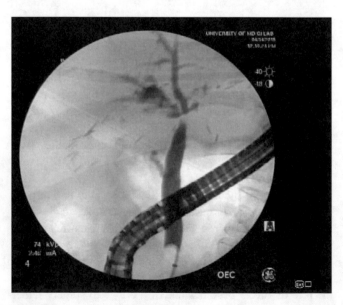

Fig. 5.12 An anastomotic stricture is seen after living donor liver transplantation

Complications

Complications rates for ERCP after OLT are generally low, with most reports showing complication rates of 2–6 % [75]. These complications include pancreatitis, bleeding, stent migration, infection, and dehiscence of the anastomosis. Management varies depending on the nature and location of injury or complication.

Pancreatic Duct Leaks

Pancreatic duct (PD) injury may result from acute or chronic pancreatitis, pancreatic and splenic surgery, pancreatic malignancy, guidewire injuries during ERCP, or abdominal trauma. Persistent PD disruption may lead to pancreatic ascites, pancreatic and peripancreatic fluid collections, or fistula formation. The clinical sequelae of PD disruption depend on a number of factors including the etiology of the disruption, the location and extent of the disruption, the presence of downstream obstruction, and the rate of pancreatic secretion.

Epidemiology

Up to 40 % of patients with acute pancreatitis will develop some type of acute fluid collection [88]. Recently, the revised Atlanta classification 2012 [89] recategorized the various types of pancreatic collections. In acute interstitial edematous pancreatitis, collections that do not have an enhancing capsule are called acute peripancreatic fluid collections (APFC); after development of a capsule, they are referred to as pancreatic pseudocysts (PP; usually after the first 4 weeks). In necrotizing pancreatitis, a collection without an enhancing capsule is called an acute necrotic collection (ANC; usually in the first 4 weeks) and once an enhancing capsule has developed, they are referred to as walled-off necrosis (WON, usually after 4 weeks). Fortunately, only a small percentage of acute fluid collections will go on to develop PP or WON. Persistent or enlarging PP suggests an ongoing ductal injury. Similarly, WON frequently involves a ductal leak. WON patients have been shown to have disconnected duct syndrome (DDS) in 35–70 % of cases [90].

Clinical Manifestations

The manifestations of PD disruption include pseudocysts, WON, pancreatic ascites, pancreatic fistula (pancreatic-cutaneous fistula, pancreatic-pleural fistula) and disconnected duct syndrome. The ductal disruption can be identified in the head, body, genu, tail and sometimes at multiple sites.

Ductal disruption can be complete or partial. Signs and symptoms are variable, but can include nausea, pain, tachycardia, ileus and hypotension. Obstruction of the biliary tree, gastric outlet and small intestine may also be seen.

Diagnosis

Computed Tomography (CT)

Cross sectional imaging with a pancreatic protocol CT is typically the best initial diagnostic test for patients with smoldering or severe pancreatitis who may have a pancreatic duct leak [90]. CT can identify the size, location, and content of fluid collections, and also determine whether there may be compression on vital organs such as the stomach, small intestine or biliary tree. CT can also help to determine the maturity of the capsule (aka rind) and whether a mature fluid collection may be amenable to endoscopic drainage. Importantly, serial CT scans can be used to date the age of a collection, an important determinant in deciding when a collection is mature enough to drain.

Endoscopic Retrograde Pancreatography (ERP)

ERP is the gold standard for the diagnosis of ductal injuries as it can provide detailed images of the pancreatic duct and define the location and nature of the injury [91]. It can be performed preoperatively, intraoperatively or postoperatively in patients with pancreatic injury, and it is also offers the potential for therapy. ERP should be considered in any patient who has evidence of a persistent or symptomatic leak. Since many acute pancreatic fluid collections related to acute pancreatitis resolve on their own, it is reasonable to defer ERP in this setting. For patients with persistent or enlarging fluid collections related to pancreatitis (ex PP or WON), ERP should be performed. Similarly, patients with evidence of persistent leaks after surgery or trauma should undergo ERP for potential diagnosis and therapy. Because of the potential of infecting sterile pancreatic fluid collections, patients with evidence of leak by ERP should be given prophylactic antibiotic therapy. A quality pancreatogram should be obtained to identify the size and location of the leak as well as any factors that may be contributing to its persistence, such as a stone or a stricture.

Magnetic Resonance Pancreatography (MRCP)

MRCP is a useful noninvasive modality that can be used as a diagnostic complement to therapeutic ERCP. Secretin-enhanced MRCP can characterize an active leak and minimizes the potential complications associated with ERCP [92]. MRCP has an added advantage of delineating the pancreatic duct upstream to complete disruption, an area not visualized on ERP. The most important limitation of MRCP is that therapeutic procedures cannot be performed [93]. Similar to cross sectional imaging with CT, MRI images can provide important information about the size, location and content of a fluid collection and whether there is impingement on important adjacent structures.

Fluid Amylase

Patients with persistent output from a JP drain after pancreatic surgery, or variable output of clear fluid following percutaneous drainage of a fluid collection may have a pancreatic duct leak. These patients should have the fluid checked for amylase levels which will be markedly elevated in the setting of a pancreatic leak [94, 95].

Management

Pseudocysts (PP)

A pancreatic pseudocyst is surrounded by a well-defined wall and contains essentially no solid material. If aspiration of cyst content is performed, there is usually a markedly increased amylase level. A low amylase content and high CEA level in the cyst may suggest an underlying mucinous neoplasm of the pancreas [96, 97]. A pancreatic pseudocyst is thought to arise from disruption of the main pancreatic duct or its intra-pancreatic branches without any recognizable pancreatic parenchymal necrosis [89].

Indications for Drainage

The indications for drainage of pancreatic pseudocysts have changed overtime. Initially, it was thought that size of pseudocyst (>6 cm) and duration of presence of pseudocyst (>6 weeks) were important indicators for pseudocyst drainage. These criteria are now obsolete [98–101]. Presently, the development of persistent symptoms thought to be related to the presence of the pseudocysts or development of a complications related to the pseudocyst such as infection, bleeding, biliary, or gastric outlet obstruction are indications for drainage.

Patient Selection for Endoscopic Drainage

The first step of determining whether the pseudocyst is endoscopically drainable is to differentiate a pseudocyst from any other types of pancreatic cysts.

Imaging

Pancreatic pseudocysts typically appear as unilocular cysts with thin walls and without internal septa, a solid component, or central cyst wall calcification (Fig. 5.13). The patient nearly always presents with a clinical history of pancreatitis. The diagnosis is supported by imaging findings of inflammation, atrophy, or calcification of pancreatic parenchyma, and dilatation of the pancreatic

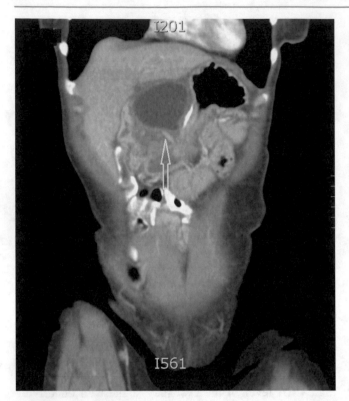

Fig. 5.13 CT scan of the abdomen showing thin walled pseudocyst compressing the stomach. Note the homogenous fluid and lack of internal septae

duct [96]. Noninvasive imaging does have limitations in distinguishing pseudocysts from cystic neoplasms, especially when there are no morphologic signs of pancreatitis and no clear communication with the duct [101, 102].

Cyst Fluid Analysis

When cross-sectional imaging does not provide a definitive diagnosis, additional information aspiration of the contents of a cyst may help the diagnosis [102]. CEA has been shown to be the most accurate marker to distinguish non-mucinous from mucinous cysts [96]. CEA does not, however, distinguish benign from malignant mucinous neoplasms [96]. Amylase is also a helpful marker, as amylase is typically very high, usually in the thousands and almost never <250 ng/mL in pseudocysts [97], but is low in serous cysts [97]. It should be understood, however, that measurement of CEA or amylase in cyst fluid has not been approved by the US Food and Drug Administration (FDA) and has never been formally validated or approved by the FDA [96].

Contraindications

Contraindications to cyst drainage include a cyst to gastrointestinal wall distance of greater than 1 cm, presence of vascular structures in the projected needle path that can't be circumvented with the aid of EUS, and pseudo-

aneurysms [103, 104]. The presence of debris is a cyst increased the risk of infection and is a relative contraindication for simple drainage. In these circumstances, more extensive procedures such as endoscopic necrosectomy (see below) should be considered.

EUS Guided Transmural Drainage (EUD) Versus Conventional Direct Transluminal Drainage by Forward-Viewing Endoscopy (CTD)

A prospective randomized controlled trial by Park et al. [105] studying CTD versus EUD revealed no significant difference in clinical outcomes between CTD and EUD [105]. However, the rate of technical success was higher for EUD (94 %) than for CTD (72 % $P=0.039$). Most of the difference in technical success was secondary to the inability of CTD to drain non-bulging cysts. A meta-analysis by Panamonta et al. comparing the technical success and clinical outcomes of EUD and CTD for bulging PPs showed EUD was not superior to CTD in terms of short-term or long-term success and the overall complications were similar in both groups [106]. EUD of PP is a preferred endoscopic option in patients who have non-bulging cysts, a small portal of entry based on computed tomography (CT), intervening vessels seen by CT, unusual locations of PPs, or coagulopathy. In cases of failed CTD, EUD should also be considered.

Endoscopic Transmural Drainage Versus Percutaneous Drainage

Retrospective studies reveal no significant differences in clinical success rates when comparing endoscopic transmural drainage to percutaneous drainage [103]. However, percutaneous transmural drainage was associated with a higher reintervention rate, longer hospital stays, and increased number of follow-up abdominal imaging studies [103]. Furthermore, percutaneous drainage of PPs may lead to pancreatico-cutaneous fistulae. Therefore, endoscopic transmural drainage is the preferred modality for the drainage of symptomatic PP compared with percutaneous drainage.

Endoscopic Transmural Drainage (ETD) Versus Surgical Drainage

A prospective randomized controlled trial by Akshintala et al. regarding surgical drainage versus ETD for symptomatic PP revealed no difference in treatment success, complications, or reinterventions between the surgical and endoscopic transmural drainage groups. However, the length of hospital stays was shorter, the physical and mental health scores were better, and the total mean costs were lower for the ETD group [104]. Surgical treatment still has an important role in terms of adjunctive or salvage therapy, if endoscopic or percutaneous intervention fails.

Transpapillary Drainage

Transpapillary drainage requires that the PP communicate with the main pancreatic duct and that it has few septations to permit complete drainage. It should be considered for small pseudocysts (typically <6 cm) that are symptomatic. An advantage of transpapillary drainage is that associated ductal pathology such as stones, strictures or fistulae can be identified and treated.

Multimodality Endoscopic Treatment of Pancreatic Duct Disruption with Stenting and Pseudocyst Drainage

Older retrospective studies have recommended assessing the main pancreatic duct at the time of PP drainage with endoscopic retrograde cholangiopancreatography (ERCP) as patients with major main pancreatic duct leaks may require stent placement to bridge the leak [107, 108]. A retrospective study by Shrode et al. [109] also demonstrated the pancreatic duct disruptions require multimodality treatment, addressing not only the integrity of the pancreatic duct but also any associated fluid collections. Based upon their results, they recommended partial ductal disruptions be managed with a bridging stent. However, complete ductal disruptions did worse with a combination of cystgastrostomy/enterostomy and transpapillary stenting than disruptions treated with cystgastrostomy/enterostomy alone [109].

Technique of Drainage

Conventional Transmural Drainage (CTD)

Either a side viewing duodenoscope or a therapeutic upper endoscope can be used for CTD. The authors prefer a duodenoscope as the elevator makes stent insertion easier. The stomach is insufflated and the area of extrinsic compression of the stomach is located. A needle knife sphincterotome is then utilized to puncture directly into the bulge created by the cyst. Blended current is utilized for the puncture. Entry into the cyst is confirmed by injecting contrast under fluoroscopy which demonstrates laminar flow. In addition, cyst fluid is aspirated and typically has a "dishwater" appearance. The fluid should be sent for amylase and culture. A guidewire is then looped inside the pseudocyst. Next, a 10–15 mm through the scope balloon is used to dilate the transmural tract. A short (5–7 cm) double pigtail 7 to 10 F plastic stent is then advanced over the guidewire and deployed with the proximal end in the gastric lumen and the distal end within the pseudocyst cavity. The steps of wire placement and stent placement can be repeated until multiple (two to four) double pigtail stents are in place.

EUS Guided Transmural Drainage (EUD)

Two-Step Approach [110]

The pseudocyst is localized using an echoendoscope. An ultrasonography examination is performed to determine characteristics and contents of the cyst and to ensure the absence of pseudoaneurysms or vascular structures within the expected trajectory of the needle. A 19-gauge needle is then used to puncture the pseudocyst. Once inside the pseudocyst, the needle is replaced with a 0.035-in. guidewire, which is looped inside the cyst. Next, the echoendoscope is withdrawn, with the wire secured in place within the pseudocyst, and the echoendoscope is replaced with a side-viewing duodenoscope. The transmural tract is then dilated and stented as described for CTD above.

One-Step Approach [110]

In this technique, the echoendoscope is used to perform the entire drainage. After identifying the pseudocyst, a needle is passed into the pseudocyst and the needle is exchanged for a guidewire (Fig. 5.14). Then, a through-the-scope balloon is used to dilate the cystogastrostomy tract. Balloon dilation of the tract is usually performed to a size that would be acceptable for delivery of either two 10 F plastic stents or a covered metal biliary stent. Typically, 8–12 mm dilating balloons suffice. After dilation of the tract, the endoprosthesis is delivered through the echoendoscope across the cystogastrostomy or cystenterostomy. The advantage of this technique over the two-step approach is that it avoids exchange of the entire

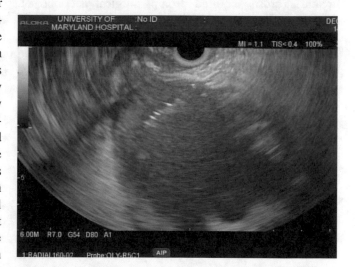

Fig. 5.14 EUS of walled off necrosis (WON) demonstrating needle puncture access. Note the heterogenous material suggesting necrotic debris

endoscope over the guidewire, and thus decreases the risk of guidewire displacement.

After performance of the endoscopic cystogastrostomy or cystenterostomy, patients are usually placed on 5–7 days of antibiotics to avoid cyst infection. Reassessment with CT abdomen in 2–4 weeks is performed to determine if the cyst has collapsed/resolved. Once the cyst has collapsed, stents may be removed.

Walled Off Necrosis (WON) and Infected Pancreatic Necrosis

WON consists of necrotic pancreatic and/or peripancreatic tissue contained within an enhancing wall of reactive tissue. By definition, it is mature, encapsulated and typically occurs ≥4 weeks after onset of necrotizing pancreatitis [89]. WON may be sterile or may become infected. Infected pancreatic necrosis has varying amounts of necrotic material and pus, and the amount of pus may increase with liquefaction of the necrosis. Clues to the presence of infected necrosis may be the development of late-onset fever, sepsis or clinical deterioration of the patient. While the presence of gas in the collection seen by cross-sectional imaging suggests infection, the diagnosis of infected necrosis requires fine needle aspiration. Infection of pancreatic necrosis develops in approximately 30 % of patients with necrosis [111]. It is important to determine whether infected necrosis is present because infected pancreatic necrosis is associated with higher mortality rate from sepsis and multiorgan failure. Historically, management of infected pancreatic necrosis required prompt surgical debridement. However this concept has been challenged by multiple reports and case series showing that antibiotics alone can lead to resolution of infection and, in select patients, avoid surgery altogether [112]. Also there is growing evidence suggesting endoscopic transmural drainage and necrosectomy is a viable alternative to percutaneous drainage and surgical intervention in the treatment of infected walled-off pancreatic and peripancreatic necrosis [113].

Endoscopic Drainage/Necrosectomy Versus Surgical Management

A prospective randomized controlled trial by Bakker et al. [114] comparing direct endoscopic drainage/necrosectomy of WON or infected WON versus surgical management demonstrated significant advantages to an endoscopic approach. These advantages included reduction of the pro-inflammatory response (serum interleukin-6), reduction in the incidence of new-onset multiple organ failure, less intra-abdominal bleeding, decreased pancreatic and enterocutaneous fistula formation, and a reduction in the incidence of iatrogenic perforation of a visceral organ.

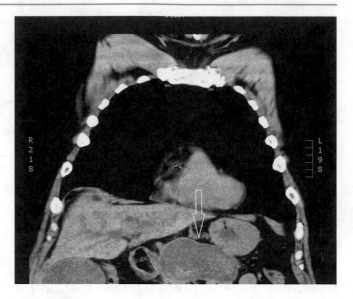

Fig. 5.15 CT scan of the abdomen showing heterogenous material within the pancreatic walled off necrosis

Endoscopic Necrosectomy

Indications

In collections with necrotic debris (Fig. 5.15), clinical success rate is poor with simple endoscopic or percutaneous drainage methods alone. The practice of utilizing a nasocystic tube to flush the necrotic debris from WON can be considered, but frequently fails and is poorly tolerated by patients. Over the last decade, endoscopic necrosectomy has emerged as a viable alternative to surgery for WON with and without infection.

A direct endoscopic necrosectomy should be considered under the following conditions [111]:

1. Necrotizing pancreatitis is present.
2. US, EUS, CT, or MRI show solid components in the fluid collection.
3. Acute inflammation suggesting an infected WON is present.

Technique

Non EUS Guided Necrosectomy

A therapeutic upper endoscope or side viewing duodenoscope is passed into the stomach. The authors prefer a straight viewing upper endoscope for endoscopic necrosectomy as it is easier to pass into the necrotic cavity. Access to the WON is obtained similar to the method described above for CTD. A guidewire is advanced into the WON and a large volume through the scope balloon is used to dilate the transmural tract to 12–15 mm. More aggressive balloon dilation can be performed in a graduated approach up to 20 mm to ease the introduction of the therapeutic upper scope into the cavity for endoscopic debridement. Necrotic debris is removed utilizing snares, baskets and vigorous flushing. Once adequate debridement is performed, the WON is stented with multiple plastic double pigtail stents or a self-expandable metallic stent (SEMS). Serial procedures are performed every few days until all necrotic tissue is removed. Usually, the patients are placed on antibiotics to avoid WON cavity infection during the course of necrosectomy.

EUS Guided Necrosectomy with New Self-Expandable Metallic Stent (SEMS) [111]

One-step EUS-guided walled-off pancreatic necrosis drainage is performed transgastrically using a 19-gauge needle. After bougie using a 4-mm dilating balloon, a self-expandable metallic stent (SEMS) is deployed under fluoroscopic and endoscopic image guidance. In further sessions, a standard upper endoscope is inserted through the SEMS into the walled-off pancreatic necrosis and the necrotic tissue is removed. Stents can be removed once there is CT confirmation of cyst collapse/resolution.

Covered Self-Expandable Metallic Stents (CSEMSs)

The use of fully covered self-expandable metallic stents (CSEMSs) may further improve the clinical success of endoscopic drainage of WON and infected necrosis (Fig. 5.16a–c). Kawakami et al. have summarized reports of 56 patients with WON infected necrosis [91]. The technical success rate was 100 % and the complete resolution rate was 87.8 %. These numbers are comparable to simple transmural pseudocyst drainage.

Treatment of Partial Main Duct Disruptions and Side Branch Disruptions

Medical management of pancreatic duct leaks utilizes conservative management with bowel rest, total parenteral nutrition (TPN), or nasojejunal tube feedings. Somatostatin analogues such as Octreotide or Pasireotide may decrease pancreatic juice extravasation [115, 116]. Many patients with small pancreatic leaks can experience resolution of their leaks without any intervention [90]. In refractory cases,

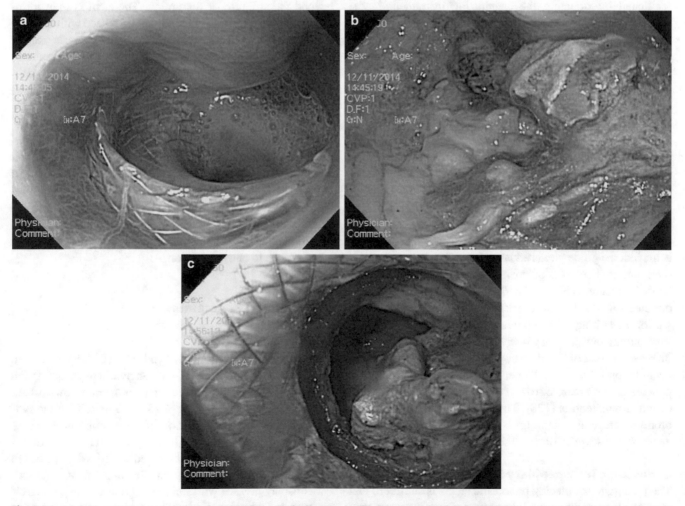

Fig. 5.16 (a) Self-expanding metal stent draining the walled off necrosis. (b) Contents of WON demonstrating necrotic material. (c) Necrotic debris being removed through the SEMS

ERCP with a transpapillary stent can facilitate the leak closure [117, 118]. Pancreatic stenting is effective in treating pancreatic leaks because the stent reduces the pancreatic ductal pressure [90, 117]. Stenting should aim to bridge the leak and is usually ineffective if the duct is completed disconnected and therefore unbridgeable [119, 120].

Pancreatic Cannulation

The main principles involved in pancreatic cannulation are similar to those of biliary cannulation. Guidewire cannulation, while often preferred for biliary cannulation, can sometimes be challenging for pancreatic cannulation in the setting of ductal injury. This is the result of an abnormal path the wire may take especially if there is a disruption in the head of the pancreas. Therefore, there should be a low threshold to inject contrast and identify the pertinent anatomy once the papilla is engaged. It is critical to understand ampullary anatomy for successful pancreatic duct cannulation. When ampulla is positioned in the middle of the endoscopic view, the pancreatic duct orients towards 1 o' clock whereas common bile duct orients towards 11 o' clock. Successful selective cannulation is facilitated by orienting the cannulating instrument in the proper orientation. If access to the main pancreatic duct is restricted by complete pancreas divisum or duct disruption in the head of the pancreas, it may be possible to access the main pancreatic duct through the minor papilla [121].

Conventional MRCP and secretin enhanced MRCP can be utilized to map out pancreatic ductal anatomy prior to ERCP. For example, its sensitivity for diagnosing divisum is 65–73 % [122, 123]. In difficult cannulation cases, IV Secretin injection can be used to facilitate cannulation of the either the major or minor papilla during endoscopic retrograde cholangiopancreatography (ERCP) [124, 125].

Pancreatic Sphincterotomy

Once successful cannulation of the pancreatic duct orifice is achieved, the guidewire is advanced into the main pancreatic duct and confirmation of position is usually obtained with contrast injection (Fig. 5.17). The sphincterotomy should be directed towards the 1 o'clock position with the very distal part of the cutting wire to prevent thermal injury to the duct. Pure cutting currents may decrease the risk of PD injury but increase the risk of bleeding compared to settings with more coagulation [126, 127]. The edema that ensues following a pancreatic sphincterotomy can cause ductal obstruction and eventual pancreatitis [128]. Therefore, following sphincterotomy, pancreatic stenting is crucial to prevent and/or decrease the severity of ERCP induced pancreatitis.

Endoscopic Transpapillary Stent Placement

The technique for placing pancreatic stents is similar to that used to place stents in the biliary tract. Once the pancreatic duct has been deeply cannulated, a hydrophilic 0.035″ guide-

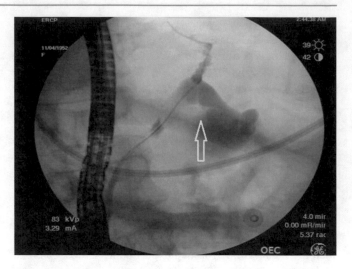

Fig. 5.17 Pancreatogram demonstrating wire extending across a partial pancreatic duct disruption. Extensive contrast extravasation is evident

wire is introduced into the duct and maneuvered if possible beyond the stricture or disruption. The stent is then introduced over the guidewire. Stents can be placed with or without pancreatic sphincterotomy. A sphincterotomy is usually preferred to facilitate drainage around the stent if it becomes clogged or dislodged, and to facilitate access in future procedures. Pancreatic stents are made primarily of polyethylene material. Pancreatic stent sizes range from 2 to 25 cm in length and 3 to 11.5 F in diameter [129] Choice of stent size depends on the caliber of the duct and the site of the disruption. Most of the pancreatic stents have side holes along their length to allow flow from side branches. In addition, most pancreatic stents have a mechanism (e.g., distal flange, pigtail) to prevent internal or external migration. If the there is a stricture in the pancreatic duct limiting the stent placement, the stricture can be dilated with a balloon or Soehendra dilator (5 or 8 F) to allow insertion.

Disconnected Pancreatic Duct Syndrome (DPDS)

Disconnected pancreatic duct syndrome (DPDS) is defined by complete discontinuity of the pancreatic duct such that a viable portion of the pancreas does not drain downstream into the duodenum [130] (Fig. 5.18). The severity of the syndrome depends on the location of the disruption. In cases where the disruption is in the head of the pancreas, the drainage of the entire pancreas is disturbed whereas disruptions in the tail affect a substantially smaller amount of pancreas. Patients may present with fluid collections, pancreatic ascites, pain and manifestations of exocrine and even endocrine insufficiency.

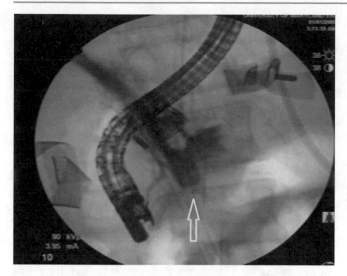

Fig. 5.18 Pancreatogram demonstrating complete disruption of the duct in the head with associated leak. Note the lack of filling of duct in the body and tail

Endoscopic Treatment

Transpapillary Stenting

Transpapillary stenting promotes drainage into the duodenum by decreasing the pressure gradient across the papilla [90, 117]. The predictors of success with this strategy depended largely on the degree of duct disruption and the ability to bridge the site of leak [120]. Because the disruption is complete in DPDS, transpapillary stenting is often unsuccessful [119]. In a study by Varadarajulu et al. of patients with complete disruption of the MPD who underwent insertion of a PD stent either to bridge the gap or into the collection, the outcome was successful in only 44 % and 26 % respectively [120]. The optimal duration of stent placement is unknown. Most endoscopists prefer stent removal and/or exchanges every 4–8 weeks [131]. A retrospective study of three patients by Telford et al. showed a longer duration of stent therapy ($P=0.002$) was associated with a more successful outcome [118].

Transmural Drainage (EUS and Non-EUS Guided)

In DPDS, collections form from drainage of the disconnected segment of pancreas. Transmural drainage can indirectly drain the disconnected pancreatic segment into the gastrointestinal tract by forming a fistula between the collection and the stomach or small intestine. The decision to choose the trans-gastric or trans-duodenal approach is based on the relationship of the collection to the stomach or the duodenum. If the collection is amenable to either, then a trans-duodenal drainage is preferred because of the theoretic greater patency of the fistula after removing the stents [131]. Transmural stents are typically removed after resolution of the peripancreatic fluid col-

lections. However, this approach has been associated with recurrence rates as high as 50 % [119, 126]. Leaving a stent permanently in place could prevent recurrence by creating a permanent fistula between the MPD and the gastrointestinal tract. In a study by Devière et al. of 13 patients with DPDS who underwent endoscopic transmural drainage, stents were left in place for a prolonged period, and no peripancreatic fluid collection recurred at a mean follow-up of 30 months [127]. A randomized control trail by Arvanitakis et al. also showed success with prolonged stent placement. None of the 15 patients in this trial developed recurrence of peripancreatic fluid collections when the stents were left in place compared with 5 of 13 patients in whom the stent was removed ($P=0.013$) [132]. Stent occlusion of small caliber plastic stents is an obvious long-term concern. Placement of fully covered self-expandable metallic stents (e.g., Axios stents) for such forms of transmural drainage could be a more favorable alternative due to better patency rates. However, data regarding success of long term covered self-expandable metallic stents in this scenario is currently lacking.

Percutaneous Drainage

Ultrasound-guided or CT-guided percutaneous drainage of fluid collections is another option to indirectly drain a disconnected pancreatic segment. The major disadvantage of percutaneous drainage is the development of external pancreatico-cutaneous fistulae [133, 134].

Surgery

The two main surgical options for DPDS are: (1) reestablishment of drainage into the gastrointestinal tract (Roux-en-Y internal drainage by pancreaticojejunostomy, pancreaticogastrostomy, fistulojejunostomy, or cystojejunostomy) and (2) Resection of the disconnected segment (distal pancreatosplenectomy) [110].

Roux-en-Y internal drainage requires much less dissection and conserves the still functioning distal pancreas and the spleen. In a study by Howard et al. [135], a Roux-en-Y procedure was associated with a significant decrease in operative time, blood loss, transfusion requirement, and duration of hospital stay.

Trauma

Pancreatic injury is uncommon because the retroperitoneal location of the pancreas offers relative protection. However, the pancreas does overly the spine and blunt trauma can cause the pancreas to "break" as it smashes into the hard bony structure. These injuries classically involve the body of the pancreas. Common blunt injuries to the pancreas include crush injuries, seat belt injuries during motor vehicle collisions, handle-bar injuries from bicycle accidents and direct blows to the pancreas from assaults. Pancreatic injuries occur in approximately 5 % of patients with blunt abdominal trauma, and 8 % of patients with penetrating abdominal injuries [136, 137]. In the setting of blunt or penetrating trauma, pancreatic injuries may be suspected at the time of exploratory laparotomy. In these instances, intraoperative ERCP can provide valuable information to the surgeon contemplating the type of repair needed. More often, ductal injuries to the pancreas become evident postoperatively due to the accumulation of amylase rich fluids in the peritoneum, retroperitoneum or external drains. ERCP plays a crucial role in the diagnosis of the location and extent of the leak.

The American Association for the Surgery of Trauma (AAST) Organ Injury Scaling Committee has described a grading system that is widely used and can guide appropriate management [138].

Grades I injuries (Minor contusion or laceration without ductal injury) and Grade II injuries (Major contusion or laceration without ductal injury) are treated with nonoperative management techniques or simple drainage. Grade III injuries (Complete transection of distal pancreas or distal pancreatic parenchymal injury with pancreatic duct injury), Grade IV injuries (Proximal pancreatic transection or injury involving proximal duct or the ampulla), or Grade V injuries (Massive disruption involving the head of pancreas) often require resection with possible reconstruction and/or drainage procedures [139].

Endoscopic Treatment

Principles of endoscopic management of traumatic ductal injuries are similar to management of ductal disruptions described in previous sections. Early ERCP within a few days of the inciting trauma is essential to the potential success of endoscopic therapy. Endoscopic transpapillary drainage has been successfully used to heal duct disruptions in the early phase of pancreatic trauma and in the delayed phase to treat the complications of pancreatic duct injuries. However, in patients with type IV or V ductal injuries not amenable to transpapillary stents, morbidity and mortality greatly increase unless surgery is undertaken within the first 24 h. Most of the published experience in endoscopic treatment of pancreatic injury is in the form of case reports, and case series are retrospective and heterogeneous with small number of patients [115, 140, 141].

Pancreatic Strictures

Pancreatic strictures (Fig. 5.19a, b) are a common endpoint of various pancreatic injuries including chronic pancreatitis, acute pancreatitis, trauma, iatrogenic injuries from pancreatic stents and wires, and surgical anastomoses. Despite, the differing etiologies of pancreatic strictures, the presentation, evaluation and management are similar.

PD strictures typically present with pain and manifestations of exocrine insufficiency late in their course. CT can be helpful by showing ductal dilation upstream of the stricture. Depending on the cause of the stricture, parenchymal and ductal calcifications can also be seen. MRCP is very helpful in delineating the anatomy. Treatment is indicated in patients who are symptomatic. Asymptomatic pts do not necessarily require therapy.

Main pancreatic strictures should always be approached with suspicion since chronic pancreatitis patients have increased risk of pancreatic cancer. It is recommended that all pancreatic duct strictures be brushed for cytology. The absence of pancreatic calcifications, the presence of exocrine insufficiency and K-ras mutation on pancreatic duct brushing were identified as additional predictive factors for the development of pancreatic adenocarcinoma [142]. Physicians should have a low threshold to perform EUS to more closely examine the pancreatic parenchyma, with fine-needle aspiration of any areas felt to be suspicious for possible malignancy [36].

Symptomatic CP patients with a single MPD stricture located in the head of the pancreas are the ideal candidates for ERCP with pancreatic endotherapy while isolated strictures in the tail or multiple strictures with a chain of lake appearance are less amenable to endotherapy [143, 144]. A pancreatic sphincterotomy, by itself, is not effective for the treatment of pancreatic strictures. However, it facilitates instrumentation, drainage around stents, and access to the pancreatic duct during future treatment sessions. For isolated short PD strictures, dilation with a balloon is effective. (sizes 4–8 mm) For diffuse strictures, dilating catheters such as a Sohendra dilator are preferred (6–10 F). The size of dilation is dictated by the caliber of the stricture and the size of the remaining duct. Care must be taken not to overdilate a stricture and risk duct disruption. Following dilation therapy, stents that bridge the stricture are utilized. Typically, plastic stents are utilized with calibers ranging from 4 to 11.5 F. Size is again determined by caliber of the stricture and diameter of the remaining PD. Large-bore (8.5–11.5 F) stents have a longer patency [145]. Pain relief after single pancreatic stenting in chronic pancreatitis has been observed in 70–94 % of the patients [143, 146]. In the absence of early symptomatic improvement, stents should be removed [147]. If the stents are effective in improving symptoms, patients undergo serial pancreatic dilation and stenting procedures every 2–3 months for 6–24 months duration. It should be noted that pancreatic duct strictures often improve in their radiographic appearance, but rarely does the pancreatogram normalize. However, data suggest

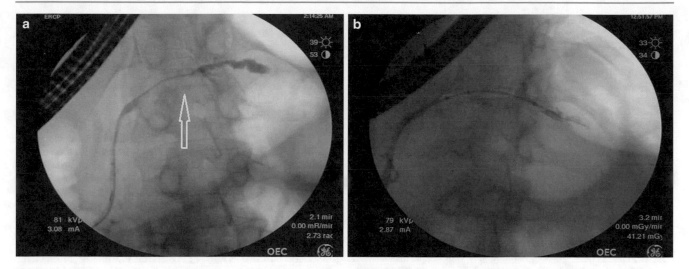

Fig. 5.19 (a) Pancreatogram showing stricture of the body of the pancreas that resulted from pancreatic trauma. Note the location of the stricture overlies the spine, a common spot for traumatic PD strictures. (b) Dilating balloon position across the PD stricture

that resolution of the stricture is not a prerequisite for symptomatic improvement since symptomatic improvement may persist after pancreatic stent removal despite persistence of the stricture [148]. After serial dilations and stenting sessions, a stent free trial should be considered. Recurrence of strictures requiring re-stenting was reported in 38 % of patients after 2 years follow-up [149]. The clinical results of pancreatic stenting are a good predictive factor for the outcome of drainage surgeries such as pancreaticojejunostomy.

Conclusions

Pancreatic and biliary injuries are commonly encountered by interventional endoscopists. A thorough understanding of the mechanisms of injury, pertinent anatomy, and patient presentation is vital for successful endotherapy. Patients with these injuries are often acutely ill and at risk for significant morbidity and mortality. ERCP can play a crucial role in treating these injuries and promoting patient recovery. Multidisciplinary approaches with surgeons and interventional radiologists are often necessary, especially in cases of complex injuries.

Video Legends

Video 5.1 Bile leak from the right intrahepatic bile system. The leak was treated with a biliary sphincterotomy and stent placement.

Video 5.2 Post liver transplant anastomotic stricture immediately distal to the bifurcation. The stricture was treated with balloon dilations and two traversing bile duct stents into the left and right hepatic ducts.

References

1. Koch M, et al. Bile leakage after hepatobiliary and pancreatic surgery: a definition and grading of severity by the International Study Group of Liver Surgery. Surgery. 2011;149:680–8. doi:10.1016/j.surg.2010.12.002.
2. Elboim CM, Goldman L, Hann L, Palestrant AM, Silen W. Significance of post-cholecystectomy subhepatic fluid collections. Ann Surg. 1983;198:137–41.
3. Kaffes AJ, et al. Impact of endoscopic intervention in 100 patients with suspected postcholecystectomy bile leak. Gastrointest Endosc. 2005;61:269–75.
4. Binmoeller KF, Katon RM, Shneidman R. Endoscopic management of postoperative biliary leaks: review of 77 cases and report of two cases with biloma formation. Am J Gastroenterol. 1991;86:227–31.
5. Davids PH, Rauws EA, Tytgat GN, Huibregtse K. Postoperative bile leakage: endoscopic management. Gut. 1992;33:1118–22.
6. Sandha GS, Bourke MJ, Haber GB, Kortan PP. Endoscopic therapy for bile leak based on a new classification: results in 207 patients. Gastrointest Endosc. 2004;60:567–74.
7. Barkun AN, et al. Postcholecystectomy biliary leaks in the laparoscopic era: risk factors, presentation, and management. McGill Gallstone Treatment Group. Gastrointest Endosc. 1997;45:277–82.
8. Tewani SK, Turner BG, Chuttani R, Pleskow DK, Sawhney MS. Location of bile leak predicts the success of ERCP performed for postoperative bile leaks. Gastrointest Endosc. 2013;77:601–8. doi:10.1016/j.gie.2012.11.026.
9. Sofi AA, Tang J, Alastal Y, Nawras AT. A simultaneous endoscopic and laparoscopic approach for management of early iatrogenic bile duct obstruction. Gastrointest Endosc. 2014;80:511–5. doi:10.1016/j.gie.2014.04.039.
10. Aksoz K, et al. Endoscopic sphincterotomy alone in the management of low-grade biliary leaks due to cholecystectomy. Dig Endosc. 2009;21:158–61. doi:10.1111/j.1443-1661.2009.00878.x.
11. Li J, et al. Intraoperative application of "white test" to reduce postoperative bile leak after major liver resection: results of a prospective cohort study in 137 patients. Langenbecks Arch Surg. 2009;394:1019–24. doi:10.1007/s00423-008-0455-7.
12. Lo CM, Fan ST, Liu CL, Lai EC, Wong J. Biliary complications after hepatic resection: risk factors, management, and outcome. Arch Surg. 1998;133:156–61.

13. Yamashita Y, et al. Bile leakage after hepatic resection. Ann Surg. 2001;233:45–50.
14. Capussotti L, et al. Bile leakage and liver resection: where is the risk? Arch Surg. 2006;141:690–4. doi:10.1001/archsurg.141.7.690. discussion 695.
15. Dechêne A, et al. Endoscopic management is the treatment of choice for bile leaks after liver resection. Gastrointest Endosc. 2014;80:626–33.e621. doi:10.1016/j.gie.2014.02.1028.
16. Croce MA, et al. Nonoperative management of blunt hepatic trauma is the treatment of choice for hemodynamically stable patients. Results of a prospective trial. Ann Surg. 1995;221:744–53. discussion 753–5.
17. Vassiliu P, Toutouzas KG, Velmahos GC. A prospective study of post-traumatic biliary and pancreatic fistuli. The role of expectant management. Injury. 2004;35:223–7.
18. Fleming KW, Lucey BC, Soto JA, Oates ME. Posttraumatic bile leaks: role of diagnostic imaging and impact on patient outcome. Emerg Radiol. 2006;12:103–7. doi:10.1007/s10140-005-0453-9.
19. Bridges A, Wilcox CM, Varadarajulu S. Endoscopic management of traumatic bile leaks. Gastrointest Endosc. 2007;65:1081–5. doi:10.1016/j.gie.2006.11.038.
20. Ball CG, et al. A decade of experience with injuries to the gallbladder. J Trauma Manag Outcomes. 2010;4:3. doi:10.1186/1752-2897-4-3.
21. Thomson BN, et al. Management of blunt and penetrating biliary tract trauma. J Trauma Acute Care Surg. 2012;72:1620–5. doi:10.1097/TA.0b013e318248ed65.
22. Sawaya DE, Johnson LW, Sittig K, McDonald JC, Zibari GB. Iatrogenic and noniatrogenic extrahepatic biliary tract injuries: a multi-institutional review. Am Surg. 2001;67:473–7.
23. Lubezky N, et al. Endoscopic sphincterotomy and temporary internal stenting for bile leaks following complex hepatic trauma. Br J Surg. 2006;93:78–81. doi:10.1002/bjs.5195.
24. Bajaj JS, Spinelli KS, Dua KS. Postoperative management of noniatrogenic traumatic bile duct injuries: role of endoscopic retrograde cholangiopancreaticography. Surg Endosc. 2006;20:974–7. doi:10.1007/s00464-005-0472-3.
25. Sugiyama M, et al. Endoscopic biliary stenting for treatment of bile leakage after hepatic resection. Hepatogastroenterology. 2001;48:1579–81.
26. D'Amours SK, Simons RK, Scudamore CH, Nagy AG, Brown DR. Major intrahepatic bile duct injuries detected after laparotomy: selective nonoperative management. J Trauma. 2001;50:480–4.
27. Sugiyama M, Atomi Y, Matsuoka T, Yamaguchi Y. Endoscopic biliary stenting for treatment of persistent biliary fistula after blunt hepatic injury. Gastrointest Endosc. 2000;51:42–4.
28. Carrillo EH, et al. Interventional techniques are useful adjuncts in nonoperative management of hepatic injuries. J Trauma. 1999;46:619–22. discussion 622–4.
29. Ward J, et al. Bile duct strictures after hepatobiliary surgery: assessment with MR cholangiography. Radiology. 2004;231:101–8. doi:10.1148/radiol.2311030017.
30. Ryu CH, Lee SK. Biliary strictures after liver transplantation. Gut Liver. 2011;5:133–42. doi:10.5009/gnl.2011.5.2.133.
31. Tuvignon N, et al. Long-term follow-up after biliary stent placement for postcholecystectomy bile duct strictures: a multicenter study. Endoscopy. 2011;43:208–16. doi:10.1055/s-0030-1256106.
32. de Reuver PR, et al. Endoscopic treatment of post-surgical bile duct injuries: long term outcome and predictors of success. Gut. 2007;56:1599–605. doi:10.1136/gut.2007.123596.
33. Kassab C, et al. Endoscopic management of post-laparoscopic cholecystectomy biliary strictures. Long-term outcome in a multicenter study. Gastroenterol Clin Biol. 2006;30:124–9.
34. Vitale GC, et al. Endoscopic management of postcholecystectomy bile duct strictures. J Am Coll Surg. 2008;206:918–23. doi:10.1016/j.jamcollsurg.2008.01.064. discussion 924–5.
35. Draganov P, Hoffman B, Marsh W, Cotton P, Cunningham J. Long-term outcome in patients with benign biliary strictures treated endoscopically with multiple stents. Gastrointest Endosc. 2002;55:680–6.
36. Adler DG, et al. ASGE guideline: the role of ERCP in diseases of the biliary tract and the pancreas. Gastrointest Endosc. 2005;62:1–8. doi:10.1016/j.gie.2005.04.015.
37. van Boeckel PG, Sijbring A, Vleggaar FP, Siersema PD. Systematic review: temporary stent placement for benign rupture or anastomotic leak of the oesophagus. Aliment Pharmacol Ther. 2011;33:1292–301. doi:10.1111/j.1365-2036.2011.04663.x.
38. Zepeda-Gómez S, Baron TH. Benign biliary strictures: current endoscopic management. Nat Rev Gastroenterol Hepatol. 2011;8:573–81. doi:10.1038/nrgastro.2011.154.
39. Costamagna G, Pandolfi M, Mutignani M, Spada C, Perri V. Long-term results of endoscopic management of postoperative bile duct strictures with increasing numbers of stents. Gastrointest Endosc. 2001;54:162–8.
40. van Boeckel PG, Vleggaar FP, Siersema PD. Plastic or metal stents for benign extrahepatic biliary strictures: a systematic review. BMC Gastroenterol. 2009;9:96. doi:10.1186/1471-230X-9-96.
41. Devière J, et al. Successful management of benign biliary strictures with fully covered self-expanding metal stents. Gastroenterology. 2014;147:385–95. doi:10.1053/j.gastro.2014.04.043. quiz e315.
42. Tsukamoto T, et al. Percutaneous management of bile duct injuries after cholecystectomy. Hepatogastroenterology. 2002;49:113–5.
43. Fiocca F, et al. Complete transection of the main bile duct: minimally invasive treatment with an endoscopic-radiologic rendezvous. Gastrointest Endosc. 2011;74:1393–8. doi:10.1016/j.gie.2011.07.045.
44. Rerknimitr R, et al. Biliary tract complications after orthotopic liver transplantation with choledochocholedochostomy anastomosis: endoscopic findings and results of therapy. Gastrointest Endosc. 2002;55:224–31. doi:10.1067/mge.2002.120813.
45. Stratta RJ, et al. Diagnosis and treatment of biliary tract complications after orthotopic liver transplantation. Surgery. 1989;106:675–83. discussion 683–4.
46. Lerut J, et al. Biliary tract complications in human orthotopic liver transplantation. Transplantation. 1987;43:47–51.
47. Akamatsu N, Sugawara Y, Hashimoto D. Biliary reconstruction, its complications and management of biliary complications after adult liver transplantation: a systematic review of the incidence, risk factors and outcome. Transpl Int. 2011;24:379–92. doi:10.1111/j.1432-2277.2010.01202.x.
48. Yazumi S, et al. Endoscopic treatment of biliary complications after right-lobe living-donor liver transplantation with duct-to-duct biliary anastomosis. J Hepatobiliary Pancreat Surg. 2006;13:502–10. doi:10.1007/s00534-005-1084-y.
49. Liu CL, Lo CM, Chan SC, Fan ST. Safety of duct-to-duct biliary reconstruction in right-lobe live-donor liver transplantation without biliary drainage. Transplantation. 2004;77:726–32.
50. Todo S, Furukawa H, Kamiyama T. How to prevent and manage biliary complications in living donor liver transplantation? J Hepatol. 2005;43:22–7. doi:10.1016/j.jhep.2005.05.004.
51. Kao D, Zepeda-Gomez S, Tandon P, Bain VG. Managing the post-liver transplantation anastomotic biliary stricture: multiple plastic versus metal stents: a systematic review. Gastrointest Endosc. 2013;77:679–91. doi:10.1016/j.gie.2013.01.015.
52. St Peter S, et al. Significance of proximal biliary dilatation in patients with anastomotic strictures after liver transplantation. Dig Dis Sci. 2004;49:1207–11.
53. Kok T, et al. Ultrasound and cholangiography for the diagnosis of biliary complications after orthotopic liver transplantation: a comparative study. J Clin Ultrasound. 1996;24:103–15. doi:10.1002/(SICI)1097-0096(199603)24:3<103::AID-JCU1>3.0.CO;2-L.

54. Zemel G, Zajko AB, Skolnick ML, Bron KM, Campbell WL. The role of sonography and transhepatic cholangiography in the diagnosis of biliary complications after liver transplantation. AJR Am J Roentgenol. 1988;151:943–6. doi:10.2214/ajr.151.5.943.

55. Jorgensen JE, et al. Is MRCP equivalent to ERCP for diagnosing biliary obstruction in orthotopic liver transplant recipients? A meta-analysis. Gastrointest Endosc. 2011;73:955–62. doi:10.1016/j.gie.2010.12.014.

56. Nair S, Lingala S, Satapathy SK, Eason JD, Vanatta JM. Clinical algorithm to guide the need for endoscopic retrograde cholangiopancreatography to evaluate early postliver transplant cholestasis. Exp Clin Transplant. 2014;12:543–7.

57. Hopkins LO, et al. Tc-99m-BrIDA hepatobiliary (HIDA) scan has a low sensitivity for detecting biliary complications after orthotopic liver transplantation in patients with hyperbilirubinemia. Ann Nucl Med. 2011;25:762–7. doi:10.1007/s12149-011-0523-x.

58. Al Sofayan MS, et al. Nuclear imaging of the liver: is there a diagnostic role of HIDA in posttransplantation? Transplant Proc. 2009;41:201–7. doi:10.1016/j.transproceed.2008.10.076.

59. Seehofer D, Eurich D, Veltzke-Schlieker W, Neuhaus P. Biliary complications after liver transplantation: old problems and new challenges. Am J Transplant. 2013;13:253–65. doi:10.1111/ajt.12034.

60. Testa G, Malagò M, Broelseh CE. Complications of biliary tract in liver transplantation. World J Surg. 2001;25:1296–9.

61. Verdonk RC, et al. Anastomotic biliary strictures after liver transplantation: causes and consequences. Liver Transpl. 2006;12:726–35. doi:10.1002/lt.20714.

62. Thuluvath PJ, Pfau PR, Kimmey MB, Ginsberg GG. Biliary complications after liver transplantation: the role of endoscopy. Endoscopy. 2005;37:857–63. doi:10.1055/s-2005-870192.

63. Rabkin JM, et al. Biliary tract complications of side-to-side without T tube versus end-to-end with or without T tube choledochocholedochostomy in liver transplant recipients. Transplantation. 1998;65:193–9.

64. López-Andújar R, et al. T-tube or no T-tube in cadaveric orthotopic liver transplantation: the eternal dilemma: results of a prospective and randomized clinical trial. Ann Surg. 2013;258:21–9. doi:10.1097/SLA.0b013e318286e0a0.

65. Vougas V, et al. A prospective randomised trial of bile duct reconstruction at liver transplantation: T tube or no T tube? Transpl Int. 1996;9:392–5.

66. Cursio R, Gugenheim J. Ischemia-reperfusion injury and ischemic-type biliary lesions following liver transplantation. J Transplant. 2012;2012:164329. doi:10.1155/2012/164329.

67. Ludwig J, Batts KP, MacCarty RL. Ischemic cholangitis in hepatic allografts. Mayo Clin Proc. 1992;67:519–26.

68. Guichelaar MM, et al. Risk factors for and clinical course of nonanastomotic biliary strictures after liver transplantation. Am J Transplant. 2003;3:885–90.

69. Graziadei IW, et al. Long-term outcome of endoscopic treatment of biliary strictures after liver transplantation. Liver Transpl. 2006;12:718–25. doi:10.1002/lt.20644.

70. Schwartz DA, Petersen BT, Poterucha JJ, Gostout CJ. Endoscopic therapy of anastomotic bile duct strictures occurring after liver transplantation. Gastrointest Endosc. 2000;51:169–74.

71. Zoepf T, et al. Balloon dilatation vs. balloon dilatation plus bile duct endoprostheses for treatment of anastomotic biliary strictures after liver transplantation. Liver Transpl. 2006;12:88–94. doi:10.1002/lt.20548.

72. Morelli J, Mulcahy HE, Willner IR, Cunningham JT, Draganov P. Long-term outcomes for patients with post-liver transplant anastomotic biliary strictures treated by endoscopic stent placement. Gastrointest Endosc. 2003;58:374–9.

73. Pasha SF, et al. Endoscopic treatment of anastomotic biliary strictures after deceased donor liver transplantation: outcomes after maximal stent therapy. Gastrointest Endosc. 2007;66:44–51. doi:10.1016/j.gie.2007.02.017.

74. Holt AP, et al. A prospective study of standardized nonsurgical therapy in the management of biliary anastomotic strictures complicating liver transplantation. Transplantation. 2007;84:857–63. doi:10.1097/01.tp.0000282805.33658.ce.

75. Sanna C, et al. Safety and efficacy of endoscopic retrograde cholangiopancreatography in patients with post-liver transplant biliary complications: results of a cohort study with long-term follow-up. Gut Liver. 2011;5:328–34. doi:10.5009/gnl.2011.5.3.328.

76. Vandenbroucke F, et al. Treatment of post liver transplantation bile duct stricture with self-expandable metallic stent. HPB (Oxford). 2006;8:202–5. doi:10.1080/13651820500501800.

77. Kahaleh M, et al. Temporary placement of covered self-expandable metal stents in benign biliary strictures: a new paradigm? (with video). Gastrointest Endosc. 2008;67:446–54. doi:10.1016/j.gie.2007.06.057.

78. Traina M, et al. Efficacy and safety of fully covered self-expandable metallic stents in biliary complications after liver transplantation: a preliminary study. Liver Transpl. 2009;15:1493–8. doi:10.1002/lt.21886.

79. Mahajan A, et al. Temporary placement of fully covered self-expandable metal stents in benign biliary strictures: midterm evaluation (with video). Gastrointest Endosc. 2009;70:303–9. doi:10.1016/j.gie.2008.11.029.

80. García-Pajares F, et al. Covered metal stents for the treatment of biliary complications after orthotopic liver transplantation. Transplant Proc. 2010;42:2966–9. doi:10.1016/j.transproceed.2010.07.084.

81. Tarantino I, et al. Endoscopic treatment of biliary complications after liver transplantation. World J Gastroenterol. 2008;14:4185–9.

82. Chaput U, et al. Temporary placement of partially covered self-expandable metal stents for anastomotic biliary strictures after liver transplantation: a prospective, multicenter study. Gastrointest Endosc. 2010;72:1167–74. doi:10.1016/j.gie.2010.08.016.

83. Alazmi WM, et al. Recurrence rate of anastomotic biliary strictures in patients who have had previous successful endoscopic therapy for anastomotic narrowing after orthotopic liver transplantation. Endoscopy. 2006;38:571–4. doi:10.1055/s-2006-925027.

84. Tabibian JH, et al. Endoscopic treatment of postorthotopic liver transplantation anastomotic biliary strictures with maximal stent therapy (with video). Gastrointest Endosc. 2010;71:505–12. doi:10.1016/j.gie.2009.10.023.

85. Zoepf T, et al. Optimized endoscopic treatment of ischemic-type biliary lesions after liver transplantation. Gastrointest Endosc. 2012;76:556–63. doi:10.1016/j.gie.2012.04.474.

86. Tsujino T, et al. Endoscopic management of biliary complications after adult living donor liver transplantation. Am J Gastroenterol. 2006;101:2230–6. doi:10.1111/j.1572-0241.2006.00797.x.

87. Hsieh TH, et al. Endoscopic treatment of anastomotic biliary strictures after living donor liver transplantation: outcomes after maximal stent therapy. Gastrointest Endosc. 2013;77:47–54. doi:10.1016/j.gie.2012.08.034.

88. Balthazar EJ, Robinson DL, Megibow AJ, Ranson JH. Acute pancreatitis: value of CT in establishing prognosis. Radiology. 1990;174:331–6. doi:10.1148/radiology.174.2.2296641.

89. Banks PA, et al. Classification of acute pancreatitis—2012: revision of the Atlanta classification and definitions by international consensus. Gut. 2013;62:102–11. doi:10.1136/gutjnl-2012-302779.

90. Larsen M, Kozarek R. Management of pancreatic ductal leaks and fistulae. J Gastroenterol Hepatol. 2014;29:1360–70. doi:10.1111/jgh.12574.

91. Kawakami H, Itoi T, Sakamoto N. Endoscopic ultrasound-guided transluminal drainage for peripancreatic fluid collections: where are we now? Gut Liver. 2014;8:341–55. doi:10.5009/gnl.2014.8.4.341.

92. Fulcher AS, et al. Magnetic resonance cholangiopancreatography (MRCP) in the assessment of pancreatic duct trauma and its sequelae: preliminary findings. J Trauma. 2000;48:1001–7.

93. Bhasin DK, Rana SS, Rawal P. Endoscopic retrograde pancreatography in pancreatic trauma: need to break the mental barrier. J Gastroenterol Hepatol. 2009;24:720–8. doi:10.1111/j.1440-1746.2009.05809.x.

94. Kozarek R. Role of ERCP in acute pancreatitis. Gastrointest Endosc. 2002;56:S231–6. doi:10.1067/mge.2002.129006.

95. Runyon BA. Amylase levels in ascitic fluid. J Clin Gastroenterol. 1987;9:172–4.

96. Pitman MB, et al. Pancreatic cysts: preoperative diagnosis and clinical management. Cancer Cytopathol. 2010;118:1–13. doi:10.1002/cncy.20059.

97. van der Waaij LA, van Dullemen HM, Porte RJ. Cyst fluid analysis in the differential diagnosis of pancreatic cystic lesions: a pooled analysis. Gastrointest Endosc. 2005;62:383–9.

98. Vitas GJ, Sarr MG. Selected management of pancreatic pseudocysts: operative versus expectant management. Surgery. 1992;111:123–30.

99. Cheruvu CVN, Clarke MG, Prentice M, Eyre-Brook IA. Conservative treatment as an option in the management of pancreatic pseudocyst. Ann R Coll Surg Engl. 2003;85:313–6. doi:10.1308/003588403769162413.

100. Andrén-Sandberg A, Dervenis C. Pancreatic pseudocysts in the 21st century. Part II: Natural history. JOP. 2004;5:64–70.

101. Singhal S, Rotman SR, Gaidhane M, Kahaleh M. Pancreatic fluid collection drainage by endoscopic ultrasound: an update. Clin Endosc. 2013;46:506–14. doi:10.5946/ce.2013.46.5.506.

102. Pinto MM, Meriano FV. Diagnosis of cystic pancreatic lesions by cytologic examination and carcinoembryonic antigen and amylase assays of cyst contents. Acta Cytol. 1991;35:456–63.

103. Akshintala VS, et al. A comparative evaluation of outcomes of endoscopic versus percutaneous drainage for symptomatic pancreatic pseudocysts. Gastrointest Endosc. 2014;79:921–8. doi:10.1016/j.gie.2013.10.032. quiz 983.e922, 983.e925.

104. Varadarajulu S, et al. Equal efficacy of endoscopic and surgical cystogastrostomy for pancreatic pseudocyst drainage in a randomized trial. Gastroenterology. 2013;145:583–90.e581. doi:10.1053/j.gastro.2013.05.046.

105. Park DH, et al. Endoscopic ultrasound-guided versus conventional transmural drainage for pancreatic pseudocysts: a prospective randomized trial. Endoscopy. 2009;41:842–8. doi:10.1055/s-0029-1215133.

106. Panamonta N, Ngamruengphong S, Kijsiricareanchai K, Nugent K, Rakvit A. Endoscopic ultrasound-guided versus conventional transmural techniques have comparable treatment outcomes in draining pancreatic pseudocysts. Eur J Gastroenterol Hepatol. 2012;24:1355–62. doi:10.1097/MEG.0b013e32835871eb.

107. Baron TH. Endoscopic drainage of pancreatic pseudocysts. J Gastrointest Surg. 2007;12:369–72. doi:10.1007/s11605-007-0334-5.

108. Varadarajulu S, Bang JY, Phadnis MA, Christein JD, Wilcox CM. Endoscopic transmural drainage of peripancreatic fluid collections: outcomes and predictors of treatment success in 211 consecutive patients. J Gastrointest Surg. 2011;15:2080–8. doi:10.1007/s11605-011-1621-8.

109. Shrode CW, et al. Multimodality endoscopic treatment of pancreatic duct disruption with stenting and pseudocyst drainage: how efficacious is it? Dig Liver Dis. 2013;45:129–33. doi:10.1016/j.dld.2012.08.026.

110. Nasr JY, Chennat J. Endoscopic ultrasonography-guided transmural drainage of pseudocysts. Tech Gastrointest Endosc. 2012;14:195–8. doi:10.1016/j.tgie.2012.07.001.

111. Itoi T, Nageshwar Reddy D, Yasuda I. New fully-covered self-expandable metal stent for endoscopic ultrasonography-guided intervention in infectious walled-off pancreatic necrosis (with video). J Hepatobiliary Pancreat Sci. 2013;20:403–6. doi:10.1007/s00534-012-0551-5.

112. Tenner S, Baillie J, DeWitt J, Vege SS. American College of Gastroenterology guideline: management of acute pancreatitis. Am J Gastroenterol. 2013;108:1400–15, 16. doi:10.1038/ajg.2013.218.

113. Schmidt PN, Novovic S, Roug S, Feldager E. Endoscopic, transmural drainage and necrosectomy for walled-off pancreatic and peripancreatic necrosis is associated with low mortality—a single-center experience. Scand J Gastroenterol. 2015;50:611–8. doi:10.3109/00365521.2014.946078.

114. Bakker OJ, et al. Endoscopic transgastric vs surgical necrosectomy for infected necrotizing pancreatitis: a randomized trial. JAMA. 2012;307:1053–61. doi:10.1001/jama.2012.276.

115. Allen PJ, et al. Pasireotide for postoperative pancreatic fistula. N Engl J Med. 2014;370:2014–22.

116. Li-Ling J, Irving M. Somatostatin and octreotide in the prevention of postoperative pancreatic complications and the treatment of enterocutaneous pancreatic fistulas: a systematic review of randomized controlled trials. Br J Surg. 2001;88:190–9. doi:10.1046/j.1365-2168.2001.01659.x.

117. Tanaka T, et al. Endoscopic transpapillary pancreatic stenting for internal pancreatic fistula with the disruption of the pancreatic ductal system. Pancreatology. 2013;13:621–4. doi:10.1016/j.pan.2013.08.006.

118. Telford JJ, et al. Pancreatic stent placement for duct disruption. Gastrointest Endosc. 2002;56:18–24.

119. Lawrence C, et al. Disconnected pancreatic tail syndrome: potential for endoscopic therapy and results of long-term follow-up. Gastrointest Endosc. 2008;67:673–9. doi:10.1016/j.gie.2007.07.017.

120. Varadarajulu S, Noone TC, Tutuian R, Hawes RH, Cotton PB. Predictors of outcome in pancreatic duct disruption managed by endoscopic transpapillary stent placement. Gastrointest Endosc. 2005;61:568–75. doi:10.1016/S0016-5107(04)02832-9.

121. Fujimori N. Endoscopic approach through the minor papilla for the management of pancreatic diseases. World J Gastrointest Endosc. 2013;5:81. doi:10.4253/wjge.v5.i3.81.

122. Mosler P, et al. Accuracy of magnetic resonance cholangiopancreatography in the diagnosis of pancreas divisum. Dig Dis Sci. 2012;57:170–4. doi:10.1007/s10620-011-1823-7.

123. Carnes ML, Romagnuolo J, Cotton PB. Miss rate of pancreas divisum by magnetic resonance cholangiopancreatography in clinical practice. Pancreas. 2008;37:151–3. doi:10.1097/MPA.0b013e318164cbaf.

124. Devereaux BM, et al. A new synthetic porcine secretin for facilitation of cannulation of the dorsal pancreatic duct at ERCP in patients with pancreas divisum: a multicenter, randomized, double-blind comparative study. Gastrointest Endosc. 2003;57:643–7. doi:10.1067/mge.2003.195.

125. Devereaux BM, et al. Facilitation of pancreatic duct cannulation using a new synthetic porcine secretin. Am J Gastroenterol. 2002;97:2279–81. doi:10.1111/j.1572-0241.2002.05982.x.

126. Baron TH, Harewood GC, Morgan DE, Yates MR. Outcome differences after endoscopic drainage of pancreatic necrosis, acute pancreatic pseudocysts, and chronic pancreatic pseudocysts. Gastrointest Endosc. 2002;56:7–17. doi:10.1067/mge.2002.125106.

127. Devière J, et al. Complete disruption of the main pancreatic duct: endoscopic management. Gastrointest Endosc. 1995;42:445–51.

128. Buscaglia JM. Pancreatic sphincterotomy: technique, indications, and complications. World J Gastroenterol. 2007;13:4064. doi:10.3748/wjg.v13.i30.4064.

129. Pfau PR, et al. Pancreatic and biliary stents. Gastrointest Endosc. 2013;77:319–27. doi:10.1016/j.gie.2012.09.026.

130. Kozarek RA, et al. Endoscopic transpapillary therapy for disrupted pancreatic duct and peripancreatic fluid collections. Gastroenterology. 1991;100:1362–70.

131. Nadkarni NA, Kotwal V, Sarr MG, Swaroop Vege S. Disconnected pancreatic duct syndrome: endoscopic stent or surgeon's knife? Pancreas. 2015;44:16–22. doi:10.1097/MPA.0000000000000216.

132. Arvanitakis M, et al. Pancreatic-fluid collections: a randomized controlled trial regarding stent removal after endoscopic transmural drainage. Gastrointest Endosc. 2007;65:609–19. doi:10.1016/j.gie.2006.06.083.

133. Seewald S, et al. Endoscopic sealing of pancreatic fistula by using N-butyl-2-cyanoacrylate. Gastrointest Endosc. 2004;59:463–70. doi:10.1016/S0016-5107(03)02708-1.

134. Labori KJ, Trondsen E, Buanes T, Hauge T. Endoscopic sealing of pancreatic fistulas: four case reports and review of the literature. Scand J Gastroenterol. 2009;44:1491–6. doi:10.3109/00365520903362610.

135. Howard TJ, et al. Roux-en-Y internal drainage is the best surgical option to treat patients with disconnected duct syndrome after severe acute pancreatitis. Surgery. 2001;130:714–9. doi:10.1067/msy.2001.116675. discussion 719–21.

136. Jurkovich GJ, Carrico CJ. Pancreatic trauma. Surg Clin North Am. 1990;70:575–93.

137. Subramanian A, Dente CJ, Feliciano DV. The management of pancreatic trauma in the modern era. Surg Clin North Am. 2007;87:1515–32, x. doi:10.1016/j.suc.2007.08.007.

138. Moore EE, et al. Organ injury scaling, II: Pancreas, duodenum, small bowel, colon, and rectum. J Trauma. 1990;30:1427–9.

139. Fisher M, Brasel K. Evolving management of pancreatic injury. Curr Opin Crit Care. 2011;17:613–7. doi:10.1097/MCC.0b013e32834cd374.

140. Houben CH, et al. Traumatic pancreatic duct injury in children: minimally invasive approach to management. J Pediatr Surg. 2007;42:629–35. doi:10.1016/j.jpedsurg.2006.12.025.

141. Canty TG, Weinman D. Treatment of pancreatic duct disruption in children by an endoscopically placed stent. J Pediatr Surg. 2001;36:345–8. doi:10.1053/jpsu.2001.20712.

142. Arvanitakis M, et al. Predictive factors for pancreatic cancer in patients with chronic pancreatitis in association with K-ras gene mutation. Endoscopy. 2004;36:535–42. doi:10.1055/s-2004-814401.

143. Tringali A, Boskoski I, Costamagna G. The role of endoscopy in the therapy of chronic pancreatitis. Best Pract Res Clin Gastroenterol. 2008;22:145–65. doi:10.1016/j.bpg.2007.10.021.

144. Tandan M, Nageshwar Reddy D. Endotherapy in chronic pancreatitis. World J Gastroenterol. 2013;19:6156–64. doi:10.3748/wjg.v19.i37.6156.

145. Ikenberry SO, Sherman S, Hawes RH, Smith M, Lehman GA. The occlusion rate of pancreatic stents. Gastrointest Endosc. 1994;40:611–3.

146. Seicean A, Vultur S. Endoscopic therapy in chronic pancreatitis: current perspectives. Clin Exp Gastroenterol. 2015;8:1–11. doi:10.2147/CEG.S43096.

147. Delhaye M, Matos C, Devière J. Endoscopic technique for the management of pancreatitis and its complications. Best Pract Res Clin Gastroenterol. 2004;18:155–81. doi:10.1016/S1521-6918(03)00077-5.

148. Adler DG, et al. The role of endoscopy in patients with chronic pancreatitis. Gastrointest Endosc. 2006;63:933–7. doi:10.1016/j.gie.2006.02.003.

149. Eleftherladis N, et al. Long-term outcome after pancreatic stenting in severe chronic pancreatitis. Endoscopy. 2005;37:223–30.

ERCP in Postsurgical Patients

Meir Mizrahi, Tyler M. Berzin, Jeffrey D. Mosko,
and Douglas Pleskow

Introduction

Over the past 40 years, endoscopic retrograde cholangiopancreatography (ERCP) has been widely used in patients with pancreaticobiliary diseases including bile duct stones, cholangiocarcinoma, primary sclerosing cholangitis, pancreatic cancer with bile duct obstruction, and chronic pancreatitis. Cotton [1] published an overview of 30 years' experience with ERCP, and describes that the use of side-viewing endoscopes for cannulation of native papilla is an efficient technique for radiologic imaging and treatment. In the "modern" biliary era, Freeman and Guda [2, 3] reported a treatment success rate of 95 % in patients with normal anatomy and native papillary anatomy, and many high volume centers can surpass even this high bar in terms of success.

In patients with surgically altered anatomy, the early treatment success rates with a conventional ERCP procedure were significantly lower. In 1984, Forbes and Cotton [4] were able to achieve diagnostic cholangiograms in only 52 % of ERCP procedures for post-Billroth II patients. Still, when the papilla is reached and successfully cannulated, high success rates for therapeutic procedures can be achieved, particularly in the hands of an experienced endoscopist. There are various explanations for the lower success rates in patients with altered anatomy including long afferent limbs, enteric anastomoses and angulations (that make endoscope passage difficult), an "upside down" or inverted position of the papilla during certain endoscopic approaches (most notably Billroth

II and Roux-en-Y gastric bypass anatomy), and the presence of a hepaticojejunostomy or pancreaticojejunostomy.

ERCP in patients with Roux-en-Y anastomosis is perhaps most challenging for the endoscopist, especially in patients after Roux-en-Y gastric bypass (RYGB) due to the length of the afferent limb and the presence of the native papilla which is encountered in a retrograde approach. Instruments other than a duodenoscope can be used to improve the success rate ERCP in patients with altered anatomy, such as forward viewing endoscopes, pediatric or adult colonoscopes, double or single balloon enteroscopy, and oblique viewing endoscopes. When ERCP via an oral route fails in the Roux-en-Y setting, surgical options such as a gastrostomy, whether created laparoscopically or through other methods can be performed to complete an ERCP procedure.

This chapter provide an overview of endoscopic approaches required to perform ERCP in the most common "altered-anatomy" conditions.

ERCP in Billroth I and II Anatomy

Partial gastrectomy using the Billroth method of reconstruction was first performed successfully in 1881 by Theodor Billroth [5, 6]. Reconstruction of the gastrointestinal tract can be performed via two approaches, Billroth I (end to end gastroduodenal anastomosis) and Billroth II (end to side

Electronic supplementary material: The online version of this chapter (doi:10.1007/978-3-319-26854-5_6) contains supplementary material, which is available to authorized users. Videos can also be accessed at http://link.springer.com/chapter/10.1007/978-3-319-26854-5_6.

M. Mizrahi, M.D. (✉)
Division of Gastroenterology, Advanced Endoscopy Center, Beth Israel Deaconess Medical Center, Harvard Medical School, 330 Brookline Avenue Stoneman 4, Boston, MA 02215, USA
e-mail: mmizrahi@bidmc.harvard.edu

T.M. Berzin, M.D., M.S.
Division of Gastroenterology, Advanced Endoscopy Center, Beth Israel Deaconess Medical Center, Harvard Medical School, 330 Brookline Avenue Stoneman 4, Boston, MA 02215, USA

J.D. Mosko, M.D., F.R.C.P.C.
Department of Medicine, University of Toronto, Toronto, ON, Canada

D. Pleskow, M.D.
Division of Gastroenterology, Advanced Endoscopy Center, Beth Israel Deaconess Medical Center, Harvard Medical School, 330 Brookline Avenue Stoneman 4, Boston, MA 02215, USA

© Springer International Publishing Switzerland 2016
D.G. Adler (ed.), *Advanced Pancreaticobiliary Endoscopy*, DOI 10.1007/978-3-319-26854-5_6

Fig. 6.1 Billroth II anatomy
(Illustration contributed by
James Slattery RN)

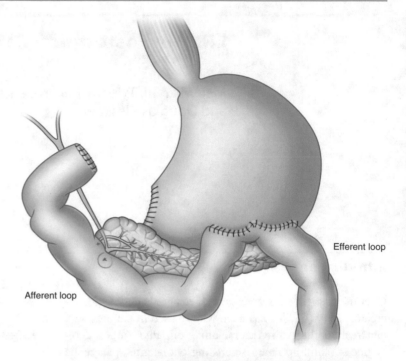

gastrojejunal anastomosis). See Fig. 6.1. There can be variations between Billroth II reconstruction as well [7, 8]. An ERCP can be performed on patients with a history of a Billroth I procedure using the same technique as for patients with normal gastrointestinal anatomy, and the success rate should be comparable to normal anatomy ERCP.

On the other hand, ERCP for patients who previously underwent a Billroth II procedure can sometimes be very challenging. Prior to proceeding with ERCP in post-Billroth II patients, the endoscopist needs to consider several issues including: time from surgery, understanding of the surgical anastomosis from surgical reports and choosing the appropriate endoscope. Once the ERCP is begun, the endoscopist must be prepared to identify and enter the afferent loop, reach the duodenal stump, recognize the papilla, perform a successful cannulation from a reverse position ("upside down") compared to patient with normal anatomy, and, finally, to perform any therapeutic interventions which requiring an endoscopic sphincterotomy.

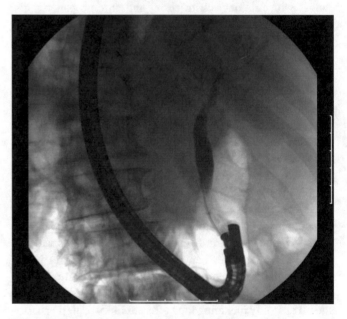

Fig. 6.2 ERCP performed with a duodenoscope in a patient with Billroth II anatomy in a patient with cholangiocarcinoma (Image courtesy of Douglas G. Adler MD)

Choosing the Appropriate Endoscope

In our practice, a duodenoscope is preferred over a front-viewing scope for ERCP in the Billroth II setting, recognizing that this is not always possible in practice (Fig. 6.2). Advantages of the duodenoscope are the side viewing lens and elevator, although the side viewing lens can make reaching the major papilla difficult.

Previously published studies by Demarquay [9], Aabakken [10, 11] and Kim [12] have suggested that a forward viewing endoscope, such as a gastroscope or

pediatric colonoscope, may help to facilitate identification of the correct, afferent loop. Older studies have suggested that in non-expert hands, the rate of jejunal perforation may be higher than expected using a duodenoscope, although if the major papilla can be reached with the duodenoscope the side viewing lens and presence of an elevator are often critical to procedural success. It has been suggested by Byun, Prat, Fylona, Lin, and Osnes [13–17] that perforation rates can be lowered by using forward viewing endoscopes, particularly in low ERCP volume centers. One study published by Kim [12] in 1997 compared the use of forward viewing endoscopes versus side viewing endoscopes and showed that cannulation of the papilla was higher in the group using the forward viewing endoscopes due to higher rate of afferent loop intubation. However, when comparing the rate of cannulation once the papilla was reached successfully there was no significant difference between the two study groups (83 % vs. 80 % respectively). The study also showed a second advantage of the forward viewing endoscope which was a lower rate of complications, such as jejunal perforation. This finding may not have been due to the view of the endoscope, but rather may be due to the fact that the side viewing endoscopes used at that time were manufactured with a hard distal end. Modern duodenoscopes now have smoother ends, likely lowering the rate of perforations during ERCP in Billroth II patients.

ERCP with forward viewing endoscopes also has disadvantages, including difficult direct visualization of the papilla and the lack of elevator that facilitates ampullary cannulation [16, 18]. With forward viewing endoscopes, the overall cannulation success rate is shown to be 63 %. Nonetheless, several studies showed that when side viewing endoscopes are used by experts for post-Billroth patients, the rate of cannulation and successful ERCP therapy is equal to patients without altered anatomy [18, 19].

Early reports using side viewing endoscopes as a first choice also had higher rates of complications in some studies, with the most common and severe being jejunal perforation developing in up to 10 % of patients undergoing the procedure [12, 20]. Again, if a duodenoscope can be used it has significant advantages over forward viewing instruments.

A recent paper describing the experience of 30 years of performing ERCPs in post-Billroth II patients showed a jejunal perforation rate of 1.8 %, a rate that is similar to the perforation rate (0.1–1 %) in patients with normal anatomy as described by others [19, 21–24]. Additionally, other complications such as post-ERCP pancreatitis, delayed bleeding, cholangitis, and cholecystitis have been described with the same incidence in patients with normal anatomy and patients post-Billroth II procedure [19, 25, 26]. Overall, instrument choice is often individualized based on personal experience and preference.

Due to the disadvantages of both conventional forward and side viewing endoscopes in post-Billroth II patients undergoing ERCP, new endoscopes have been developed in an effort to make ERCP in Billroth II patients easier. One such endoscope is the anterior oblique viewing endoscope (AOE). As described by Nakahara, in the AOE scope, the intact papilla can be seen in the 5 o'clock position and the channel outlet is at the 11 o'clock position, which facilitates cannulation in patients with Billroth II anatomy [27]. A second advantage of the AOE is the presence of an elevator, which helps facilitate

both cannulation and sphincterotomy in patients with native papillary anatomy. One disadvantage of the AOE is the lack of availability of the instrument outside of Asia.

In the rare setting of a very long afferent loop, balloon enteroscopy can be considered to reach the papilla in the Billroth II [28]. The disadvantages of this approach include a forward viewing lens and the lack of an elevator on the endoscope, as well as limited endoscopic accessories with which to perform ERCP.

Procedure Technique

After choosing an appropriate endoscope, the ERCP procedure is initiated. The endoscopist almost always faces the challenge of identifying the afferent loop and advancing the endoscope to the major papilla. This can be difficult due to the potential presence of adhesions, distorted anatomy within the duodenojejunal angle, and acute anastomosis angles [29].

The first challenge the endoscopist encounters in Billroth II anatomy is at the gastrojejunal anastomosis. Two jejunal limbs are seen, and the endoscopist must select the afferent limb in order to reach the papilla. The appearance of bile in either limb is not a reliable indicator of the correct direction for scope passage. The afferent loop should generally be towards the lesser curvature of the stomach, but the angle of entry can be difficult to identify with a side-viewing scope, and it is possible to repeatedly enter the incorrect limb. When this occurs, a front-viewing scope may be helpful to identify the correct limb, followed by exchanging to a duodenoscope over a wire left in place by the forward viewing instrument. After the duodenoscope enters the apparent afferent limb, fluoroscopy can be used to confirm that the scope is advancing towards the right upper quadrant. Changing the patient's position may also facilitate afferent loop intubation, although the major papilla can often be accessed with patients in the prone position.

If endoscope maneuvers and repositioning the patient do not assist in achieving afferent loop intubation, other options are still available. The adjunctive use of biliary catheters and balloons, coupled with contrast injection and soft-tipped guidewires (to help identify local anatomy and the length to the major papilla), has also been suggested to attain afferent loop intubation along with switching to a forward-viewing endoscope [19]. Some endoscopists who use forward-viewing endoscopes recommend the use of transparent plastic caps that may simplify the intubation of the afferent loop by improving visualization when the afferent limb is at an acute angle to the anastomosis. The use of a plastic cap may also help in advancing the endoscope to the papilla by displacing jejunal folds and decreasing the need for air insufflation. Such caps can potentially also reduce loop formation during ERCP [30–32].

Biliary and Pancreatic Cannulation

Cannulation of the papilla, even with normal intestinal anatomy, may be difficult due to the presence of redundant folds, periampullary diverticula, and a variety of other reasons. Unlike in patients with normal gastrointestinal anatomy, where the duodenoscope views the papilla in a standard *en face* position, in patients with Billroth II anatomy the papilla will be encountered in an inverted position, with the biliary orifice towards the 5–6 o'clock position. In this setting, the standard "upward flexion" of the sphincterotome does not provide a proper path for biliary cannulation, and thus cannulation devices must be aimed, bent, or rotated in order to facilitate cannulation in a "downwards" direction [18]. In our practice, a rotatable sphincterotome is the preferred method for biliary cannulation in this setting, and a straight biliary catheter is also sometimes used.

When a forward viewing endoscope is used cannulation may be even more difficult or, in some cases, impossible. Some data suggests that the use of transparent plastic cap assist in visualization of the native papilla, stabilize the endoscope tip, and line up the ampulla towards the scope may help when using forward viewing instruments [32–34].

Sphincterotomy in Billroth II Patients

When the papilla is encountered in the inverted position, sphincterotomy may be more difficult and the risk of complications (including perforation) may be higher. The primary issue is that the cutting wire in a standard sphincterotome is oriented to cut in the 11–12 o'clock direction when flexed. In order to facilitate sphincterotomy in this setting, a variety of sphincterotome designs have been proposed and made commercially available, ranging from a device with a sigmoid shape and long distal tip, a dedicated Billroth II papillotome, and an inverted sphincterotome [17, 35–37]. It should be stressed that, despite these devices, most patients with Billroth II anatomy can undergo sphincterotomy with a standard sphincterotomy simply by rotating it into an inverted position (See Chap. 1 for details on this technique).

Another common sphincterotomy technique to consider in patients with Billroth II anatomy is to place a biliary stent, and then to perform a needle knife sphincterotomy over the biliary stent, cutting towards the 5–6 o'clock direction [38] (Fig. 6.3). Additionally, biliary sphincteroplasty, usually used in conjunction with biliary sphincterotomy, can be used to open the papillary orifice, particularly if large stones must be cleared (Fig. 6.4) [39].

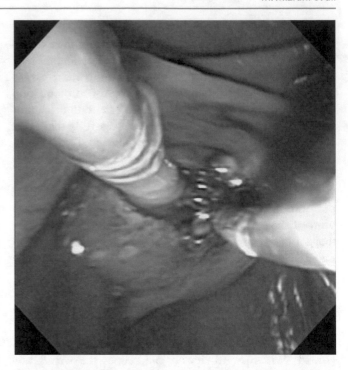

Fig. 6.3 Endoscopic image of biliary sphincterotomy being performed with a needle knife over a plastic stent in a patient with Billroth II anatomy

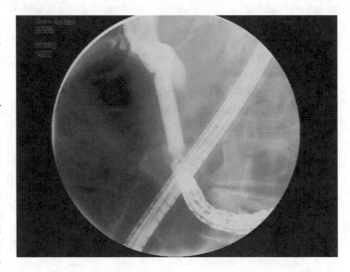

Fig. 6.4 Biliary balloon sphincteroplasty being performed in a patient with Billroth II anatomy

ERCP in Patients Following Pancreaticoduodenectomy

Pancreaticoduodenectomy (The Whipple procedure) is one of the most complicated operations in general surgery. It was first described in 1909 by Kausch, a German surgeon, but was widely performed by Whipple during the first part of the nineteenth century [40]. The conventional Whipple procedure for treating a pancreatic head malignancy consists of resection of the pancreatic head, a distal gastrectomy and duodenectomy, and resection of the initial 15 cm of the jejunum, the common bile duct and gallbladder, with reanastomosis of the remaining structures. This results in a gastrojejunostomy, a hepaticojejunostomy, and a pancreaticojejunostomy (Fig. 6.5). During the 1970s, when the Whipple procedure was also being performed as treatment for chronic pancreatitis, a modified "pylorus preserving" technique was developed to preserve the gastric antrum, pylorus and the initial 2–3 cm of the duodenum [41]. This was done to ensure continuity of the GI tract and, at least in theory, provide a more "physiologic" result. The pylorus-preserving Whipple procedure is now being used for both benign and malignant etiologies.

Patients who previously underwent a Whipple procedure may have variations with respect to the pancreatic anastomo-

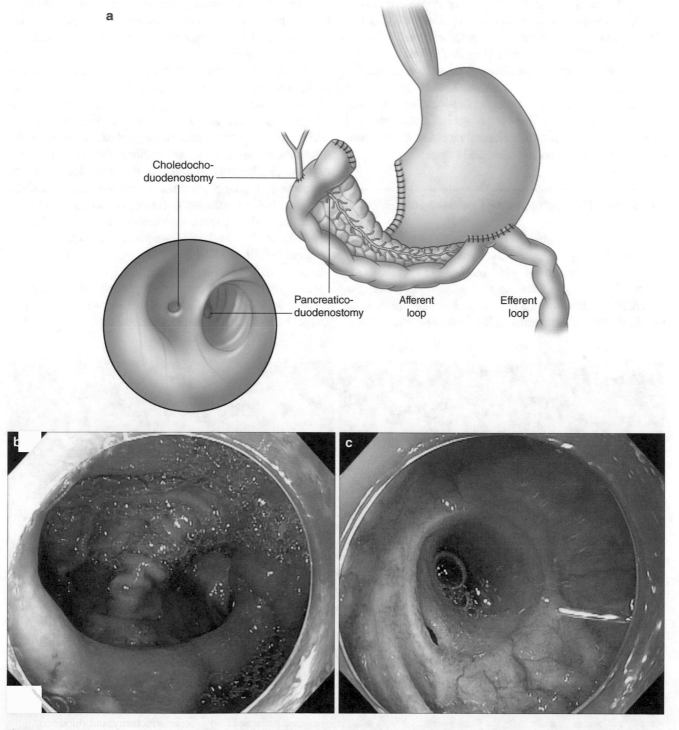

Fig. 6.5 (a) Pancreaticoduodenectomy (Whipple Procedure) anatomy (Illustration contributed by James Slattery RN). (b) Endoscopic view of gastrojejunostomy following pancreaticoduodenectomy (Whipple Procedure). Note orifices for the afferent and efferent limbs. (c) Endoscopic view of a typical hepaticojejunostomy following pancreaticoduodenectomy (Whipple Procedure)

sis or the hepaticojejunal anastomosis. Prior to performing an ERCP procedure the endoscopist needs to make every effort to understand the altered anatomy and the new anastomosis, although in practice such efforts may be fruitless as the surgery may have been performed at an outside institution and records may not be available.

The ideal pancreatic anastomosis after Whipple procedure is a matter of debate and there are several methods in clinical use including: pancreaticogastrostomy (PG), pancreaticojejunostomy (PJ) with end to end or side to end anastomosis, duct-to-mucosa pancreaticojejunostomy (DMPJ), binding pancreaticojejunostomy (BPJ), and ligation of the pancreatic duct without anastomosis (IPD). Various studies [42–46] have compared the different methods of anastomosis and one meta-analysis [47] attempted to evaluate the rate of complications among the various anastomoses. The meta-analysis concluded that there is no specific method that can be performed to reduce complication rates and that the various anastomosis can be considered equivalent.

Choosing the Appropriate Endoscope

Few studies have evaluated ERCP in patients who underwent Whipple procedure. One study, using primarily side-viewing duodenoscopes, included 51 patients in whom 38 patients had an end to side, mucosa to mucosa pancreaticojejunostomy [48]. In patients in whom intubation of the afferent loop failed, a second attempt was performed with a forward-viewing endoscope. Thirty-eight patients in the study underwent 44 ERCP attempts for pancreatic indications such as pancreatitis, pancreatic pain, malabsorption and pancreatic duct dilatation. Twenty-four patients underwent 51 ERCP attempts for biliary indications such as biliary obstruction. Technical success for pancreatic indications was only 8 %, vs. a much higher 84 % for biliary indications. The high rate of failure for pancreatic procedures is likely related to the high rate of severe structuring at the pancreaticojejunostomy, which is unfortunately common. If the pancreaticojejunostomy is not stenosed, it can usually be accessed endoscopically (Fig. 6.6).

In recent years some studies have examined the use of balloon enteroscopy to perform ERCP in patients following pancreaticoduodenectomy [32, 49–52]. Reaching the biliary and pancreatic anastomosis is generally easier with a front-viewing endoscope technique but a major disadvantage of both single balloon (SBE) and double balloon (DBE) enteroscopes is the long length of the endoscope working channels, necessitating specially designed biliary catheters and long guidewires. In recent years, several studies have demonstrated the utility of novel short DBE and SBE enteroscopes, with a working channel length of 152 cm and the possibility to use conventional ERCP instruments [53, 54].

One of the largest cohorts of patients who underwent ERCP after Whipple was reported by Itokawain in 2014 [55]. Using both long and short DBE and SBE, the authors

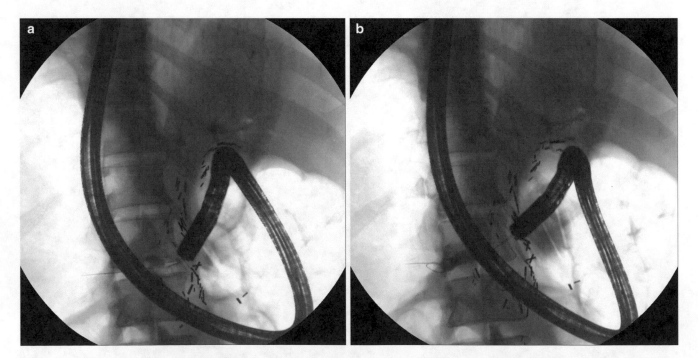

Fig. 6.6 (a) Fluoroscopic View of guidewire cannulation of the pancreatic duct following pancreaticoduodenectomy (Whipple Procedure) (Image courtesy of Douglas G. Adler MD). (b) Same patient as A, now with pancreatogram performed (Image courtesy of Douglas G. Adler MD)

achieved an afferent loop insertion rate of 89.3 %. The authors of this study also showed a diagnostic ERCP success rate of 96 % and therapeutic success rate of 95 %. Most of the patients in this cohort presented with strictures at the hepaticojejunostomy, rather than at the pancreaticojejunal anastomosis, contributing to the high success rate. As mentioned above, the pancreaticojejunostomy often strictures completely closed and often cannot be opened endoscopically in this event [48].

Other Technical Considerations for ERCP in Whipple Anatomy

Identifying the location of the biliary and/or pancreatic anastomosis is crucial for cannulation and overall procedural success. Once the desired anastomosis is identified a balloon catheter or a sphincterotome can be used to access the duct in question. If a forward viewing endoscope is used (i.e., a colonoscope or enteroscope) endoscopic accessories will exit the endoscope and become visible towards the 6 o'clock position. Rotating the endoscope to move the anastomosis towards this position can sometimes facilitate cannulation. Once cannulation is achieved, standard pancreaticobiliary techniques can be used for the management of anastomotic strictures and or stones/debris. Cancer recurrence at the anastomosis requiring permanent metal stenting

can be harder to manage endoscopically, particularly if a colonoscope or enteroscope is used to reach the anastomosis, as some self-expanding metal stents cannot be placed if the endoscope length is too long or the working channel is too narrow, although a colonoscope will almost always allow metal biliary stent placement.

ERCP in Roux-en-Y Patients

The Roux-en-Y anastomosis (Fig. 6.6) was first developed by a Swiss surgeon named César Roux. The most common indications for Roux-en-Y anastomosis include: (1) gastric bypass for obesity, (2) Roux-en-Y reconstruction following partial or complete gastrectomy in gastric carcinoma, (3) Roux-en-Y hepaticojejunostomy (Fig. 6.7) for the treatment of bile duct obstruction from cholangiocarcinoma or biliary injury.

When available, the endoscopist should review available surgical reports and imaging in order to understand the new anatomy and be aware of the time interval from the surgery (Fig. 6.8). If possible, the endoscopist should be aware of the length of the Roux and afferent limb and the presence of a native papilla vs. surgical biliary or pancreatic anastomosis. A major decision for the endoscopist is whether to attempt endoscopy through the standard per-oral route, or whether laparoscopic assistance is required.

Fig. 6.7 Roux-en-Y gastric bypass anatomy (Illustration contributed by James Slattery RN)

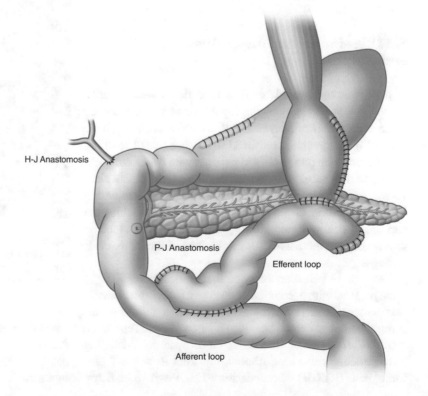

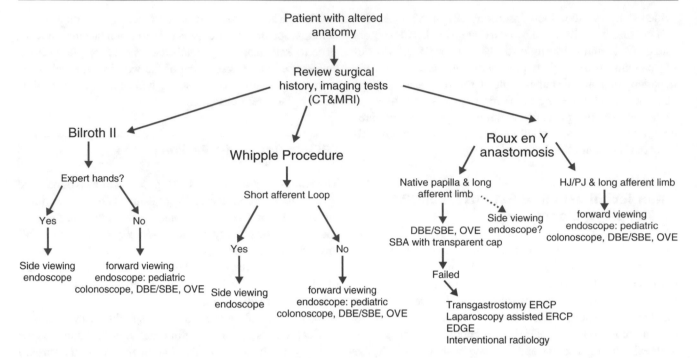

Fig. 6.8 Proposed schema for planning ERCP in patients with altered anatomy

Choosing the Appropriate Endoscope

Choosing the appropriate endoscope depends mostly on two parameters: the type of papilla (native or presence of biliojejunal or pancreaticojejunal anastomosis), and the length of the afferent loop [56] (Table 6.1).

Side Viewing Versus Forward Viewing Endoscopes

A duodenoscope would be ideal in patients with a native papilla due to its side viewing capabilities and the presence of an elevator. However, in the Roux-en-Y setting, Hintze et al. [36] demonstrated only a 33 % success rate of reaching the afferent loop and papilla in patients with a short afferent loop, and the success rate in reaching the papilla with a side-viewing endoscope should be even lower in patients with a long afferent loop. Given the low success rate of reaching the papilla, a standard side-viewing duodenoscope cannot be universally recommended for routine use in the Roux-en-Y setting.

Gostout and Bender were the first to describe ERCP in three patients with a Roux-en-Y anatomy (for gastrectomy in two patients and hepaticojejunostomy in a third patient) using a pediatric colonoscope [57]. Elton E et al. reported a series of 18 patients with Roux-en-Y anatomy, including three patients with a long afferent limb after Roux-en-Y gastric bypass (RYGB) who underwent ERCP with a pediatric

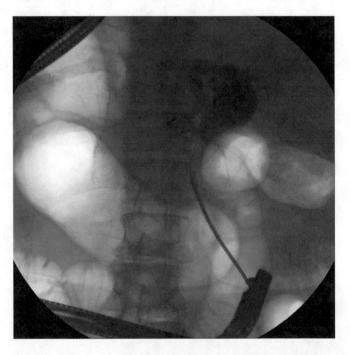

Fig. 6.9 Fluoroscopic image of ERCP being performed for stone extraction with a duodenoscope in a patient with Roux-en-Y gastric bypass, showing that a duodenoscope can reach the major papilla in this situation (Image courtesy of Douglas G. Adler MD)

colonoscope or an enteroscope [58]. These authors reported a success rate in reaching the papilla of 84 % and overall papilla cannulation success rate was 83.3 % in patients with intact papilla. Wright et al. described a combined method

Table 6.1 Comparison of the different approaches for ERCP in patients with surgically altered anatomy

Instrument or technique	Advantages	Disadvantages	Best application
Duodenoscope—anatomic route	Side viewing endoscope	Time consuming	Native papilla
	Higher cannulation rate for native papilla	Often unsuccessful in long limb anatomy	Short afferent loop
	Minimally invasive		Billroth I or Billroth II
			Hepaticojejunostomy
			RYGB
Colonoscope or enteroscope—anatomic route	Minimally invasive	Time consuming	Hepaticojejunostomy or pancreaticojejunostomy anastomosis
		Often unsuccessful in long afferent loop	Short afferent loop
		Lack of elevator	Billroth II
			RYGB
Long Single/Double balloon enteroscope	Minimally invasive	Forward viewing	Hepaticojejunostomy or pancreaticojejunostomy anastomosis
	High afferent intubation success rate	Limited availability of instruments	Short and long afferent loop
		Lack of elevator	Billroth II
			RYGB
Short Single/Double balloon enteroscope	Minimally invasive	Forward viewing	Hepaticojejunostomy or pancreaticojejunostomy anastomosis
	High afferent intubation success rate	Lower rate of afferent loop intubation	Short afferent loop
		Lack of elevator	RYGB
Oblique viewing endoscope	Minimally invasive	Difficulty with very long afferent limbs	Short afferent loop
	High afferent intubation success rate	Not available in most countries	Any type of papilla
			Billroth II
Single balloon enteroscope with transparent cap	Minimally invasive	Forward viewing	Hepaticojejunostomy or pancreaticojejunostomy anastomosis
	High afferent intubation success rate	Lack of elevator	Short and long afferent loop including patients with RYGB
	High therapeutic rate		
Transgastrostomy ERCP	Side viewing	Invasive method	RYGB patients with native papilla
	Standard accessories		Repeated procedures
	Access for repeated procedures		
Laparoscopy-assisted ERCP	Side viewing	Invasive method	RYGB patients with native papilla
	Standard accessories	Endoscopic and surgical team	Presence of internal hernias
	Diagnosis and treatment of internal hernias		
EUS guided transgastric ERCP	Side viewing	Experimental	RYGB patients with native papilla
	Standard accessories	Limited use	Repeated procedures
	Access for repeated procedures	Separate procedure	
Interventional radiology	Less invasive than surgery	Morbidity—external drains	Patients with biliary tract pathology who are poor candidate for surgery
	Allows biliary drainage	No pancreatic access	
		No ability to perform sphincterotomy	

using both forward viewing and side viewing endoscopes [59]. The procedure begins with the forward viewing endoscope and if cannulation of the papilla is unsuccessful a guidewire was left in place, sometimes with assistance of a guidewire balloon. A side viewing endoscope was then inserted over the guidewire in an attempt to reach the major papilla. With this technique the overall ERCP success rate was 72 %.

It is fair to say that in some patients a colonoscope, standard enteroscope, or duodenoscope can reach the major

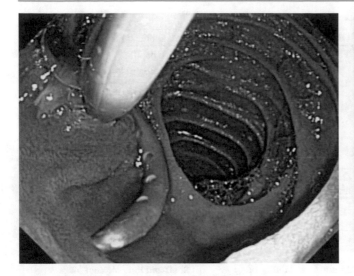

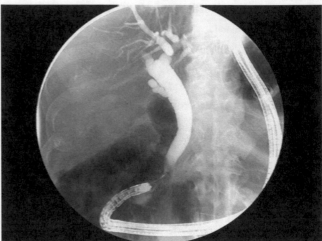

Fig. 6.10 Endoscopic image of the major papilla in a patient with Roux-en-Y gastric bypass. In this case the major papilla could be reached with a standard adult colonoscope. A percutaneous biliary drain had been previously placed and is visible exiting the biliary orifice (Image courtesy of Douglas G. Adler MD)

Fig. 6.11 Fluoroscopic view of an enteroscope used to access the bile duct in a patient with a Roux-en-Y gastric bypass

papilla and that balloon enteroscopy is not always required to perform successful ERCP in Roux-en-Y patients (Fig. 6.10).

Deep Enteroscopy Technique for ERCP

The use of longer endoscopes, such as balloon enteroscopes, allows for an increased rate of reaching the papilla (Fig. 6.11). However, long endoscopes also have disadvantages once the papilla is encountered, because of the front-viewing nature of the scope, the lack of an elevator, and the need for longer endoscopic accessories.

In reviewing the technical success rates of studies using various techniques, one must first recognize that studies including "Roux-en-Y" patients often have widely varying percentages of patients with a hepaticojejunostomy vs. an intact papilla, the former being much easier to cannulate than the latter. This single difference can often explain wide differences in the diagnostic and cannulation success rates in published Roux-en-Y ERCP series.

Multiple studies have reported their results in using balloon enteroscopes (Video 6.1) to facilitate ERCP in patients with Roux-en-Y anatomy (Table 6.2). Most of the studies most of the reports are very small, heterogeneous, and retrospective. Reports on large groups of patients with RYGB are still lacking. The overall success rate of therapeutic ERCP in patients with native papilla is 66 % (range 33 % vs. 89 %) while the overall success rate of therapeutic ERCP in patients with a hepaticojejunostomy is 81.3 % (range 47 % vs. 100 %).

Oblique-Viewing Endoscope

Kikuyama et al. described a new method to perform ERCP in patients with Roux-en-Y anastomosis using an over the tube oblique viewing endoscope [60]. This study described 11 patients who underwent ERCP. The authors successfully reach the biliary orifice in 91 % of patients and had a therapeutic success rate of 100 % once this orifice was reached. The major disadvantage of this method is that particular scope design is not widely available.

Surgical Approaches

When an oral approach to ERCP fails in the setting of a Roux-en-Y gastric bypass, patients may be referred to a combined surgical and endoscopic approach. Schreiner et al. [61] demonstrated that if the combined length of the Roux limb and pancreaticobiliary limb was >150 cm (specifically the Roux limb length added to the length of ligament of Treitz to the jejunojeunal anastomosis), then enteroscope assisted ERCP technique was unlikely to be successful. In the most commonly performed version of this procedure a duodenoscope is used to enter the remnant stomach through a surgically or endoscopically created gastrostomy. This approach allows the endoscopist to use the side viewing endoscope with conventional accessories, and without needing to traverse long limbs of jejunum.

ERCP Through Gastrostomy or Jejunostomy

Baron and Vickers in 1998 were the first to describe ERCP via gastrostomy [62]. In this technique, a gastrostomy was performed

Table 6.2 Summary of key studies on ERCP in surgically altered anatomy

Author	No. of patients	Technique	Native papilla vs. H-J	Success rate	Study limitation
Parlak [65]	14	DBE	0 vs. 14	100 % in H-J	No patients with native papilla
Ncumann [66]	13	SBE	6 vs. 7	33 % vs. 57 % Native Papilla vs. H-J	Very small study groups
Itokawa [55]	34	Standard SBE/Short SBE/ Short DBE	0 vs 34	89 % vs. 50 % standard vs. short	No patients with native papilla, compare different technique
Yutaka Tomizawa [67]	14	SBE	1 vs. 9	68 % success reaching the papilla, 73 % intervention rate	No comparison between native papilla and H-J done
Ke Li [68]	5	SBE	0 vs. 5	87.5 % success reaching the papilla, 57 % intervention rate	No long limb afferent loop patients No patients with native papilla
Skinner [28]	489	SBE/DBE/Short SBE and DBE/Spiral SBE	240 vs 249	88 % vs. 92 % Native Papilla vs. H-J	Review study, variation of patients: RYGB, Whipple, BII, R-Y
Trindade [32]	56	SBE + Transparent CAP	44 vs. 12	65.9 % vs. 91.6 % Tx rate	44 patients with very long limb RYGB
Shah [69]	124	SBE/DBE/Spiral SBE	69 vs. 55	Tx success if papilla identified SBE 87 % DBE 85 % Spiral SBE 88 %	No distinguishing between native papilla and H-J
Tako Itoi [70]	11	SBE	9 vs. 2	66 % vs. 100 % native papilla vs. H-J	Small population study No patients with RYGB
Saleem [71]	56	SBE	15 vs. 41	47 % vs. 47 % native papilla vs. H-J	Small group population with RYGB with native papilla
Azeem [72]	36	SBE	0 vs. 36	75.90 %	Post OLT H-J very selective study group

DBE double balloon enteroscopy, *SBE* single balloon enteroscopy, *H-J* hepaticojejunostomy, *RYGB* Roux-en-Y gastric bypass, *BII* Billroth II, *OLT* liver transplantation

surgically and a 24 French tube was inserted for 2 weeks. Once the gastrostomy tract matured the authors used a forward viewing pediatric colonoscope for the ERCP itself. After this initial report other studies on variations of this technique were conducted. Gutierrez JM et al. reported their results in intraoperative ERCP through gastrostomy in 26 patients [63]. In this study, the procedure was performed in one step. Immediately following the creation of the gastrostomy, a side viewing endoscope was inserted and the ERCP was performed. The overall clinical success rate in this study was 100 %. If repeat ERCP is felt to be needed in the near future, a large caliber feeding tube can be left in place to retain access to the gastric remnant. The gastrostomy tract may require dilation before future reuse. Primary disadvantages of gastrostomy-based ERCP is the invasive nature of the procedure and the risk of anesthesia complications.

Laparoscopy Assisted ERCP

ERCP via laparoscopy is performed via the creation of a surgical gastrostomy access into gastric remnant and the inser-

tion of a duodenoscope through the pylorus to the duodenum. With this procedure, high therapeutic success rate can be achieved. The disadvantages are that surgery is required, and in certain cases conversion to open laparotomy may be necessary. Schreiner et al. in 2012 compared laparoscopic assisted ERCP with a duodenoscope to balloon enteroscopy in 56 patients [64]. Rate of papilla identification was 100 % versus 72 %, and therapeutic success was 100 % versus 59 % respectively. ERCP in patients with Roux-en-Y anastomosis continues to be a great challenge for the endoscopist and additional studies and innovations are clearly needed.

Conclusion

ERCP in patients with altered anatomy remains challenging to the endoscopist. Novel endoscopic techniques have led to higher success rates over the last several years, and further refinement of techniques and devices should continue to make altered anatomy ERCP more and more accessible. In general, Billroth I patients can undergo ERCP with a standard duodenoscope. Billroth II patients can often undergo ERCP with a duodenoscope or a forward viewing instrument. Patients who have undergone a pancreaticoduodenectomy are often best approached via the use of a colonoscope or, rarely, and enteroscope. Roux-en-Y patients present special challenges and may require extensive resources to undergo ERCP, including surgical intervention.

Video Legends
Video 6.1 Single balloon enteroscopy assisted ERCP (MP4 149,575 kb).

References

1. Cotton PB. Digestive endoscopy in five decades. Clin Med. 2005;5(6):614–20.
2. Freeman ML, Guda NM. Endoscopic biliary and pancreatic sphincterotomy. Curr Treat Options Gastroenterol. 2005;8(2):127–34.
3. Freeman ML, Guda NM. ERCP cannulation: a review of reported techniques. Gastrointest Endosc. 2005;61(1):112–25.
4. Forbes A, Cotton PB. ERCP and sphincterotomy after Billroth II gastrectomy. Gut. 1984;25(9):971–4.
5. Santoro E. The history of gastric cancer: legends and chronicles. Gastric Cancer. 2005;8(2):71–4.
6. Pach R, Orzel-Nowak A, Scully T. Ludwik Rydygier--contributor to modern surgery. Gastric Cancer. 2008;11(4):187–91.
7. Porter HW, Claman ZB. A preliminary report on the advantages of a small stoma in partial gastrectomy for ulcer. Ann Surg. 1949;129(4):417–28.
8. Petri G. Our surgical heritage: the tragic destiny of the surgeon. Eugen Alexander Polya (1876-1944). Zentralbl Chir. 1985;110(1):46–52.
9. Demarquay JF, Dumas R, Buckley MJ, Conio M, Zanaldi H, Hastier P, et al. Endoscopic retrograde cholangiopancreatography in patients with Billroth II gastrectomy. Ital J Gastroenterol Hepatol. 1998;30(3):297–300.
10. Aabakken L, Holthe B, Sandstad O, Rosseland A, Osnes M. Endoscopic pancreaticobiliary procedures in patients with a Billroth II resection: a 10-year follow-up study. Ital J Gastroenterol Hepatol. 1998;30(3):301–5.
11. Aabakken L, Chak A. Internet for endoscopists: surf or drown? Gastrointest Endosc. 1998;47(5):423–5.
12. Kim MH, Lee SK, Lee MH, Myung SJ, Yoo BM, Seo DW, et al. Endoscopic retrograde cholangiopancreatography and needle-knife sphincterotomy in patients with Billroth II gastrectomy: a comparative study of the forward-viewing endoscope and the side-viewing duodenoscope. Endoscopy. 1997;29(2):82–5.
13. Byun JW, Kim JW, Sung SY, Jung HY, Jeon HK, Park HJ, et al. Usefulness of forward-viewing endoscope for endoscopic retrograde cholangiopancreatography in patients with Billroth II gastrectomy. Clin Endosc. 2012;45(4):397–403.
14. Prat F, Fritsch J, Choury AD, Meduri B, Pelletier G, Buffet C. Endoscopic sphincteroclasy: a useful therapeutic tool for biliary endoscopy in Billroth II gastrectomy patients. Endoscopy. 1997;29(2):79–81.
15. Faylona JM, Qadir A, Chan AC, Lau JY, Chung SC. Small-bowel perforations related to endoscopic retrograde cholangiopancreatography (ERCP) in patients with Billroth II gastrectomy. Endoscopy. 1999;31(7):546–9.
16. Lin LF, Siauw CP, Ho KS, Tung JC. ERCP in post-Billroth II gastrectomy patients: emphasis on technique. Am J Gastroenterol. 1999;94(1):144–8.
17. Osnes M, Rosseland AR, Aabakken L. Endoscopic retrograde cholangiography and endoscopic papillotomy in patients with a previous Billroth-II resection. Gut. 1986;27(10):1193–8.
18. Costamagna G, Loperfido S, Familiari P. Endoscopic retrograde cholangiopancreatography ERCP after Billroth II reconstruction. Howell DA, Travis AC (eds). UpToDate Available from: http://www.uptodate.com/contents/endoscopic-retrograde-cholangiopancreatography-ercpafter-billroth-ii-reconstruction2014
19. Bove V, Tringali A, Familiari P, Gigante G, Boskoski I, Perri V, et al. ERCP in patients with prior Billroth II gastrectomy: report of 30 years' experience. Endoscopy. 2015;47:611.
20. Cicek B, Parlak E, Disibeyaz S, Koksal AS, Sahin B. Endoscopic retrograde cholangiopancreatography in patients with Billroth II gastroenterostomy. J Gastroenterol Hepatol. 2007;22(8):1210–3.
21. Freeman ML, Nelson DB, Sherman S, Haber GB, Herman ME, Dorsher PJ, et al. Complications of endoscopic biliary sphincterotomy. N Engl J Med. 1996;335(13):909–18.
22. Loperfido S, Angelini G, Benedetti G, Chilovi F, Costan F, De Berardinis F, et al. Major early complications from diagnostic and therapeutic ERCP: a prospective multicenter study. Gastrointest Endosc. 1998;48(1):1–10.
23. Colton JB, Curran CC. Quality indicators, including complications, of ERCP in a community setting: a prospective study. Gastrointest Endosc. 2009;70(3):457–67.
24. Khan MH, Howard TJ, Fogel EL, Sherman S, McHenry L, Watkins JL, et al. Frequency of biliary complications after laparoscopic cholecystectomy detected by ERCP: experience at a large tertiary referral center. Gastrointest Endosc. 2007;65(2):247–52.
25. Huibregtse K. Complications of endoscopic sphincterotomy and their prevention. N Engl J Med. 1996;335(13):961–3.
26. Cohen SA, Siegel JH, Kasmin FE. Complications of diagnostic and therapeutic ERCP. Abdom Imaging. 1996;21(5):385–94.
27. Nakahara K, Horaguchi J, Fujita N, Noda Y, Kobayashi G, Ito K, et al. Therapeutic endoscopic retrograde cholangiopancreatography using an anterior oblique-viewing endoscope for bile duct stones in patients with prior Billroth II gastrectomy. J Gastroenterol. 2009;44(3):212–7.
28. Skinner M, Popa D, Neumann H, Wilcox CM, Monkemuller K. ERCP with the overtube-assisted enteroscopy technique: a systematic review. Endoscopy. 2014;46(7):560–72.
29. Costamagna G, Mutignani M, Perri V, Gabrielli A, Locicero P, Crucitti F. Diagnostic and therapeutic ERCP in patients with Billroth II gastrectomy. Acta Gastroenterol Belg. 1994;57(2):155–62.
30. Park CH, Lee WS, Joo YE, Kim HS, Choi SK, Rew JS. Cap-assisted ERCP in patients with a Billroth II gastrectomy. Gastrointest Endosc. 2007;66(3):612–5.
31. Lee YT. Cap-assisted endoscopic retrograde cholangiopancreatography in a patient with a Billroth II gastrectomy. Endoscopy. 2004;36(7):666.
32. Trindade AJ, Mella JM, Slattery E, Cohen J, Dickstein J, Garud SS, et al. Use of a cap in single-balloon enteroscopy-assisted endoscopic retrograde cholangiography. Endoscopy. 2015;47:453.
33. Osoegawa T, Motomura Y, Akahoshi K, Higuchi N, Tanaka Y, Hisano T, et al. Improved techniques for double-balloon-enteroscopy-assisted endoscopic retrograde cholangiopancreatography. World J Gastroenterol. 2012;18(46):6843–9.
34. Choi YR, Han JH, Cho YS, Han HS, Chae HB, Park SM, et al. Efficacy of cap-assisted endoscopy for routine examining the ampulla of Vater. World J Gastroenterol. 2013;19(13):2037–43.
35. Cremer M, Gulbis A, Touissaint J, de Toeuf J, van Laethem A, Hermanus A, et al. Endoscopic sphincterotomy. A Belgian experience (1976) (author's transl). Acta Gastroenterol Belg. 1977;40(1-2):41–54.
36. Hintze RE, Adler A, Veltzke W, Abou-Rebyeh H. Endoscopic access to the papilla of Vater for endoscopic retrograde cholangiopancreatography in patients with Billroth II or Roux-en-Y gastrojejunostomy. Endoscopy. 1997;29(2):69–73.
37. Costamagna G, Gabrielli A, Mutignani M, Perri V, Buononato M, Crucitti F. Endoscopic diagnosis and treatment of malignant biliary

strictures: review of 505 patients. Acta Gastroenterol Belg. 1993;56(2):201–6.

38. Ricci E, Bertoni G, Conigliaro R, Contini S, Mortilla MG, Bedogni G. Endoscopic sphincterotomy in Billroth II patients: an improved method using a diathermic needle as sphincterotome and a nasobiliary drain as guide. Gastrointest Endosc. 1989;35(1):47–50.

39. Maydeo A, Bhandari S. Balloon sphincteroplasty for removing difficult bile duct stones. Endoscopy. 2007;39(11):958–61.

40. Peters JH, Carey LC. Historical review of pancreaticoduodenectomy. Am J Surg. 1991;161(2):219–25.

41. Traverso LW, Longmire Jr WP. Preservation of the pylorus in pancreaticoduodenectomy. Surg Gynecol Obstet. 1978;146(6):959–62.

42. Bassi C, Falconi M, Molinari E, Salvia R, Butturini G, Sartori N, et al. Reconstruction by pancreaticojejunostomy versus pancreaticogastrostomy following pancreatectomy: results of a comparative study. Ann Surg. 2005;242(6):767–71. discussion 71–73.

43. Duffas JP, Suc B, Msika S, Fourtanier G, Muscari F, Hay JM, et al. A controlled randomized multicenter trial of pancreatogastrostomy or pancreatojejunostomy after pancreatoduodenectomy. Am J Surg. 2005;189(6):720–9.

44. Berger AC, Howard TJ, Kennedy EP, Sauter PK, Bower-Cherry M, Dutkevitch S, et al. Does type of pancreaticojejunostomy after pancreaticoduodenectomy decrease rate of pancreatic fistula? A randomized, prospective, dual-institution trial. J Am Coll Surg. 2009;208(5):738–47. discussion 47–49.

45. Tran K, Van Eijck C, Di Carlo V, Hop WC, Zerbi A, Balzano G, et al. Occlusion of the pancreatic duct versus pancreaticojejunostomy: a prospective randomized trial. Ann Surg. 2002;236(4):422–8. discussion 8.

46. Reissman P, Perry Y, Cuenca A, Bloom A, Eid A, Shiloni E, et al. Pancreaticojejunostomy versus controlled pancreaticocutaneous fistula in pancreaticoduodenectomy for periampullary carcinoma. Am J Surg. 1995;169(6):585–8.

47. Yang SH, Dou KF, Sharma N, Song WJ. The methods of reconstruction of pancreatic digestive continuity after pancreaticoduodenectomy: a meta-analysis of randomized controlled trials. World J Surg. 2011;35(10):2290–7.

48. Chahal P, Baron TH, Topazian MD, Petersen BT, Levy MJ, Gostout CJ. Endoscopic retrograde cholangiopancreatography in post-Whipple patients. Endoscopy. 2006;38(12):1241–5.

49. Maaser C, Lenze F, Bokemeyer M, Ullerich H, Domagk D, Bruewer M, et al. Double balloon enteroscopy: a useful tool for diagnostic and therapeutic procedures in the pancreaticobiliary system. Am J Gastroenterol. 2008;103(4):894–900.

50. Itoi T, Ishii K, Sofuni A, Itokawa F, Kurihara T, Tsuchiya T, et al. Single balloon enteroscopy-assisted ERCP using rendezvous technique for sharp angulation of Roux-en-Y limb in a patient with bile duct stones. Diagn Ther Endosc. 2009;2009:154084.

51. Chua TJ, Kaffes AJ. Balloon-assisted enteroscopy in patients with surgically altered anatomy: a liver transplant center experience (with video). Gastrointest Endosc. 2012;76(4):887–91.

52. Monkemuller K, Fry LC, Bellutti M, Neumann H, Malfertheiner P. ERCP with the double balloon enteroscope in patients with Roux-en-Y anastomosis. Surg Endosc. 2009;23(9):1961–7.

53. Itoi T, Ishii K, Sofuni A, Itokawa F, Tsuchiya T, Kurihara T, et al. Long- and short-type double-balloon enteroscopy-assisted therapeutic ERCP for intact papilla in patients with a Roux-en-Y anastomosis. Surg Endosc. 2011;25(3):713–21.

54. Cho S, Kamalaporn P, Kandel G, Kortan P, Marcon N, May G. 'Short' double-balloon enteroscope endoscopic retrograde cholangiopancreatography in patients with a surgically altered upper gastrointestinal tract. Can J Gastroenterol. 2011;25(11):615–9.

55. Itokawa F, Itoi T, Ishii K, Sofuni A, Moriyasu F. Single- and double-balloon enteroscopy-assisted endoscopic retrograde cholangiopancreatography in patients with Roux-en-Y plus hepaticojejunostomy anastomosis and Whipple resection. Dig Endosc. 2014;26 Suppl 2:136–43.

56. Lopes TL, Wilcox CM. Endoscopic retrograde cholangiopancreatography in patients with Roux-en-Y anatomy. Gastroenterol Clin North Am. 2010;39(1):99–107.

57. Gostout CJ, Bender CE. Cholangiopancreatography, sphincterotomy, and common duct stone removal via Roux-en-Y limb enteroscopy. Gastroenterology. 1988;95(1):156–63.

58. Elton E, Hanson BL, Qaseem T, Howell DA. Diagnostic and therapeutic ERCP using an enteroscope and a pediatric colonoscope in long-limb surgical bypass patients. Gastrointest Endosc. 1998;47(1):62–7.

59. Wright BE, Cass OW, Freeman ML. ERCP in patients with long-limb Roux-en-Y gastrojejunostomy and intact papilla. Gastrointest Endosc. 2002;56(2):225–32.

60. Kikuyama M, Sasada Y, Matsuhashi T, Ota Y, Nakahodo J. ERCP after Roux-en-Y reconstruction can be carried out using an oblique-viewing endoscope with an overtube. Dig Endosc. 2009;21(3):180–4.

61. Schreiner MA, Chang L, Gluck M, Irani S, Gan SI, Brandabur JJ, et al. Laparoscopy-assisted versus balloon enteroscopy-assisted ERCP in bariatric post-Roux-en-Y gastric bypass patients. Gastrointest Endosc. 2012;75(4):748–56.

62. Baron TH, Vickers SM. Surgical gastrostomy placement as access for diagnostic and therapeutic ERCP. Gastrointest Endosc. 1998;48(6):640–1.

63. Gutierrez JM, Lederer H, Krook JC, Kinney TP, Freeman ML, Jensen EH. Surgical gastrostomy for pancreatobiliary and duodenal access following Roux en Y gastric bypass. J Gastrointest Surg. 2009;13(12):2170–5.

64. Schreiner MA, Chang L, Gluck M, Irani S, Gan SI, Brandabur JJ, Thirlby R, Moonka R, Kozarek RA, Ross AS. Laparoscopy-assisted versus balloon enteroscopy-assisted ERCP in bariatric post-Roux-en-Y gastric bypass patients. Gastrointest Endosc. 2012 Apr;75(4):748-56. doi: 10.1016/j.gie.2011.11.019. Epub 2012 Jan 31. PubMed PMID: 22301340.

65. Parlak E, Çiçek B, Dişibeyaz S, et al. Endoscopic retrograde cholangiography by double balloon enteroscopy in patients with Roux-en-Y hepaticojejunostomy. Surg Endosc. 2010;24(2):466–70. doi:10.1007/s00464-009-0591-3.

66. Neumann H, Fry LC, Meyer F, Malfertheiner P, Monkemuller K. Endoscopic retrograde cholangiopancreatography using the single balloon enteroscope technique in patients with Roux-en-Y anastomosis. Digestion. 2009;80(1):52–7.

67. Tomizawa Y, Sullivan CT, Gelrud A. Single balloon enteroscopy (SBE) assisted therapeutic endoscopic retrograde cholangiopancreatography (ERCP) in patients with roux-en-y anastomosis. Dig Dis Sci. 2014;59(2):465–70.

68. Li K, Huang YH, Yao W, Chang H, et al. Adult colonoscopy or single-balloon enteroscopy-assisted ERCP in long-limb surgical bypass patients. Clin Res Hepatol Gastroenterol. 2014;38(4):513–9.

69. Shah RJ, Smolkin M, Yen R, Ross A, Kozarek RA, Howell DA, et al. A multicenter, US experience of single-balloon, double-balloon, and rotational overtube-assisted enteroscopy ERCP in patients with surgically altered pancreaticobiliary anatomy (with video). Gastrointest Endosc. 2013;77(4):593–600.

70. Itoi T, Ishii K, Sofuni A, Itokawa F, Tsuchiya T, Kurihara T, et al. Single-balloon enteroscopy-assisted ERCP in patients with Billroth II gastrectomy or Roux-en-Y anastomosis (with video). Am J Gastroenterol. 2010;105(1):93–9.

71. Saleem A, Baron TH, Gostout CJ, Topazian MD, Levy MJ, Petersen BT, et al. Endoscopic retrogradecholangiopancreatography using a single-balloon enteroscope in patients with altered Roux-en-Y anatomy. Endoscopy. 2010;42(8):656–60.

72. Azeem N, Tabibian JH, Baron TH, Orhurhu V, Rosen CB, Petersen BT, et al. Use of a single-balloon enteroscope compared with variable-stiffness colonoscopes for endoscopic retrograde cholangiography in liver transplant patients with Roux-en-Y biliary anastomosis. Gastrointest Endosc. 2013;77(4):568–77.

ERCP On-Call Emergencies

Anand R. Kumar and Jeffrey L. Tokar

Introduction

Advanced endoscopists are often called upon to perform endoscopic retrograde cholangiopancreatography (ERCP) in the emergency setting, often for patients that are critically ill. In this chapter, we focus our attention on two of the more common indications for urgent ERCP—acute cholangitis and biliary pancreatitis. These two indications have been studied extensively, and subsequent meta-analyses and practice guidelines have been published to further describe the utility and timing of ERCP in these, often urgent and emergent, settings. This chapter also discusses other urgent and emergent ERCP-related scenarios encountered by endoscopists in clinical practice such as stent migration, trapped or broken retrieval baskets, hemobilia, perforation, and cholecystitis.

Acute or Ascending Cholangitis

Charcot's triad (fever, right upper quadrant pain, and jaundice) or Reynolds' pentad (Charcot's triad plus hypotension and altered mental status) describes classic presentations of acute cholangitis [1]. However, the high specificity of these clinical findings comes with a low sensitivity for the diagnosis of acute cholangitis [2]. A combination of systemic inflammation

Electronic supplementary material: The online version of this chapter (doi:10.1007/978-3-319-26854-5_7) contains supplementary material, which is available to authorized users. Videos can also be accessed at http://link.springer.com/chapter/10.1007/978-3-319-26854-5_7.

A.R. Kumar, M.D., M.P.H. (✉)
Center for Digestive Health, Drexel University,
219 N. Broad Street, 5th Floor, Philadelphia, PA 19107, USA

Hahnemann University Hospital, Philadelphia, PA USA
e-mail: Anand.Kumar@DrexelMed.edu

J.L. Tokar, M.D., F.A.S.G.E., A.G.A.F.
Department of Medicine, Fox Chase Cancer Center,
Philadelphia, PA USA

(fever/chills, leukocytosis), cholestasis (jaundice and/or abnormal liver associated enzymes), and abnormal imaging (ductal dilatation or evidence of biliary disease such as stricture, stone, or stent) has been shown to improve pre-procedure diagnostic sensitivity [3]. Objective assessment criteria for the severity of cholangitis were described as mild (Grade I), moderate (Grade II), and severe (Grade III) in an International Consensus meeting in Tokyo in 2006 [4] and later revised in 2013 Tokyo guidelines [5]. Severe disease is defined by the presence of organ dysfunction while moderate disease is defined by abnormalities in two of the five parameters (WBC >12,000 or <4000/mm^3, Fever ≥39 °C, age ≥75, bilirubin ≥5 mg/dl, and albumin <0.7×lower limit of normal).

Cholangitis can occur spontaneously (e.g., in patients with bile duct stones), or following prior biliary interventions in patients and/or in patients with impaired bile duct emptying (e.g., when previously placed biliary stents occlude, postoperatively, following liver biopsy performed in patients with biliary obstruction) (Videos 7.1 and 7.2). To show how common this is in clinical practice, a retrospective observational study showed that more than one-third of patients with indwelling plastic biliary stents placed for pancreatic adenocarcinoma treated with neoadjuvant chemoradiation required a premature stent exchange due to stent occlusion, often with associated infection [6].

Initial management of acute cholangitis is directed toward control of accompanying sepsis or systemic inflammatory response. Fluid resuscitation, hemodynamic support as needed, and systemic antibiotics constitute the foundation of initial management. Antimicrobial coverage for gram-negative bacilli (such as *E. coli*, Klebsiella, and Enterobacter) and anaerobic organisms is recommended. In Grade III or severe disease, broader antibiotic coverage may be warranted [7]. It should be emphasized that biliary drainage is more important than antibiotics as the patient needs definitive biliary drainage to fully recover. Simultaneous discussions regarding the method and timing of achieving biliary drainage are also of paramount importance in the management of cholangitis. In practice, most patients with acute or ascending cholangitis urgent or emergent ERCP can be delayed until the patient has undergone appropriate fluid resuscitation and initiation of antibiotic therapy. While there may be great pressure to do an ERCP immediately, it is often a mistake to take an under-resuscitated patient to a procedure requiring moderate or deep sedation.

Biliary drainage can be achieved endoscopically (ERCP), percutaneously (percutaneous transhepatic biliary drainage, PTBD, or, rarely, surgically (T-tube insertion). ERCP is the recommended modality because it enables definitive therapy (e.g., stone removal or stricture dilation) in a minimally invasive manner, while minimizing post-procedural discomfort that can accompany PTBD or surgery [8]. As mentioned above, the timing of endoscopic therapy (ERCP) is determined by the severity of clinical presentation and the response to resuscitative efforts [5, 9]. An urgent (as soon as clinically feasible) ERCP is indicated for Grade II (moderate) or Grade III (severe) disease especially in a patient that fails to adequately respond to intravenous fluids and antibiotics. An early ERCP (typically defined as <72 h from presentation) is indicated in most other clinical scenarios. Standard biliary cannulation and sphincterotomy techniques are used to access the biliary tree and perform biliary interventions with an eye towards providing adequate biliary drainage. Emphasis should be placed on minimizing the procedure length if possible. There is a general perception that one should avoid over-filling the biliary system with contrast with the idea that this could predispose patients to bacteremia, but there is little clinical data to support this notion.

When definitive clearance of bile duct stones or other causes of biliary obstruction cannot be achieved expeditiously or safely (usually in a patient on active anticoagulation therapy or with altered coagulation status or low platelets as a consequence of sepsis), placement of a temporary biliary stent almost always results in rapid improvement in clinical parameters of cholangitis. Placing a biliary stent without sphincterotomy is completely acceptable, technically simple and expeditious, reduces bleeding risk in coagulopathic patients, and may also shorten procedure duration for critically ill patients that are medically unstable and unable to tolerate prolonged anesthesia [10]. The potential advantages of a plastic stent are offset by the need for a future ERCP to remove the stent and provide definitive duct clearance in the case of a stone, the most common cause of cholangitis [11].

Placement of a prophylactic pancreatic duct stent and/or administration of 100 mg rectal indomethacin can reduce the risk of post-ERCP pancreatitis [12], though their role in preventing post-ERCP pancreatitis specifically in the setting of placing a biliary stent without first performing a sphincterotomy is not well studied. In patients with cholangitis and surgically altered anatomy, such as Roux-en-Y anatomy or duodenal obstruction, PTBD can be a more efficient temporizing method of biliary drainage given the very real possibility

that the major papilla may be endoscopically inaccessible. EUS-guided bile duct access has been used for biliary obstruction with increasing frequency, but data on its use specifically in the setting of acute cholangitis are lacking [13].

Biliary Pancreatitis

The most common cause of acute pancreatitis is biliary pancreatitis, often referred to as "gallstone pancreatitis" [14]. A dilated common bile duct, jaundice and slow or no improvement (or worsening) in the clinical course of a patient with suspected gallstone pancreatitis should raise the suspicion for persistent choledocholithiasis that may warrant biliary intervention. The American Society of Gastrointestinal Endoscopy (ASGE) Standards of Practice guidelines propose a prediction model for choledocholithiasis in patients with symptomatic gallstones [15]. Presence of one very strong predictive factor (bilirubin >4 mg/dl or acute cholangitis or common bile duct (CBD) stone seen on ultrasound) or two strong predictive factors (bilirubin 1.8–4 mg/dl and dilated CBD on ultrasound in a non-cholecystectomy patient) suggest a high probability (>50 %) of choledocholithiasis, although these guidelines have been evaluated clinically in only a limited manner and they cannot be interpreted as ironclad. Gallstone pancreatitis with abnormal liver enzymes other than bilirubin elevation in a female older than 55 years with a non-dilated CBD constitutes only an intermediate probability (10–50 %) of choledocholithiasis. Absence of any of the above risk factors constitutes a low probability of choledocholithiasis (<10 %). Patients with high probability of choledocholithiasis are acceptable candidates for ERCP, whereas patients with low probability are managed expectantly without additional testing. Patients with intermediate probability should undergo additional diagnostic testing to confirm choledocholithiasis. Diagnostic tests include CT, magnetic resonance cholangiopancreatography (MRCP), and endoscopic ultrasound (EUS), with an emphasis on MRCP and EUS. Helical CT has 65–88 % sensitivity and 73–97 % overall specificity for choledocholithiasis [15]. However, the sensitivity falls below 60 %, when the size of the stone is less than 5 mm [16]. MRCP has higher sensitivity (85–92 %) and specificity (93–97 %) than helical CT [15] but it also performs poorly (33–70 % sensitivity) in the detection of small (<5 mm) CBD stones [17, 18]. Close proximity of the CBD to the duodenum makes endoscopic ultrasound an ideal test to examine for choledocholithiasis. One meta-analysis including 36 studies and 3532 patients estimated 89 % sensitivity and 94 % specificity for choledocholithiasis [19]. A subsequent meta-analysis including 27 studies and 2673 patients estimated 94 % sensitivity and 95 % specificity for choledocholithiasis [20]. Smaller (<6 mm) stones, missed on CT or MRCP, can still be detected on EUS [21, 22]. A prospective cohort study comparing the utility of EUS and MRCP in patients referred for ERCP with suspected biliary disease concluded that a strategy incorporating initial EUS prior to ERCP was the most cost-effective approach, although EUS may not be available at all centers [23].

Most patients with gallstone pancreatitis do not need ERCP if there is no evidence of persistent biliary obstruction or choledocholithiasis. Those with ongoing biliary obstruction or bilirubin >5 mg/dl should be considered to undergo early (<72 h) ERCP, and patients with accompanying acute cholangitis should undergo ERCP within 24 h when possible with regards to clinical stabilization [14]. In other patients with gallstone pancreatitis, early ERCP is usually not indicated and may be associated with higher rate of serious complications [14, 24, 25].

Stent Migration

Biliary stent migration is reported to occur with a frequency of 3.5–10 %, with equal rates being reported for distal and proximal migration [26, 27]. Similar rates were reported for pancreatic stent migration (5.2 % proximal and 7.5 % distal) [26]. Various risk factors for stent migration have been reported including stent length, stent diameter, number of stents placed, benign or malignant indications, distal or proximal stricture, and stent material (plastic stents vs. metal stents, variations in metal stent design—covered vs. uncovered, radial/axial force, presence or absence of anti-migration struts), etc. [26–29] Information regarding the relative importance of each of these factors is conflicting, except for the type of metal stents (covered/partially covered vs. uncovered) and the indication (benign or malignant). Covered or partially covered metal stents migrate more often than uncovered metal stents [30, 31]. Stents placed for benign indications such as strictures from autoimmune cholangitis or chronic pancreatitis and for bile leak or large CBD stones tend to migrate more often than stents placed for malignant indications [26, 27, 29].

Stent migration can lead to various complications or may be asymptomatic. Migration of the stent above the level of the stricture can lead to recurrent cholestasis, jaundice, and cholangitis [32, 33], and less commonly to sequelae such as stent impaction into the liver resulting in hemobilia or hepatic abscess [34], biliary-pulmonary [35] or broncho-pleuro-biliary fistulae [36], penetration into the IVC [37], and pericardial-biliary fistula [38]. Distal migration of biliary stents may be asymptomatic, recognized only at scheduled stent change, or may result in recurrent cholestasis with or without associated ascending cholangitis and the need for early reintervention. Distally migrated stents frequently pass spontaneously in the patient's stool, but intestinal perforation

[34, 39–41], bowel obstruction [42], or entero-cutaneous fistula [43] have been reported. These are all very rare events. The extent of distal migration determines the type of endoscope used and the procedure performed to extract a stent that fails to pass spontaneously. Enteroscopes, including device-assisted (e.g., balloon-assisted) enteroscopes, may be required for stents retained in the jejunum or ileum, but, again, most pass spontaneously.

Endoscopic removal of a stent that migrates proximally into the duct can be technically challenging but success rates of 80–100 % have been reported [29, 44–47]. Several reasons for the difficulty have been cited, such as stent migration into the intrahepatic ducts, the mobility of the distal end of a stent that floats freely within a dilated bile duct, presence of a tight stricture distal to the stent but between the stent and the endoscope, impaction of the distal end of the stent against the bile duct wall or within a ductal stricture, or mismatched orientation of the bile duct and stent axes [45, 47].

Removal of migrated pancreatic stents is technically similar to the removal of migrated biliary stents. However, interventions should be selected with greater caution to minimize injury to the pancreatic duct. Table 7.1 summarizes case reports and series in which various endoscopic tools were used for removal of migrated biliary and pancreatic stents. Popular tools for retrieval of plastic stents include rat-tooth forceps, biopsy forceps, polypectomy snares, retrieval baskets, and extraction balloon catheters. Pancreatoscopy-based approaches are sometimes requires if the stent cannot be grasped by other means.

Forceps (biopsy forceps, rat-tooth forceps, or three-prong grasping forceps [48]) can be used to directly grasp the distal end of the stent (Video 7.3). Occasionally, biopsy forceps can be advanced through the lumen of a migrated stent and opened either at the proximal end of the stent or inside the flange of a plastic stent, and pulled back to retrieve the stent. Commonly used, standard style forceps cannot be advanced over a guidewire.

Extraction balloon catheters can be used to remove a migrated stent in several ways (Fig. 7.1) [49]. The balloon can be inflated alongside the stent (Fig. 7.1a) or at the proximal end of the stent (Fig. 7.1b) and dragged down towards, and hopefully across, the papilla. If a guidewire passes through the stent, a balloon catheter can be advanced through the stent (provided the migrated stent's lumen is large enough to accommodate the balloon catheter) and the balloon can be then inflated at the proximal end of the stent (Fig. 7.1c) or inside the stent (Fig. 7.1d), fixing the two devices together and allowing them to be removed in tandem.

Polypectomy snares and stone retrieval baskets can also facilitate retrieval of migrated biliary or pancreatic stents. They can be advanced independent of the guidewire and used to grab the distal end of the stent—we term this *the direct grasping technique* (Fig. 7.2). Under fluoroscopy, the

Table 7.1 Summary of published literature on endoscopic techniques for removal of migrated stents

Author (year, country)	Design (*N*)	Stent	Migration	Indication	Endoscopic technique
Katsinelos [44] (2009, Greece)	Retrospective (51)	Plastic	Proximal (21)	Malignant (20)	*Proximal + distal*
			Distal (30)	Benign (31)	Retrieval basket (4 + 6)
					Snare (1 + 11)
					Forceps (7)
					Balloon intra-stent (1)
					Soehendra stent retriever (2)
Arhan [29] (2009, Turkey)	Retrospective (45)	Plastic	Proximal (24)	Malignant (17)	*Proximal*
			Distal (21)	Benign (28)	Extraction Balloon (12)
					Biopsy forceps (12)
					Distal
					Spontaneous (14)
					Snare (6)
					Biopsy forceps (1)
Chaurasia [45] (1999, Netherlands)	Retrospective (46)	Plastic	Proximal	Malignant (28)	Retrieval basket (22)
				Benign (18)	Extraction balloon (4)
					Balloon and basket (3)
					Balloon and ball tip catheter (2)
					Forceps (3)
					Soehendra stent retriever (2)
					Unknown (5)
					Unsuccessful (4)
					Not attempted (5)
Lahoti [46] (1998, USA)	Retrospective	Plastic	Proximal	Biliary:	*Biliary + pancreatic*
	Biliary (33)			Malignant (15)	Basket (10 + 10)
	PD (26)			Benign (18)	Balloon (3 + 5)
					In-stent balloon (5 + 2)
					Snare (3 + 2)
					Forceps (2 + 1)
					Soehendra (4 + 0)
					Unknown (1 + 0)
					Surgery (0 + 3)
					Unsuccessful (3 + 6)
					Lost to f/u (2 + 0)
Tarnasky [47] (1995, USA)	Retrospective (44)	Plastic	Proximal	Malignant (17)	Soehendra (13)
				Benign (27)	Balloon (7)
					Basket (5)
					Forceps (5)
					In-stent basket (2)
					In-stent balloon (1)
					Sphincterotome (2)
					In-stent forceps (1)
					Unsuccessful (6)
Goetz [48] (2014, Germany)	Case report	Plastic	Proximal	Benign	Three-prong grasping forceps
Okabe [49] (2009, Japan)	Case series (3)	Plastic	Proximal	Malignant (1)	Snare over guidewire
				Benign (2)	Biopsy forceps
					Retrieval basket
Lee [50] (2014, Taiwan)	Case report	Plastic	Proximal	Benign	Guidewire loop in a retrieval basket
Shah [51] (2014, India)	Retrospective (28)	Plastic	Proximal	Benign	No sphincteroplasty (18/28)
					Sphincteroplasty (8/28)
					Surgery or lost to f/u (2/28)
Cho [33] (2013, Korea)	Case report	Metal	Proximal	Malignant	Stricture dilation and basket
Vasquez Rey [52] (2011, Spain)	Case report	Plastic	Proximal	Malignant	Covered metallic stent followed by rat-tooth forceps

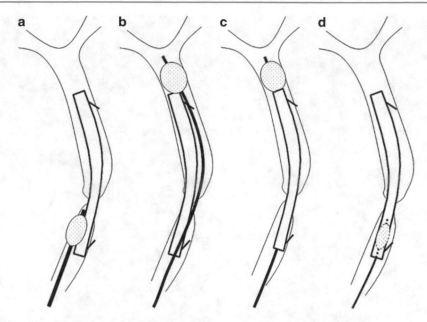

Fig. 7.1 Use of extraction balloon catheter for removal of proximally migrated biliary plastic stent. If the guidewire passes adjacent to the stent, balloon can be inflated beside the stent (**a**), or at the proximal end of the stent (**b**). If the guidewire passes through the stent and the stent's lumen is large enough to accommodate the balloon catheter, balloon can be inflated at the proximal end of the stent (**c**) or inside the stent (**d**).

Once balloon is inflated, pulling the catheter can drag the stent distally across the papilla. *Reproduced from Japan Gastroenterological Endoscopy Society; Okabe Y, Tsuruta O, Kaji R, et al. Endoscopic retrieval of migrated plastic stent into bile duct or pancreatic pseudocyst. Dig Endosc. 2009 Jan; 21(1):1–7. Courtesy of John Wiley and Sons*

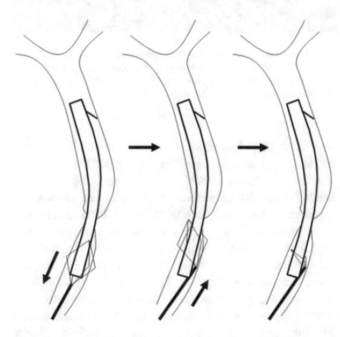

Fig. 7.2 Direct grasping technique using a basket catheter: as the distal end is grasped, the catheter pushes up. A snare could be used in a similar way. *Reproduced from Japan Gastroenterological Endoscopy Society; Okabe Y, Tsuruta O, Kaji R, et al. Endoscopic retrieval of migrated plastic stent into bile duct or pancreatic pseudocyst. Dig Endosc. 2009 Jan; 21(1):1–7. Courtesy of John Wiley and Sons*

catheter may be seen to "push up" when the stent is successfully grasped [49]. O*ver-the-guidewire techniques* may be performed in cases when a guidewire can be advanced

through the lumen of the migrated stent. The polypectomy snare is loosely closed around the guidewire such that the loop of the snare is nearly completely closed, but open just enough to avoid tightly "grabbing" the wire. The snare is then advanced down the duodenoscope channel over the wire and into the bile or pancreatic duct. With this technique, the snare and the stent are perfectly aligned which obviates the need to "fish" around inside the bile duct attempting to ensnare the stent. After the migrated stent is ensnared, it can be pulled up the duodenoscope channel, leaving the guidewire in place within the bile duct in case additional interventions need to be performed (often, ironically, the placement of another stent).

Another stent removal technique has been called *the guidewire loop technique* [50]. A retrieval basket or snare is used to grasp the end of a guidewire before either is inserted into the duodenoscope. After this device–wire complex is advanced into the duct, the guidewire is advanced further, effectively forming a guidewire loop which can then be manipulated until the migrated stent is captured. Okabe et al. describe a *ropeway technique*, which is useful when the distal end of a migrated stent is impacted against the bile duct wall or when the duct and stent axes are misaligned [49]. To perform the technique, the proximal (upper) end of the stent is captured within a retrieval basket. The basket is then "walked down" along the length of the stent until it is in a position to grasp the distal (lower) portion of the stent. Downward traction causes the distal

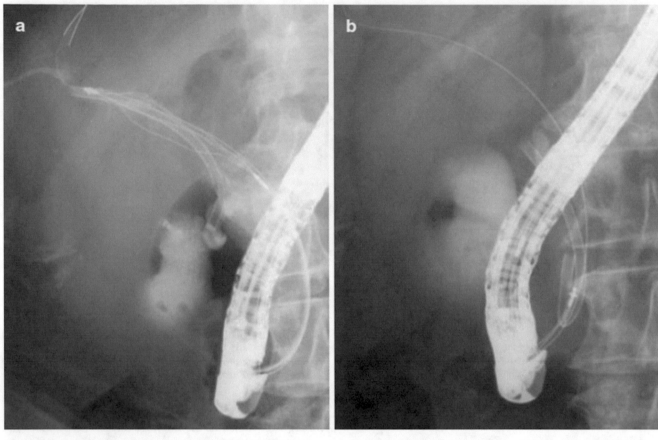

Fig. 7.3 Ropeway technique using a basket catheter: Proximal end is captured (**a**) but the basket is kept open and walked distally along the length of the stent. The basket is closed near the distal end of the stent and pulled (**b**). The distal end of the stent folds on itself. *Reproduced* *from Japan Gastroenterological Endoscopy Society*; *Okabe Y, Tsuruta O, Kaji R, et al. Endoscopic retrieval of migrated plastic stent into bile duct or pancreatic pseudocyst. Dig Endosc. 2009 Jan; 21(1):1–7. Courtesy of John Wiley and Sons*

end of the stent to fold upon itself, allowing it to be removed across the ampulla (Fig. 7.3).

The Soehendra stent retriever is another endoscopic tool that can be used to retrieve migrated plastic stents, but usually requires successful placement of a guidewire through the lumen of the stent, which can sometimes be difficult to achieve. The device has a "threaded screw" on its tip. If guidewire cannulation of the stent can be accomplished, the Soehendra stent retriever is advanced over the guidewire until it reaches the lower end of the migrated stent. While applying gentle inward force, the catheter portion of the Soehendra stent retriever is rotated in a clockwise direction, until the device is "screwed" into the distal end of the migrated stent, effectively creating a Soehendra–stent complex that can be withdrawn up the duodenoscope channel. If performed carefully, biliary access with the wire can be preserved during removal of the stent.

Balloon sphincteroplasty can also facilitate removal of migrated stents [51], as can dilation of biliary stricture(s) located below the stent. After balloon sphincteroplasty is performed, the normally conical portion of the biliary sphincter

and distal CBD becomes cylindrical, which may facilitate extraction of stent(s) from the bile duct. The maximum diameter of dilation should be "sized" to the bile duct, to minimize the risk of perforation. A variety of dilation balloons are commercially available for use in the biliary tree and esophageal or pyloric/colonic balloons can be used as well. Duration of dilation is largely empirical, but should be done at least until the "waist" is obliterated on fluoroscopy. Most endoscopists dilate for 30–120 s. Bleeding following dilation is uncommon and rarely severe, and can be managed with standard techniques used for post-sphincterotomy bleeding, such as holding the inflated balloon in position to tamponade the bleeding, injecting epinephrine, and/or using other mechanical or thermal modalities for hemostasis. Placement of a fully covered metal stent across a biliary stenosis may also facilitate removal of the migrated stent and can tamponade bleeding if it develops [33, 52].

Migration of self-expandable metal biliary stents (SEMS) occurs more often with covered SEMS than uncovered SEMS. Distally migrated fully covered or partially covered SEMS can usually be removed using a snare or a rat-tooth

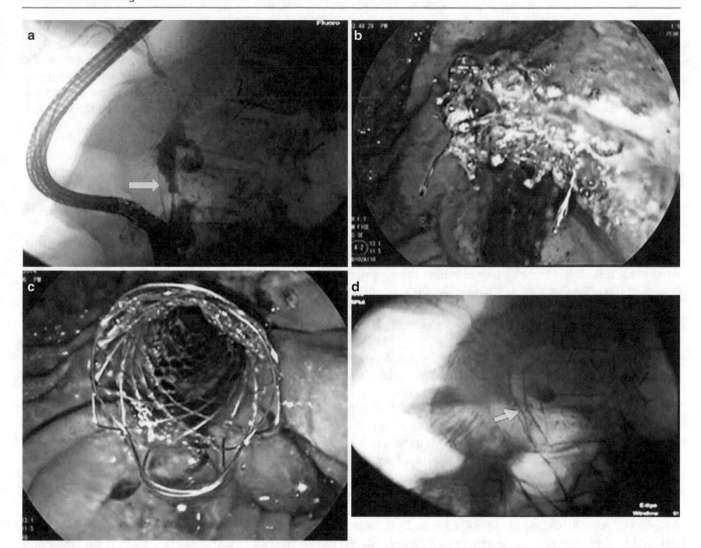

Fig. 7.4 (**a**) Tumor ingrowth at the proximal end of a metal stent (*arrow*). (**b**) The distal portion of the stent was trimmed (shortened) using argon plasma coagulation (APC) at 80–100 W to facilitate cannulation of the stent lumen. Cholangiogram revealed tissue ingrowth within the body of the original uncovered metal stent, and thus a new fully covered metal stent was deployed inside the cut stent (**c**, **d**)

forceps, even when a portion of the SEMS remains in the biliary tree. However, significant resistance encountered during attempt to remove a partially covered SEMS suggests that tissue ingrowth and/or overgrowth has occurred. If the area with ingrowth/overgrowth can be visualized directly or via peroral choledochoscopy, tissue fulguration (e.g., argon plasma coagulation) may free the stent adequately to allow its removal. Alternatively, temporary placement of an overlapping fully covered SEMS within the first stent "sandwiches" the ingrown tissue and causes it to necrose, enabling the ingrown/overgrown SEMS to be removed along with the newer SEMS during a subsequent ERCP.

SEMS that have migrated partially out of the duct can impact the opposite wall of the duodenum and can cause ulceration, bleeding, or duodenal perforation. If the SEMS cannot be removed, it can sometimes be cut/trimmed using argon plasma coagulation. Some stents are made of metal with a higher melting point than APC can generate. High power settings may be required to cut/trim a metal stent. The case depicted in Fig. 7.4 required 80–100 W to cut through the stent completely.

Trapped or Broken Baskets

Retrieval of pancreatic and biliary stones can occasionally be very difficult and/or complex. An impacted ("trapped") or broken retrieval basket is reported to occur in ~4 % of cases when mechanical lithotripsy is attempted [53]. Rates of trapped basket are higher for pancreatic lithotripsy (10 %) compared to biliary cases (3 %) [53]. The approach to a trapped basket requires an understanding of the design of the basket being used. Some baskets, such as the Trapezoid basket (Boston Scientific, Natick MA), are manufactured in such a way as to "break" or partly "disassemble" when sufficient force is applied to the basket handle during basket closure. For example, the Trapezoid basket has a "ball" at its tip where the basket wires join. If a threshold force is exceeded while attempting to crush a stone, the "ball" pops off, freeing the upper ends of the wires, allowing the basket to be removed and any stone in the basket to be released (but not removed).

An important "rescue" option remains for baskets that do not possess a release mechanism or when the release mechanism fails. This involves the use of an emergency lithotripter device. First, the basket catheter is cut and completely transected close to the handle (using wire-cutters or comparable shears) and the duodenoscope is removed, with or without the plastic sheath from the trapped basket, over the basket wires. This leaves only the wire elements from the trapped basket in place (or the wire and plastic sheath) emerging from the patient's mouth. The wires (+/− plastic sheath) are then threaded into a "crank" style lithotripter, such as a Soehendra mechanical lithotripter, which is composed of two main parts: a rotatable handle ("crank") attached to a flexible but very strong metal sheath. Fluoroscopic guidance is typically used at this point as there is no endoscope in the patient at this point. The handle of the crank is turned, which advances the metal sheath perorally over the wires of the trapped basket until the end of the metal sheath abuts the trapped basket and stone. Once the lithotripter reaches the trapped basket–stone complex, further rotation of the crank handle effectively releases the trapped basket by either stone fragmentation, breaking of the trapped basket wires, or both. At this point the trapped basket can be removed from the patient and further attempts to remove the stone and/or provide biliary drainage can commence.

Other techniques to remove a trapped or impacted basket have been described as well. In one report, a "through-the-scope" technique comparable to the Soehendra technique was employed. The plastic sheath of the trapped basket was cut and removed, but the duodenoscope was left in place. Then, a proprietary "through-the-scope" mechanical lithotripter with a spiral metal sheath (Medi-Globe, Grassau, Germany) was advanced over the bare wires from the trapped basket, under direct endoscopic visualization (unlike the Soehendra lithotripter, which is not "through-the-scope") [54]. In turn, the basket wire was tightened using the handle of lithotripter, and stone fragmentation or wire breakage and removal ensued, similar to the Soehendra lithotripter technique. Extracorporeal shock-wave lithotripsy (ESWL), electrohydraulic lithotripsy (EHL), and use of a second retrieval basket to grasp and extract a trapped/impacted basket have also been reported as rescue measures to release a trapped basket [53, 55–57].

If the basket cannot be removed, or the emergency device is broken or unavailable, another option is to simply leave the basket in the bile duct, coil the wires of the basket catheter in the stomach, and reinsert the endoscope and place a plastic stent in the bile duct next to the basket–stone complex to provide drainage. There is also a chance that the stent may help to break up the trapped stone in the basket prior to the next procedure.

Hemobilia and Post-sphincterotomy Bleeding

Hemobilia is a rare cause of upper gastrointestinal bleeding. Jaundice may accompany the bleeding secondary to biliary obstruction from blood clots or may be due to separate (but often related) biliary obstruction, usually from malignancy. Etiologies of hemobilia include tumors involving the liver or biliary tree and various iatrogenic causes, such as liver biopsy, biliary sphincterotomy, or dilation of malignant biliary strictures. Overall, most hemobilia is due to iatrogenic causes from prior procedures or instrumentation.

Sphincterotomy associated hemorrhage occurs in less than 2 % of ERCP procedures. Risk factors include coagulopathy, thrombocytopenia, hemodialysis, and initiation of anticoagulants within 3 days of sphincterotomy [58]. Bleeding during sphincterotomy is also a risk factor for delayed post-ERCP hemorrhage. Treatment includes injection of dilute epinephrine (frequently directed at the "apex" sphincterotomy, just above the incision), balloon tamponade, thermal therapy or placement of clips. Care should be taken to avoid injury to the pancreatic orifice during endoscopic treatment of post-sphincterotomy bleeding.

Tumor-associated hemobilia is usually difficult to control endoscopically. Mild to moderate hemobilia that can occasionally result from trauma to biliary tumors during ERCP procedures often resolve spontaneously (in the absence of significant underlying coagulopathy). In this setting, placement of biliary stents with their proximal end well above the location of the bile duct blood clots can ensure adequate biliary drainage and prevent cholangitis until the bleeding resolves. If the bleeding is more significant or persistent, the blood clots can occlude the stents, and cholangitis may ensue. Placement of a nasobiliary catheter to facilitate biliary irrigation may prevent clots from occluding the biliary system and allow for endoscopic reintervention once bleeding stops [59]. Vascular imaging may be required in cases of unexplained or significant hemobilia to assess for tumor invasion into the portal vein or hepatic artery, or presence of a vascular fistula. Anecdotally, biliary metal stents (SEMS) may provide tamponade for bleeding tumors within the large-caliber portions of the biliary tree and result in cessation of tumor-associated hemobilia (Figs. 7.5, 7.6, and 7.7) [60]. However, failure to achieve hemostasis with biliary SEMS is not uncommon, and data to support this as a preferred modality are lacking. If bleeding is clinically significant and cannot be controlled endoscopically, angiographic intervention (such as embolization or intravascular stent placement) and/or radiation therapy may be required [61].

Guidewire and Luminal Perforation

Guidewire-associated bile duct injury and endoscope or sphincterotomy-associated perforations are reported to occur in less than 1 % of ERCP procedures. Intrahepatic bile duct injury may be manifested by a blush of contrast within the hepatic parenchyma during cholangiography. When ductal injury is recognized, management is similar to treatment of other causes of transmural bile duct injury (e.g., postsurgical bile leaks) with biliary sphincterotomy, stent placement, or both. Adequate ductal drainage should be confirmed. Most patients with guidewire perforations recover quickly with only conservative treatment.

Bowel perforations during ERCP happen more often in patients with surgically altered anatomy such as Roux-en-Y and Billroth II anatomy although they can certainly occur in patients with normal anatomy. Perforations can also occur at the gastroesophageal junction due to buckling of the endoscope as it is advanced into extreme "long positions." Duodenal perforation can occur during biliary or pancreatic sphincterotomy and can be difficult to detect during the procedure. Many patients with duodenal perforations from sphincterotomy can be treated conservatively if the perforation is recognized in a reasonable time frame by NPO status, antibiotics, and serial abdominal exams to look for signs of worsening clinical performance.

Occasionally, endoscopists that perform ERCP receive telephone calls regarding small amounts of retroperitoneal or even intraperitoneal air that is found incidentally on an imaging study performed within days following ERCP in an otherwise asymptomatic patient. Microperforations from ERCP with sphincterotomy can be seen in up to 30 % of patients [62], and frequently have neither clinical significance nor long-term sequelae. Close observation with periodic clinical monitoring and/or repeat imaging is often all that is required in such situations.

Duodenal perforations can occur when balloon dilation of a duodenal stenosis is performed to enable advancement to the ampulla. If perforation is recognized during ERCP, endoscopic clipping for small to medium sized defects, using through-the-scope and over-the-scope clips can be considered, but large perforations often require surgical repair.

Cholecystitis

Acute cholecystitis has been described as a rare (less than 1–3 %) complication associated with biliary interventions such as stent placement but can occur following any biliary ERCP [63]. The exact mechanism is unclear, but obstruction of cystic duct by a stone or stent and gallbladder distension with resultant ischemia are proposed mechanisms [64]. Contrast injection into the gallbladder, especially in patients with primary sclerosing cholangitis (PSC), may be enough to seed an infection.

The rate of cholecystitis may be higher with metal stents (SEMS) compared to plastic stents, probably even higher when bilateral SEMS are placed [65]. Following metal stent placement, cholecystitis rates of 1.9–12 % have been reported, including cases of emphysematous cholecystitis, gallbladder abscess, and transmural gallbladder perforation, usually if the cystic duct orifice is partially or fully obstructed by the stent [66]. Malignant involvement of the cystic duct orifice also appears to be a risk factor for cholecystitis [67, 68].

Conceptually, placing a covered SEMS over the cystic duct insertion (particularly if the cystic orifice is involved in the malignant obstruction) should pose a greater risk of cholecystitis compared to an uncovered SEMS (which should allow gallbladder contents to drain through the uncovered SEMS interstices), but meta-analyses describe similar (low) rates of cholecystitis regardless of the type of SEMS used [31, 69]. Despite this, at least one small series described successful treatment of SEMS (fully covered) related cholecystitis by replacing the covered SEMS with either an uncovered SEMS or plastic stent [66]. Alternative management strategies include cholecystectomy, percutaneous drainage (cholecystostomy), or EUS-guided transmural drainage (below). When the cystic duct orifice is clearly compromised by tumor, as demonstrated by cholangiography, the decision regarding whether to place any metal SEMS (versus plastic), and which to place (covered versus uncovered) becomes more complex, and varies from institution to institution. In many centers, the risk of causing cholecystitis with SEMS for malignant distal biliary obstruction (~2–12 %) is felt to be offset by the multiple benefits of using SEMS in this setting (longer patency, fewer repeat ERCP procedures required, and cost-effectiveness compared to plastic stents). Thus, at centers where this is the dominant factor, SEMS are placed in all patients, regardless of whether the cystic duct is involved by tumor. In other centers, uncovered SEMS are chosen in this setting to try to prevent cholecystitis, though this approach is not supported by the meta-analyses mentioned earlier. Plastic stents which do not expand and are thus less likely to further compromise a partially occluded cystic duct orifice, might mitigate the cholecystitis risk and

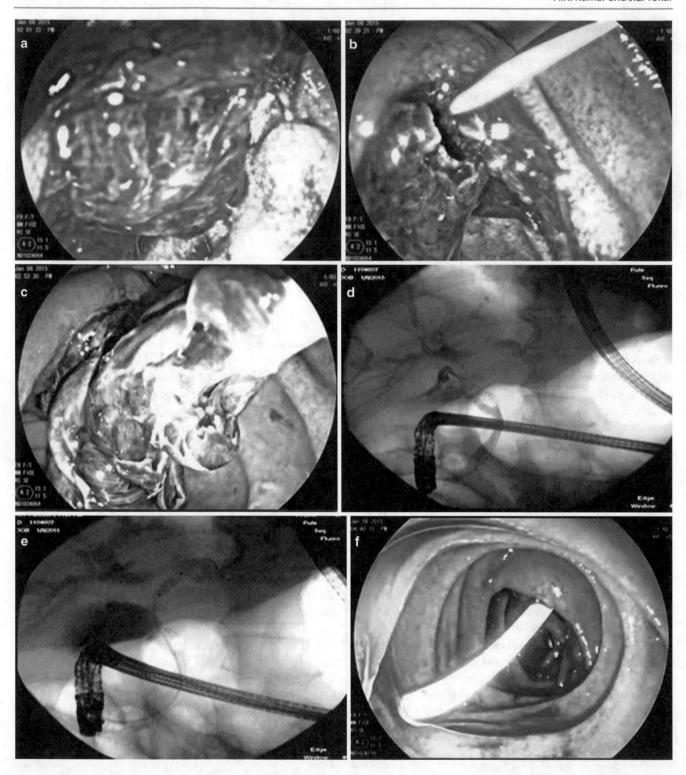

Fig. 7.5 A case of refractory hemobilia from intrahepatic cholangio-carcinoma treated with bilateral uncovered biliary metal stents. Patient had plastic stents placed 2 weeks earlier but re-presented with fever, chills, and recurrent jaundice. (**a**) Large clot was seen covering the prior stent. (**b**) The plastic stents were removed and biliary cannulation with guidewire access was achieved. (**c**) Large clots were swept from the bile duct. (**d**) Residual clot burden and strictures seen on cholangiogram, including a stricture in the left main hepatic duct. (**e**) The hepatic duct stricture was dilated and (**f**) a long plastic stent was placed to the level of the intrahepatic bile ducts

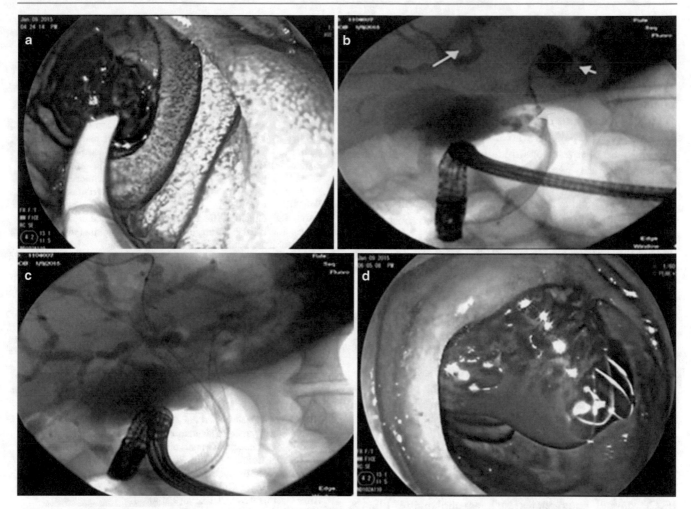

Fig. 7.6 A case of refractory hemobilia from intrahepatic cholangiocarcinoma treated with bilateral uncovered biliary metal stents. Due to persistent fevers and jaundice, repeat ERCP revealed clot around the stent (**a**). The stent was removed and cholangiogram showed multiple clots throughout the biliary tree (*arrows*, **b**). Bilateral uncovered metal stents were deployed (**c**, **d**), resulting in excellent drainage and subsequently successful resolution of the hemobilia and cholangitis

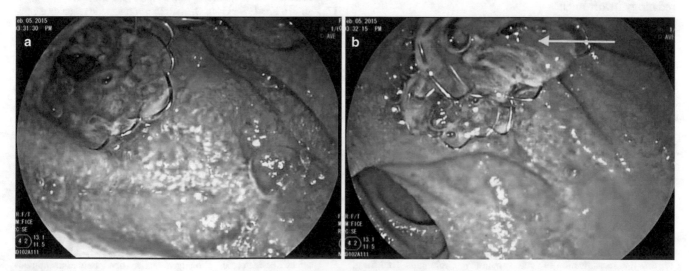

Fig. 7.7 A case of refractory hemobilia from intrahepatic cholangiocarcinoma treated with bilateral uncovered biliary metal stents. A follow-up ERCP 1 month later confirmed resolution of hemobilia. Panel (**a**) demonstrates the right hepatic duct stent. Panel (**b**) demonstrates both the metal stents with the *arrow* pointing at the left hepatic duct stent

its subsequent sequelae (e.g., delaying chemoradiation or surgery for the underlying malignancy). However, they lack the aforementioned advantages of SEMS. If SEMS are used, we try to place them below the insertion of cystic duct, if possible, recognizing that the literature on this point is far from definitive.

Acute cholecystitis of various etiologies has been treated endoscopically in patients who are not ideal surgical candidates because of severe comorbidities (such as cirrhosis with ascites) and elderly patients with limited life expectancy who are perceived to have higher risk of adverse events with aggressive surgical management [70]. Transpapillary gallbladder stenting [71] is the approach described most often, though endoscopic ultrasound guided transgastric or transduodenal gallbladder drainage [72] has been reported, most recently using novel lumen-apposing self-expanding metal stents [73]. In expert hands, transpapillary gallbladder stenting using 7 Fr or 10 Fr double pigtail plastic stents can be successful in over 75 % of patients and effective in preventing recurrence of cholecystitis [71]. However, there is limited data on long-term outcomes with endoscopic gallbladder drainage, and a paucity of comparisons of endoscopic drainage to percutaneous cholecystostomy, thus the procedure is currently only performed at centers with expertise in advanced therapeutic EUS and ERCP.

Conclusion

ERCP on-call emergencies such as cholangitis, biliary pancreatitis, stent migrations, perforations, and hemobilia are all commonly encountered in clinical practice. Most of these situations can be managed endoscopically, but some require multimodality therapy with surgery or interventional radiology involvement.

Video Legends

Video 7.1 Cholangitis after prior biliary intervention with a plastic stent (MP4 6163 kb).

Video 7.2 Occluded biliary metal stent with sludge and debris resulting in cholangitis (MP4 17,547 kb).

Video 7.3 Proximally migrated PD stent retrieved using a rat-tooth forceps (MP4 19,624 kb).

References

1. Reynolds BM, Dargan EL. Acute obstructive cholangitis a distinct clinical syndrome. Ann Surg. 1959;150(2):299–303.
2. Csendes A, Diaz JC, Burdiles P, Maluenda F, Morales E. Risk factors and classification of acute suppurative cholangitis. Br J Surg. 1992;79:655–8.
3. Kiriyama S, Takada T, Strasberg SM, Solomkin JS, et al. New diagnostic criteria and severity assessment of acute cholangitis in revised Tokyo Guidelines. J Hepatobiliary Pancreat Sci. 2012;19:548–56.
4. Mayumi T, Takada T, Kawarada Y, et al. Results of the Tokyo consensus meeting Tokyo guidelines. J Hepatobiliary Pancreat Sci. 2007;14(1):114–21.
5. Kiriyama S, Takada T, Strasberg SM, et al. TG13 guidelines for diagnosis and severity grading of acute cholangitis (with videos). J Hepatobiliary Pancreat Sci. 2013;20(1):24–34.
6. Ge PS, Hamerski CM, Watson RR, et al. Plastic biliary stent patency in patients with locally advanced pancreatic adenocarcinoma receiving downstaging chemotherapy. Gastrointest Endosc. 2015;81(2):360–6.
7. Gomi H, Solomkin JS, Takada T, et al. TG13 antimicrobial therapy for acute cholangitis and cholecystitis. J Hepatobiliary Pancreat Sci. 2013;20(1):60–70.
8. Itoi T, Tsuyuguchi T, Takada T, et al. TG13 indications and techniques for biliary drainage in acute cholangitis (with videos). J Hepatobiliary Pancreat Sci. 2013;20(1):71–80.
9. ASGE Standards of Practice Committee. The role of endoscopy in the management of choledocholithiasis. Gastrointest Endosc. 2011;74(4):731–44.
10. Horiuchi A, Kajiyama M, Ichise Y, et al. Biliary stenting as alternative therapy to stone clearance in elderly patients with bile duct stones. Acta Gastroenterol Belg. 2014;77(3):297–301.
11. Okano N, Igarashi Y, Kishimoto Y, Mimura T, Ito K. Necessity for endoscopic sphincterotomy for biliary stenting in cases of malignant biliary obstruction. Dig Endosc. 2013;25 Suppl 2:122–5.
12. Elmunzer BJ, Scheiman JM, Lehman GA, et al. A randomized trial of rectal indomethacin to prevent post-ERCP pancreatitis. N Engl J Med. 2012;366(15):1414–22.
13. Khashab MA, Valeshabad AK, Modayil R, et al. EUS-guided biliary drainage by using a standardized approach for malignant biliary obstruction: rendezvous versus direct transluminal techniques (with videos). Gastrointest Endosc. 2013;78(5):734–41.
14. Tenner S, Baillie J, DeWitt J, Vege SS. American College of Gastroenterology Guideline: Management of acute pancreatitis. Am J Gastroenterol. 2013;108(9):1400–15.
15. ASGE Standards of Practice Committee. The role of endoscopy in the management of suspected choledocholithiasis. Gastrointest Endosc. 2010;71(1):1–9.
16. Tseng CW, Chen CC, Chen TS, et al. Can computed tomography with coronal reconstruction improve the diagnosis of choledocholithiasis? J Gastroenterol Hepatol. 2008;23(10):1586–9.
17. Zidi SH, Prat F, Le Guen O, et al. Use of magnetic resonance cholangiography in the diagnosis of choledocholithiasis: prospective comparison with a reference imaging method. Gut. 1999;44:118–22.
18. Sugiyama M, Atomi Y, Hachiya J. Magnetic resonance cholangiography using half-Fourier acquisition for diagnosing choledocholithiasis. Am J Gastroenterol. 1998;93:1886–90.
19. Garrow D, Miller S, Sinha D, et al. Endoscopic ultrasound: a meta-analysis of test performance in suspected biliary obstruction. Clin Gastroenterol Hepatol. 2007;5:616–23.
20. Tse F, Liu L, Barkun AN, et al. EUS: a meta-analysis of test performance in suspected choledocholithiasis. Gastrointest Endosc. 2008;67:235–44.
21. Sugiyama M, Atomi Y. Endoscopic ultrasonography for diagnosing choledocholithiasis: a prospective comparative study with ultrasonography and computed tomography. Gastrointest Endosc. 1997;45:143–6.
22. Kondo S, Isayama H, Akahane M, et al. Detection of common bile duct stones: comparison between endoscopic ultrasonography, magnetic resonance cholangiography, and helical-computed-tomographic cholangiography. Eur J Radiol. 2005;54:271–5.
23. Scheiman JM, Carlos RC, Barnett JL, et al. Can endoscopic ultrasound or magnetic resonance cholangiopancreatography

replace ERCP in patients with suspected biliary disease? A prospective trial and cost analysis. Am J Gastroenterol. 2001;96(10): 2900–4.

24. Folsch UR, Nitsche R, Ludtke R, et al. Early ERCP and papillotomy compared with conservative treatment for acute biliary pancreatitis. N Engl J Med. 1997;336:237–42.

25. Oria A, Cimmino D, Ocampo C, et al. Early endoscopic intervention versus early conservative management in patients with acute gallstone pancreatitis and biliopancreatic obstruction: a randomized clinical trial. Ann Surg. 2007;245:10–7.

26. Johanson JF, Schmalz MJ, Geenen JE. Incidence and risk factors for biliary and pancreatic stent migration. Gastrointest Endosc. 1992;38:341–6.

27. Kawaguchi Y, Ogawa M, Kawashima Y, et al. Risk factors for proximal migration of biliary tube stents. World J Gastroenterol. 2014;20(5):1318–24.

28. Nakai Y, Isayama H, Kogure H, et al. Risk factors for covered metallic stent migration in patients with distal malignant biliary obstruction due to pancreatic cancer. J Gastroenterol Hepatol. 2014;29(9):1744–9.

29. Arhan M, Odemis B, Parlak E, et al. Migration of biliary plastic stents: experience of a tertiary center. Surg Endosc. 2009;23:769–75.

30. Telford JJ, Carr-Locke DL, Baron TH, et al. A randomized trial comparing uncovered and partially covered self-expandable metal stents in the palliation of distal malignant biliary obstruction. Gastrointest Endosc. 2010;72(5):907–14.

31. Saleem A, Leggett CL, Murad MH, Baron TH. Meta-analysis of randomized trials comparing the patency of covered and uncovered self-expandable metal stents for palliation of distal malignant bile duct obstruction. Gastrointest Endosc. 2011;74(2):321–7.

32. Al-Zubaidi AM, Al-Zubaidi AH, Qureshi LA, AL-Haroon EE. Full length migration of plastic biliary stent into the left lobe of liver and its endoscopic retrieval. J Coll Physicians Surg Pak. 2014;24(11):861–2.

33. Cho NJ, Lee TH, Park SH, et al. Endoscopic removal of a proximally migrated metal stent during balloon sweeping after stent trimming. Clin Endosc. 2013;46(4):418–22.

34. Santos A, Leitao C, Vieira A, Pereira E. Endoscopic and percutaneous extraction of two biliary stents migrated to distinct abdominal locations. BMJ Case Rep. 2014 Dec 19;2014.

35. Antonsen J, Preisler L, Skram U, Klein M. Fatal biliary-pulmonary fistula due to a proximally migrating biliary stent. Endoscopy. 2013;45(Suppl 2 UCTN):E265–6.

36. Dasmahapatra HK, Pepper JR. Bronchopleurobiliary fistula. A complication of intrahepatic biliary stent migration. Chest. 1988;94(4):874–5.

37. Kumar V, Rajalingam R, Saluja SS, Chander Sharma B, Mishra PK. Unusual proximal migration of biliary plastic endoprostheses into the inferior vena cava. Am Surg. 2012;78(12):E520–2.

38. Lee V, Woldman S, Meier P. Biliary stent migration as a cause of cardiac tamponade. J Cardiovasc Med (Hagerstown). 2013;14(10):750–2.

39. Barut I, Tarhan OR. Cecum perforation due to biliary stent migration. Saudi Med J. 2014;35(7):747–9.

40. El Zein MH, Kumbhari V, Tieu A, et al. Duodenal perforation as a consequence of biliary stent migration can occur regardless of stent type or duration. Endoscopy. 2014;46:E281–2.

41. Kittappa K, Maruthachalam K, Brookstein R, Debrah S. Migrated biliary stent presenting as a sigmoid diverticulitis – case report. Indian J Surg. 2013;75 Suppl 1:253–4.

42. Toth P, Dvorak J, Marz J. Biliary stent as a cause of bowel obstruction. Rozhl Chir. 2014;93(1):28–30.

43. Mavrogenis G, Lalot M, Hoebeke Y, et al. Biliary stent migration presenting as a recurrent pilonidal abscess with underlying rectocutaneous fistula. Endoscopy. 2013;45(S 02):E301–2.

44. Katsinelos P, Kountouras J, Paroutoglou G, et al. Migration of plastic biliary stents and endoscopic retrieval: an experience of three referral centers. Surg Laparosc Endosc Percutan Tech. 2009;19(3):217–21.

45. Chaurasia OP, Rauws EA, Fockens P, Huibregtse K. Endoscopic techniques for retrieval of proximally migrated biliary stents: the Amsterdam experience. Gastrointest Endosc. 1999;50(6):780–5.

46. Lahoti S, Catalano MF, Geenen JE, Schmalz MJ. Endoscopic retrieval of proximally migrated biliary and pancreatic stents: experience of a large referral center. Gastrointest Endosc. 1998; 47(6):486–91.

47. Tarnasky PR, Cotton PB, Baillie J, et al. Proximal migration of biliary stents: attempted endoscopic retrieval in forty-one patients. Gastrointest Endosc. 1995;42(6):513–20.

48. Goetz M, Walther U, Malek N, Fuchs J, et al. Transpapillary retrieval of a proximally migrated stent using a three-prong polyp retrieval device in a 2-years-old girl. Z Gastroenterol. 2014; 52(4):351–3.

49. Okabe Y, Tsuruta O, Kaji R, et al. Endoscopic retrieval of migrated plastic stent into bile duct or pancreatic pseudocyst. Dig Endosc. 2009;21(1):1–7.

50. Lee JH, Yan SL, Chen CH, Yeh YH, Yueh SK. Endoscopic retrieval of a proximally migrated biliary plastic stent using a guidewire loop technique. Endoscopy. 2014;46(Suppl 1 UCTN):E232–3.

51. Shah DK, Jain SS, Somani PO, Rathi PM. Biliary sphincteroplasty facilitates retrieval of proximally migrated plastic biliary stent. Trop Gastroenterol. 2014;35(2):103–6.

52. Vázquez Rey MT, González Conde B, Alonso Aguirre PA, et al. Retrieval of proximally migrated plastic biliary stents using a metal stent. Endoscopy. 2011;43(Suppl 2 UCTN):E376.

53. Thomas M, Howell DA, Carr-Locke D, et al. Mechanical lithotripsy of pancreatic and biliary stones: complications and available treatment options collected from expert centers. Am J Gastroenterol. 2007;102(9):1896–902.

54. Draganov P, Cunningham JT. Novel "through-the-endoscope" technique for removing biliary stones trapped in a retrieval basket. Endoscopy. 2002;34(2):176.

55. Hu LH, Du TT, Liao Z, Zou WB, Ye B, Li ZS. Extracorporeal shock wave lithotripsy as a rescue for a trapped stone basket in the pancreatic duct. Endoscopy. 2014;46(Suppl 1 UCTN):E332–3.

56. Ng EK, Lau JY, Chung SC, Li AK. Retrieval of an impacted mechanical lithotripsy basket. Endoscopy. 1997;29(2):128.

57. Schutz SM, Chinea C, Friedrichs P. Successful endoscopic removal of a severed, impacted Dormia basket. Am J Gastroenterol. 1997;92(4):679–81.

58. Freeman ML, Nelson DB, Sherman S, et al. Complications of endoscopic biliary sphincterotomy. N Engl J Med. 1996;335:909–18.

59. Conio M, Caroli-Bosc FX, Buckley M, et al. Massive hematobilia after extraction of plastic biliary endoprosthesis. J Clin Gastroenterol. 1997;25(4):706.

60. Goenka MK, Harwani Y, Rai V, Goenka U. Fully covered self-expandable metal biliary stent for hemobilia caused by portal biliopathy. Gastrointest Endosc. 2014;80(6):1175.

61. Marynissen T, Maleux G, Heye S, et al. Transcatheter arterial embolization for iatrogenic hemobilia is a safe and effective procedure: case series and review of the literature. Eur J Gastroenterol Hepatol. 2012;24(8):905–9.

62. Genzlinger JL, McPhee MS, Fisher JK, et al. Significance of retroperitoneal air after endoscopic retrograde cholangiopancreatography with sphincterotomy. Am J Gastroenterol. 1999;94:1267–70.

63. Kitano M, Yamashita Y, Tanaka K, et al. Covered self-expandable metal stents with an anti-migration system improve patency duration without increased complications compared with uncovered stents for distal biliary obstruction caused by pancreatic carcinoma: a randomized multicenter trial. Am J Gastroenterol. 2013;108(11): 1713–22.

64. Itah R, Bruck R, Santo M, Skornick Y, Avital S. Gangrenous chole-cystitis - a rare complication of ERCP. Endoscopy. 2007;39 Suppl 1:E223–4.

65. Kim DU, Kang DH, Kim GH, et al. Bilateral biliary drainage for malignant hilar obstruction using the 'stent-in-stent' method with a Y-stent: efficacy and complications. Eur J Gastroenterol Hepatol. 2013;25(1):99–106.

66. Saxena P, Singh VK, Lennon AM, et al. Endoscopic management of acute cholecystitis after metal stent placement in patients with malignant biliary obstruction: a case series. Gastrointest Endosc. 2013;78(1):175–8.

67. Isayama H, Kawabe T, Nakai Y, et al. Cholecystitis after metallic stent placement in patients with malignant distal biliary obstruc-tion. Clin Gastroenterol Hepatol. 2006;4(9):1148–53.

68. Shimizu S, Naitoh I, Nakazawa T, et al. Predictive factors for pan-creatitis and cholecystitis in endoscopic covered metal stenting for distal malignant biliary obstruction. J Gastroenterol Hepatol. 2013;28(1):68–72.

69. Almadi MA, Barkun AN, Martel M. No benefit of covered vs uncovered self-expandable metal stents in patients with malignant distal biliary obstruction: a meta-analysis. Clin Gastroenterol Hepatol. 2013;11(1):27–37.

70. Tsuyuguchi T, Itoi T, Takada T, et al. TG13 indications and tech-niques for gallbladder drainage in acute cholecystitis (with videos). J Hepatobiliary Pancreat Sci. 2013;20(1):81–8.

71. Maekawa S, Nomura R, Murase T, Ann Y, Oeholm M, Harada M. Endoscopic gallbladder stenting for acute cholecystitis: a retro-spective study of 46 elderly patients aged 65 years or older. BMC Gastroenterol. 2013;13:65.

72. Widmer J, Singhal S, Gaidhane M, Kahaleh M. Endoscopic ultrasound-guided endoluminal drainage of the gallbladder. Dig Endosc. 2014;26(4):525–31.

73. Teoh AY, Binmoeller KF, Lau JY. Single-step EUS-guided punc-ture and delivery of a lumen-apposing stent for gallbladder drain-age using a novel cautery-tipped stent delivery system. Gastrointest Endosc. 2014;80(6):1171.

Endoscopic Treatment of Simultaneous Malignant Biliary and Gastric Outlet Obstruction

Brian P. Riff and Christopher J. DiMaio

Background

Symptomatic obstruction of the stomach, duodenum, and biliary tract can occur in many malignant diseases. The most common scenario is seen in patients with pancreatic ductal adenocarcinoma which rarely (<25 % of the time) presents with localized resectable disease [1]. In addition to pancreatic neoplasms, other primary malignancies can be present with obstructive symptoms including gastric cancers, small bowel cancer including lymphoma and adenocarcinoma, gastrointestinal stromal tumors (GIST), extra-intestinal lymphoma, cholangiocarcinoma, ampullary cancer, and metastatic disease [2–4]. While malignant disease is the predominant etiology for obstruction, benign processes such as acute pancreatitis and sclerosing mesenteritis, or rarely from large calculi (Bouveret's syndrome) can present with intestinal and biliary obstructions [5–7] (Table 8.1).

Much has been written on endoscopic management of isolated malignant gastrointestinal or biliary obstruction; however, simultaneous obstruction is increasingly managed endoscopically with excellent symptomatic palliation. Historically, surgical bypass (involving the creation of choledochojejunal and gastrojejunal anastomoses in one procedure) was the procedure of choice and has a wealth of literature documenting safety, efficacy, and long-term patency rates [11, 12]. Unfortunately, many of these patients are poor surgical candidates with limited life expectancy. Patients presenting with a malignant gastroduodenal obstruction have a mean survival of 12.1 weeks after presentation [13]. As such, alternative palliative techniques are preferred.

Recently, there has been increasing use of self-expanding metal stents (SEMS) for management of malignant enteric and biliary obstruction. Many series have established the utility of SEMS as a safe and effective tool for symptomatic palliation in advanced gastroduodenal and hepaticobiliary malignancy [14–16]. While a surgical bypass was the traditional palliation technique and progress has been made in laparoscopic approaches to biliary bypass, endoscopic stenting has been shown to be at least as effective with resultant shorter hospital stays, decreased costs and have lower procedural related mortality (endoscopy: 0 % vs. surgical bypass 2.5–19 %) [17–22] (Fig. 8.1).

In addition to the utility of SEMS in managing malignant strictures, the application of endoscopic ultrasound (EUS) when endoscopic retrograde cholangiopancreatography (ERCP) fails in gaining biliary access has allowed for endoscopic management in situations that previously needed surgical or interventional radiology interventions [23].

Surgical bypass may still be preferred in certain centers depending on local experience and expertise. Multidisciplinary discussion between gastroenterology, surgery and oncology should be routine in management of these patients.

Gastroduodenal Obstruction

While recognizing biliary obstruction can be more obvious because of the laboratory abnormalities, many of the symptoms of the primary malignancy can overlap with symptoms of luminal obstruction leading to a delay in diagnosis. Because of this, it is important to keep luminal obstruction in the differential diagnosis. Gastric outlet obstruction (GOO) is a proximal obstruction either at the level of the distal stomach or proximal small bowel leading to inability of the stomach to properly empty its contents into the small bowel. This obstruction leads

Electronic supplementary material: The online version of this chapter (doi:10.1007/978-3-319-26854-5_8) contains supplementary material, which is available to authorized users. Videos can also be accessed at http://link.springer.com/chapter/10.1007/978-3-319-26854-5_8.

B.P. Riff, M.D. • C.J. DiMaio, M.D. (✉)
The Dr. Henry D. Janowitz Division of Gastroenterology,
Icahn School of Medicine at Mount Sinai, One Gustave L. Levy Place,
Box 1069, New York, NY 10029, USA
e-mail: Christopher.DiMaio@mountsinai.org

Table 8.1 Malignant types presenting with simultaneous obstruction [8–10]

Malignancy type	Percentage
Pancreatic	71
Biliary	15
Gastric	6
Metastatic (breast, colon, kidney)	5
Other (Lymphoma, small bowel)	3

to symptoms of nausea, vomiting, dehydration, weight loss, abdominal pain, and an inability to tolerate oral feeding with resultant anorexia. The decreased oral intake often leads to the presentation with dehydration, hypovolemia, and malnourished states [24]. Early presentation may be subtle, with only early satiety and/or loss of appetite present.

GOO can be seen with many malignancies but is most commonly seen in advanced pancreatic cancer. At the time

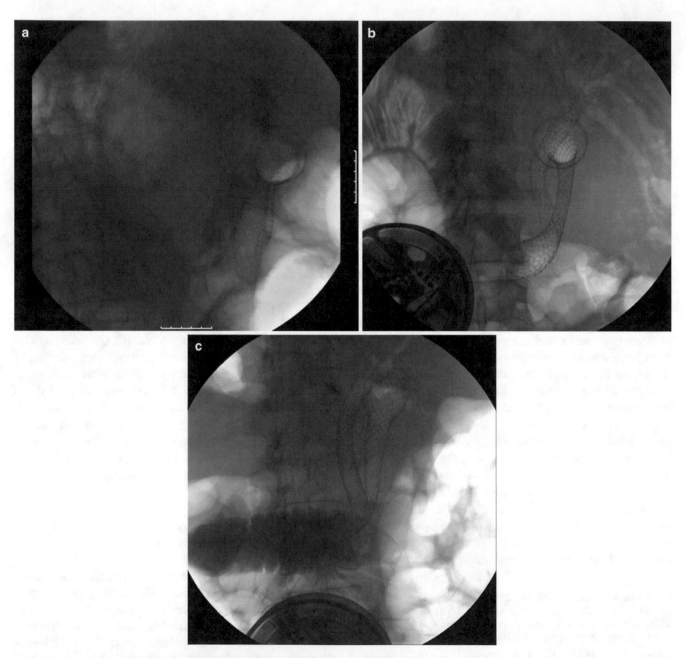

Fig. 8.1 Different views of patients with combined biliary and gastric outlet obstruction treated by endoscopic techniques. (**a**) Enteric and Biliary SEMS in a patient with pancreatic cancer where the duodenal stenosis is proximal to the Ampulla of Vater. (**b**) Enteric and Biliary SEMS placement in a patient with cholangiocarcinoma. Enteric obstruction occurs at the level of the ampulla. Note that the patient required four biliary stents to restore patency of his biliary tree. (**c**) Enteric and Biliary SEMS placement in a patient with pancreatic cancer. The enteric obstruction in just distal to the ampulla (Images courtesy of Douglas G. Adler MD)

of diagnosis, 30–50 % of patients with pancreatic cancer will report symptoms of nausea and vomiting but a rare minority will present with frank obstruction. However, in the setting of unresectable disease, many retrospective and prospective series have reported that 10–20 % of patients with pancreatic cancer and other periampullary tumors will develop GOO over the course of their disease process [12, 21]. After pancreatic cancer, in a large multicenter retrospective series of patients presenting with GOO, metastatic disease (colon, breast, kidney) was the next common etiology (19 % of patients in the series), followed by primary gastric cancer (11 %), cholangiocarcinoma (8 %), ampullary cancer (5 %), gallbladder cancer (2 %). The site of obstruction was most common in the proximal duodenum (71 % of cases) followed by the distal stomach (10 %) and synchronous lesions in the distal stomach and duodenum (10 %) [25].

Biliary Obstruction

In contrast to GOO, biliary obstruction is easier to recognize given the objective findings of elevated bilirubin and alkaline phosphatase that occur secondary to obstruction of the biliary tree. Jaundice is seen in up to 70 % of patients at the time of diagnosis of a periampullary malignancy [26]. In addition to the cosmetic problem of jaundice, patients report pruritus, nausea, pain, loss of appetite, fatigue, and steatorrhea in the setting of obstruction that can result in significant decrease in quality of life. Relief of biliary obstruction even in nonsurgically resectable disease has been shown to improve symptoms of pruritus, anorexia, fat malabsorption, and dyspepsia [27].

Combined Biliary and Gastric Obstruction

The most common presentation is not simultaneous obstruction but rather sequential. In one of the original trials looking at plastic biliary stents for biliary obstruction, 6–9 % of the patients that presented with obstructive jaundice ultimately developed a duodenal obstruction that required a gastrojejunostomy [28]. Larger surgical series showed that 20 % of patients who had previously undergone biliary bypass developed GOO at a median of 2 months post-op. One study randomizing patients to hepaticojejunostomy alone to combined hepaticojejunostomy and gastrojejunostomy was stopped early by the safety monitoring committee due a high rate of symptomatic GOO in the single bypass group [12, 29].

In a study of patients who ultimately required management of both enteral and biliary obstruction, 72 % of the patients presented with a biliary obstruction at median time of 107 days (range: 15–1825 days) prior to the enteral obstruction, 22 % of the patients presented with simultaneous obstruction and

only in the minority of patients did the duodenal obstruction precede the biliary obstruction by a median time of 121 days (range 21–377 days). Patients presenting with simultaneous biliary and gastric outlet obstruction had the shortest survival time compared to those with a sequential presentation [10].

It is well established that almost half of patients that require a duodenal stent will either have or develop a biliary obstruction at some point [14]. Because of this, it is prudent to consider biliary evaluation in any patient presenting with a malignant gastroduodenal obstruction given the high likelihood of a future biliary obstruction.

Anatomical Classification

In 2006, Mutignani et al. published a classification scheme of the three possible locations of the duodenal obstruction relative to the papilla [10] (Fig. 8.2). This bilioduodenal stricture classification is useful in preparing endoscopic approach and most importantly predictive of endoscopic success. Biliary strictures tend to occur in the mid or distal common bile duct when presenting with simultaneous obstruction much more commonly than at more proximal locations.

Patients with Type I combined biliary and duodenal stenosis develop bowel obstruction at the level of the duodenal bulb or the duodenal genu (D1) without involvement of the papilla. In Type II patients the bowel stenosis occurs at the second portion of the duodenum (D2) with direct involvement of the papilla. Patients with Type III stenosis develop bowel obstruction in the third portion of the duodenum (D3), distal and removed from the papilla itself.

Because the bowel obstruction is distal to the papilla, type III stenosis is technically the easiest of the three subtypes to remediate followed by type I then type II. Type II is the most technically challenging because the obstruction occurs directly at the level of the papilla obscuring native anatomy and sometimes making standard biliary access difficult. The type of stricture is also predictive of clinical success (Table 8.2).

Pre-procedural Evaluation

Diagnosis of a simultaneous biliary and duodenal obstruction is based on a combination of clinical history including a known malignancy with potential for obstruction, physical exam, radiographic evaluation, and endoscopy as the gold standard test. It is important that the possibility of a simultaneous obstruction be recognized to help guide not only endoscopic approach but also patient consent and expectations.

Physical examination usually will be notable for scleral icterus and/or jaundice consistent with history of biliary

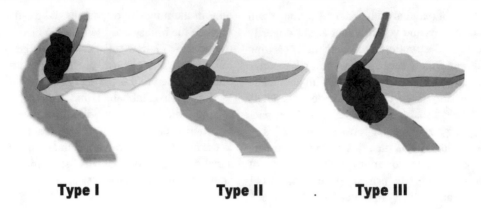

Type I   **Type II**   .   **Type III**

Fig. 8.2 Mutignani bilioduodenal strictures. Type I: Enteric stenosis occurs in D1 proximal to the papilla without papillary involvement Type II: Enteric stenosis occurs in D2 at the level of the biliary stenosis

Type III: Stenosis occurs distal to the papilla [10]. These also correlate with the images shown above in Fig. 8.1a–c, respectively

Table 8.2 Frequency and endoscopic success based on bilioduodenal stricture type [8–10, 13]

	Type I (%)	Type II (%)	Type III (%)
Frequency	40	45	15
Efficacy	94–100	80–86	100

obstruction. Abdominal examination may range from a benign exam to distended abdomen that is tympanic to percussion. The classic finding of a succession splash was only seen in 31 % of patients presenting with endoscopic proven GOO [30].

Radiographic examination prior to endoscopy is helpful for procedural planning and also to determine if endoscopic remediation is possible. If GOO is suspected, a computed tomography (CT) scan of the abdomen with both oral and intravenous (IV) contrast is recommended. Radiographic findings of marked gastric or duodenal dilation proximal to focal transition point are usually diagnostic of a GOO. In addition to establishing the diagnosis, the CT scan can provide information on the stricture itself including length as well as provide details on contraindications for endoscopic management including necrosis, perforation and distal and/or multifocal stricture. It should be cautioned that if no specific transition point is seen, alternate diagnosis such as delayed gastric emptying or diffuse small bowel hypomotility, often seen in the setting of opioids or peritoneal carcinomatosis, should be considered.

There is debate on the value of a pre-procedural fluoroscopic contrast study such as an upper gastrointestinal (UGI) series or small-bowel follow-through (SBFT). A SBFT with either water soluble or barium contrast can sometimes help to define the level of the obstruction and if not completely obstructed gives details about the stricture including length,

complexity and if multifocal strictures are presents. If a diagnosis of a GOO is in doubt, direct examination with an endoscope should be performed to evaluate the anatomy directly.

Patient Preparation

Given the suspected or known GOO with a high likelihood of retained gastric contents, a nasogastric tube with suction is often placed prior to endoscopy in patients with evidence of significant clinical obstruction. This will decrease the risk of aspiration of gastric contents during procedural sedation as well as improve visualization [31]. Additionally, anesthesia support should be considered with general anesthesia and endotracheal intubation to further limit the risk of aspiration. Patients can be positioned supine, prone, or in the left lateral decubitus position depending on operator preference.

Equipment and Room Setup

Gastroduodenal and biliary stent placement require fluoroscopy for safe and accurate placement. The procedure should be performed in a fluoroscopy-ready ERCP room. Patients should be consented for endoscopy with enteral stenting as well as ERCP with biliary stenting.

The endoscopy should be performed with a therapeutic endoscope or duodenoscope as these have a large enough working channel to allow passage of the enteral and biliary stents. The choice of enteral and biliary stent is dependent on the length of the stricture. All currently available enteral SEMS are deployed via a through-the-scope (TTS) over-the-wire system.

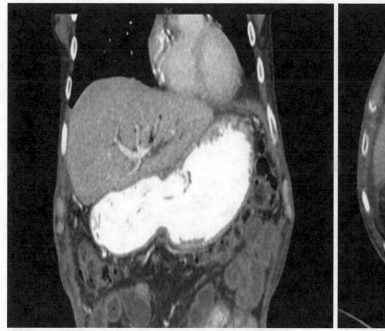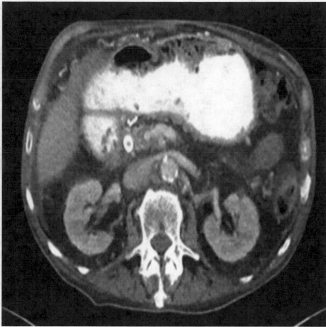

Fig. 8.3 Case example of Type I: 76 year old male with known stage IV pancreatic cancer with indwelling biliary SEMS presenting to the ED with nausea, vomiting, jaundice. CT A/P obtained in the ED showing GOO with intrahepatic biliary dilation

Patients with Preexisting Biliary Stricture

The most common presentation especially with pancreatic cancer is biliary obstruction followed by the development of enteral obstruction. As such, many patients will already have either a plastic or metal biliary stent already in place (Fig. 8.3). If there is a preexisting biliary SEMS in place without signs/symptoms of stent occlusion, then an enteral stent can be placed without concern for obstructing the papilla as currently available enteral stents are all uncovered. If a plastic biliary stent is in place, the stent should be exchanged for a biliary SEMS prior to placement of the enteral stent. If the plastic stent cannot be removed because of the severity of the enteric stricture, interventional radiology should be consulted for percutaneous removal of the plastic stent with placement of a biliary SEMS in an anterograde fashion.

Technical Approach

Type I: It is preferred to perform the ERCP portion of the procedure prior to placing the enteral so as to avoid "jailing" the papilla with the "enteral stent" [14]. One approach to these patients is to pass the duodenoscope to the level of the obstruction and use gentle pressure to pass through the stricture to gain access to the papilla (Fig. 8.4). This is not always possible, of note.

More likely, gentle pressure will not allow passage of the duodenoscope. At this point, there are a number of options. An acceptable initial approach is to perform balloon dilation using a TTS balloon through the duodenoscope from 15 to 18 mm or even up to 20 mm [32–34]. As the balloon is being deflated, the duodenoscope can be advanced through the stricture [35]. Dilation of the stricture itself does carry a small risk of perforation; as such the balloon can be used as an anchor to help the duodenoscope advance into position beyond the stricture. The balloon is advanced distal to the stricture, inflated so as to hold position allowing the duodenoscope to advance forward during reduction techniques rather than get pushed back against the stricture. There is less radial force applied since the balloon is inflated against normal caliber duodenum rather than the area of stenosis.

Alternatively if visualization is limited with the side viewing endoscope, balloon dilation may be performed via a forward viewing endoscope which is then withdrawn and replaced with the duodenoscope. Often the dilation effect can be transitory and that by the time the duodenoscope is inserted, the lumen may not allow passage. As such, a variation of this approach is to place a guidewire through the endoscope beyond the gastroduodenal obstruction. The gastroscope is then exchanged over the guidewire. Finally, the guidewire is then backloaded into the duodenoscope (via a catheter in the accessory channel). Once the duodenoscope is inserted per os, the guidewire can assist in identifying the

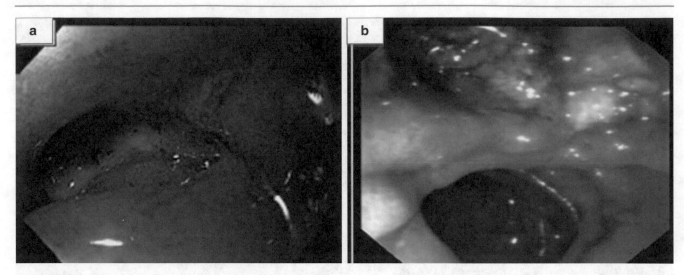

Fig. 8.4 Same patients as Fig. 8.3: Upper endoscopy was performed which was notable for post bulbar stricture (**a**). This was able to be traversed with gentle pressure to reveal the obstructed indwelling biliary SEMS (**b**)

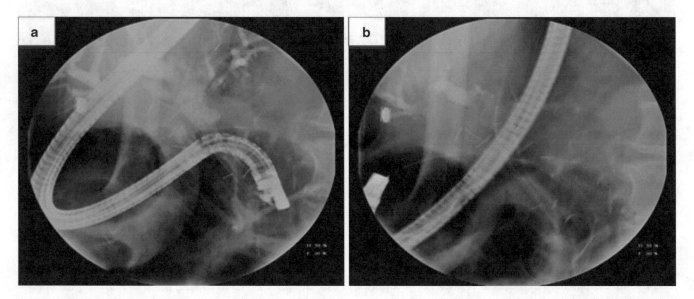

Fig. 8.5 Case continued: ERCP was performed with biliary decompression via a new Biliary SEMS (**a**) followed by placement of an enteric SEMS with distal release (**b**)

compromised lumen and thus allow for a safer and effective scope passage.

At this point, standard biliary cannulation is performed with placement of an expandable metal stent in the bile duct. Once adequate biliary drainage is obtained, a guide wire is passed through the working channel of the duodenoscope and advanced to the distal duodenum under fluoroscopic guidance. The duodenoscope is withdrawn into the stomach and then the enteral stent is deployed in the standard transendoscopic fashion. Care should be taken to ensure that the proximal end of the stent traverses the pylorus, as this will minimize the risk of the duodenal stent becoming impacted against the wall of the duodenal bulb (Fig. 8.5).

In the event that the enteral stricture cannot be traversed, an alternate option is to simply place the enteral stent in one procedure (with the distal end of the stent above the ampulla) and then to do ERCP at a later date by passing the duodenoscope through the Enteral stent to reach the second duodenum. This approach avoids the risk of endoscopic dilation entirely and may be optimal for some patients.

The goal, if possible, is to try to have the distal end of the enteral stent positioned just proximal to the papilla to avoid the "jailed papilla" phenomena. This location can be estimated using real time fluoroscopy if there is an indwelling plastic stent in place or by using spot images when the duodenoscope was in its most distal point of insertion.

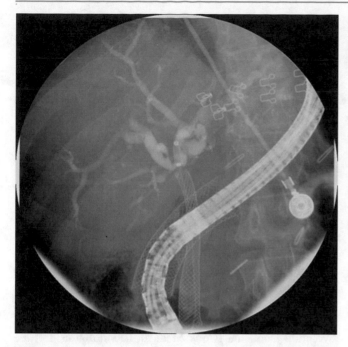

Fig. 8.6   Placement of a biliary SEMS via an enteric SEMS

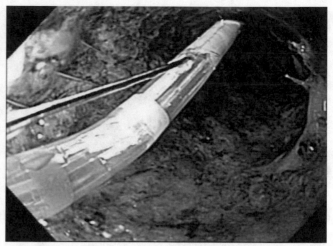

Fig. 8.7   Cannulation of the bile duct through the interstices of a previously placed enteral stent using a sphincterotome (Image courtesy of Douglas G. Adler MD)

Balloon dilation typically to 15 mm inside the stent can be performed to expedite stent expansion and allow passage of the endoscope, although balloon dilation of a stent does increase the risk of perforation [36]. Alternatively, one can give the stent 48–72 h to spontaneously expand and then perform the ERCP portion of the procedure at a separate endoscopic session. It is possible to pass the duodenoscope through a duodenal SEMS in 98 % cases 24 h after the stent was placed without needing balloon dilation [10] (Fig. 8.6). If there is overlap of the sent over the papilla, techniques to access the papilla do exist and are discussed below.

Type II: This is the most challenging configuration of the combined biliary and enteric strictures. The papilla is typically distorted or in many cases not identifiable due to periampullary tumor invasion. In cases where the papilla can be visualized, difficulty accessing it can be a challenge as luminal narrowing limits the maneuverability of the duodenoscope and accessories. When encountering a Type II obstruction, dedicated attempts at standard biliary cannulation and biliary SEMS placement should be pursued. If this is successful then an enteral stent can be placed immediately after. Given that the enteral stent will cross the periampullary region, it would be expected that the biliary SEMS will drain through the side holes of the uncovered enteral stent (Video 8.1).

In situations where standard ERCP cannot be performed, then alternate biliary access techniques will need to be considered. In cases of failed ERCP, there are a number of options to manage this situation. A standard enteral stent can be placed across the stricture, with the understanding that

this crosses the periampullary region. The endoscopist can then attempt to perform standard ERCP through the enteral stent [37]. While this can be attempted at the same session, it is our practice to wait 24–48 h to allow the enteral stent to fully expand and situate itself, thus minimizing the risk of stent migration once the ERCP scope is inserted. Once the duodenal stent is in place, it may be possible to identify the papilla through the interstices of the stent. If that is the case there are a number of different techniques to facilitate ERCP and passage of the biliary SEMS through the interstices (Fig. 8.7). If cannulation can be achieved, a biliary dilating balloon can be used to dilate the metallic mesh to allow for easier passage of the biliary SEMS. Besides dilating the mesh, physical holes can be created in the mesh using a rat tooth foreign body forceps (Olympus FG-42L-1) [10].

Argon plasma coagulation (ICC 200/APC300; ERBE USA, Atlanta, GA) using a standard end-fire APC probe has been described to create an access hole in the enteral SEMS [38, 39]. The APC is set at a power of 99 W and argon flow 1.0 L/min has been used to create a hole in the stent by placing the probe directly against the stent with care to avoid direct contact with the papilla. The endoscope tip should be deflected against the contralateral wall to try to lift the enteral stent off the medial wall. Once the duodenal stent is adequately fenestrated, ERCP can be performed with placement of a biliary SEMS. In addition to the mechanical means of creating more room in the interstices of the stent, a new duodenal uncovered SEMS (BONASTENT M-DUODENAL; Standard Sci-Tech Inc, Seoul, South Korea) was developed specifically for this indication. The central portion of the stent has a cross-wired unfixed portion in the central 3 cm to facilitate biliary cannulation through the stent with a reported efficacy rate of 87.5 % in cannulation and placement of a biliary SEMS through this specific duodenal SEMS [40]. It

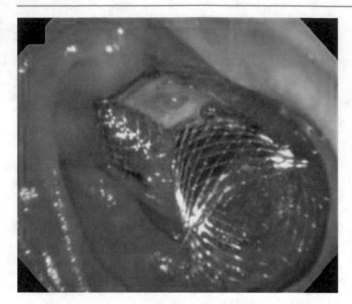

Fig. 8.8 Type III bilioduodenal stricture. The biliary SEMS was placed first followed by enteral SEMS to avoid overlap of the papilla by the enteral SEMS

is noted that this duodenal stent is not currently FDA approved in the United States.

If the papilla cannot be visualized or accessed following placement of the enteral stent, there are a number of different approaches for biliary access including EUS-guided or percutaneous as discussed below.

Type III: Due to the location of the duodenal stricture being distal to the papilla, type III strictures are considered the easiest to remediate. As is seen in Fig. 8.1, the tumor often arises from the uncinate process, thus extending in an inferior fashion and resulting in a distal duodenal obstruction (D2 or D3). The decision of which stent to place first is not critical given that they are removed from each other. Typically, we perform the ERCP portion first followed by the enteral stent to ensure that there is no overlap of the enteral stent over the papilla (Fig. 8.8).

Clinical Outcomes

There have been a number of single center case series that have evaluated the clinical effectiveness, patency rates and associated complications following combined biliary and duodenal stenting without requiring EUS assisted biliary drainage. A Korean group retrospectively evaluated 24 patients who underwent combined stenting [8]. They reported a technical success rate of 100 % in relieving both obstructions; however, 11 patients (45 %) required percutaneous drainage via a percutaneous transhepatic catheter (PTC) followed by biliary SEMS placement via the PTC tract. All the patients in their cohort were able tolerate an oral

diet 2.7 ± 1.2 days following duodenal stent placement. Another group reported success in 17 out of 18 patients presenting with simultaneous obstruction [9]. Mutignani et al., who developed the original bilioduodenal stricture classification, reported that the type of stricture was predictive of success in a cohort of 64 patients with 100 % of Type I and III being able to be remediated while only 86 % in Type II [10]. In this series, only 10 % of patients needed percutaneous biliary drainage.

Enteral Stent Placement

The enteral stent that is chosen should be long enough to have a 2 cm margin at both the proximal and distal end. In addition, most enteral SEMS typically foreshorten by 25 % after deployment, so this should be taken into consideration as well [25, 36, 41]. The Wallflex Duodenal, Wallstent Enteral (Boston Scientific/Microvasive, Natick, MA) and Evolution Duodenal (Cook Medical, Bloomington, IN) are the currently available enteral stents that have approval for palliation of malignant gastric outlet obstruction in the USA; all enteral stents available in the USA are uncovered, and thus considered permanent [42, 43].

Once the appropriate SEMS is chosen, a guidewire, usually in a biliary catheter, is advanced across the stricture under direct endoscopic visualization and fluoroscopy. Once guidewire access to the distal small bowel has been achieved, the catheter can be exchanged over the wire for the stent itself. Enteral stents are currently all of the distal release variety. Visualization of the proximal end of the stent should be maintained endoscopically to ensure that there is an adequate coverage of the stricture. When deployed, a goal should be to center the stent around the stricture, recognizing that some eccentricity is clinically acceptable in most patients. If necessary, additional stents can be placed in a stent-within-stent fashion to extend distal coverage.

Alternative Biliary Access Techniques

In the event that one cannot achieve biliary access as is most common in type II strictures, there are a number of alternative approaches for biliary drainage including endoscopic ultrasound guided-biliary drainage (EUS-BD), surgical bypass and percutaneous drainage. ERCP for biliary decompression secondary to malignant disease is successful in greater than 75 % of the cases; however, a simultaneous duodenal obstruction is an acknowledged risk factor for failed ERCP [44]. Because of that risk, endoscopists should be aware of the risk for failure and knowledgeable of alternative techniques. The most commonly recommended step following any failed ERCP is a repeat attempt by another endoscopist at a high volume center [45]. Following that, the optimal approach to biliary drainage should be considered on a patient by patient basis in the context of the expertise of the endoscopist.

Percutaneous Approach

Biliary drainage can be achieved in consultation with an interventional radiologist via percutaneous transhepatic cholangiography (PTC). This technique predates ERCP and was the historical preferred method for biliary drainage [46]. Traditional PTC is performed using ultrasound assistance to cannulate peripheral biliary radicles after a percutaneous puncture followed by fluoroscopic guided wire manipulation. Once biliary access is gained, an external drain can be placed that allows for upstream (relative to the malignant obstruction) biliary drainage into an external drainage bag [47]. While the percutaneous approach is highly successful (greater than 95 %) in relieving the obstruction, there is a reported complication rate of 8–33 % along with a quality of life issue related to having an external drainage device [48–50].

Alternatively, it is possible to place an internal biliary drain across the obstruction into the duodenum in an anterograde fashion using the initial PTC access with reported success rates of 90 %. This can be done with an enteral stent in place. Unfortunately, many catheter exchanges can be required using this approach, often necessitating multiple procedure sessions to obtain an adequate sized drain [51, 52]. Lastly, many experienced interventional radiology departments are now able to offer antegrade placement of metal biliary stents, thus eliminating the need for an external drainage tube or collection bag.

Because of the technical demand with increased risk for complication of placing an internal drain via a PTC tract, the rendezvous technique was developed. In this technique, PTC is performed with fluoroscopic guided wire placement across the papilla in an anterograde fashion. The wire which will come through the interstices of the previously placed enteral stent is then grasped using a polypectomy snare withdrawn into the accessory channel. ERCP is then performed in the normal fashion with over-the-wire cannulation [53, 54].

Endoscopic Ultrasound Guided Biliary Drainage

EUS guided cholangiopancreatography (EUCP) was first described in 1996 and since then has been well established as an alternative technique to obtain biliary access in the setting of a failed cannulation [55]. The procedure can be performed either by a single skilled operator or by two endoscopists with individual expertise in ERCP and interventional EUS. EUS-BD can be performed through a rendezvous technique via transgastric or transduodenal routes or creation of a choledochoduodenostomy or hepaticogastrostomy as described below [56]. It must be noted that EUS-BD is a technically challenging procedure with higher complication rates compared to ERCP and should only be performed by an experienced endoscopist in a tertiary center with appropriate surgical and radiological support in the event of a complication [57, 58].

EUS-BD with a rendezvous technique is similar in idea to the PTC rendezvous but utilizes endoscopic ultrasound to obtain biliary access. This technique requires access to the papilla and is possible to perform through a previously placed enteral stent [37, 59, 60]. The curved linear array echoendoscope positioned in the antrum or the duodenum and utilized to visualize the bile duct. A 19 or 22 gauge fine needle aspiration (FNA) needle is used to puncture the bile duct either as a transgastric approach into the intrahepatic portion of the duct or a transduodenal puncture into the extrahepatic portion of the duct. The intrahepatic puncture is performed with the echoendoscope positioned in the cardia or the lesser curvature of the stomach allowing for visualization of the left intrahepatic duct system. The extrahepatic puncture is performed from the duodenum or distal antrum. Following puncture, aspiration is performed to confirm ductal access and then a cholangiogram is performed using a contrast injection. A long hydrophilic ERCP wire (0.18–0.35 in.) is advanced in an anterograde fashion across the stricture and across the papilla. Excess wire should be passed across the papilla so as to ensure the wire will maintain position. At this point, the echoendoscope is removed and replaced with a duodenoscope allowing for capture of the papillary end of the wire with a snare. The wire is withdrawn into the duodenoscope via the working channel, ultimately allowing for over-the-wire cannulation. There is a reported success rate of 50–100 % in obtaining biliary drainage using this technique [61–66]. Complications include perforation, pneumoperitoneum and bile leaks but at a low rate (4 %) compared to the other EUS-BD techniques [66].

EUS-guided choledochoduodenostomy (EUS-CD) was first described in 2001 and involves the creation of a biliary enteric fistula to allow for biliary drainage upstream of the malignant obstruction [67]. The echoendoscope is position in the duodenal bulb and the bile duct is punctured in the extrahepatic portion using a 19 or 22 gauge FNA needle with bile aspiration and contrast injection to confirm location. Following biliary access, a guidewire is advanced into the intrahepatic portion of the bile duct under fluoroscopy. In order to facilitate placement of a stent across the newly choledochoduodenostomy tract, various dilation accessories are used. These include use of biliary dilating balloons (typically 4–6 mm), and/or the use of bougie-type dilating catheters (typically to 6 Fr). Following tract dilation, stent placement is then performed. Choice of stent may include the use of straight plastic biliary stents, partially covered biliary SEMS, fully covered biliary SEMS, or some combination thereof. Biliary SEMS have gained popularity given their relatively larger diameter and favorable patency rates compared to plastic stents. One caveat is that there may be a high migration rate when placing a covered biliary SEMS across the choledochoduodenostomy tract. The use of a partially covered biliary SEMS may improve stent anchoring. In addition, some practitioners will place a double pigtail biliary stent through the biliary SEMS as a way to minimize risk of migration. EUS-CD has a reported much higher success rate in obtaining biliary drainage 80–100 % compared to the EUS rendezvous technique but with a higher complication rate of approximately 15 % [68–71].

EUS-guided hepaticogastrostomy (EUS-HG) was first described in 2003 and is similar in many ways to EUS-CD in that a biliary enteral fistula is created to allow upstream drainage [72]. In this technique, the echoendoscope is position in the stomach in the cardia or along the lesser curvature with puncture into the left intrahepatic system. The remainder of the technique is similar to EUS-CD. Because biliary puncture occurs in the stomach, EUS-guided hepaticogastrostomy can be performed independent of the enteric stent or in cases of altered anatomy. Success rates for biliary drainage are high 90–100 % but again at the expense of increased complication rates of 14–18 % including pneumoperitoneum, bile leak, cholangitis and stent migration [64, 68, 73–75].

In both the EUS-CD and EUS-HG technique, the original description was for placement of a stent across the fistula tract. However, the techniques have also advanced to allow for placement of a SEMS across the papilla in an anterograde fashion for downstream biliary drainage. Biliary access is obtained as described above and the wire is preferentially placed anterograde across the papilla under fluoroscopy. The puncture tract is dilated followed by biliary dilation of the stricture with either rigid or balloon dilators. Following dilation, a SEMS is placed across the stricture in a position that is comparable to stent placement in conventional ERCP. EUS guided anterograde placement of a transpapillary stent has been reported to be successful in 86–100 % of patients who had previously failed conventional ERCP in obtaining biliary drainage with a complication rate of 10.5 % including bleeding, cholangitis and perforation [23, 76].

When EUCP techniques are needed for biliary access, the success rates drop compared to conventional ERCP. In the largest EUCP series, by very experienced providers, success of the intrahepatic approach to obtain biliary access is 83 % and the extrahepatic approach is 86 % [77]. A pooled analysis of all EUCP studies report a success rate of 87 % in achieving biliary drainage [57]. Similar to traditional ERCP, the plastic stent used in the CDS or HGS tract can become obstructed. A multicenter series in Japan reports a 3 month patency rate of 80 % for EUS-CD and 50 % for EUS-HG [58]. It should be

noted that the majority of these studies were not exclusively performed in patients with simultaneous obstruction but rather failed ERCP so the reported success rate may not accurately reflect this particular presentation.

Surgical Bypass

Surgical biliary bypass, a choledochojejunostomy or a choledochoduodenostomy typically concurrently with a gastrojejunostomy, is highly effective (76–100 %) in obtaining biliary decompression in metastatic noncurable disease. In a meta-analysis comparing surgical bypass to endoscopic management, there was no difference in efficacy or mortality (malignancy driven) between surgery and endoscopy. However, surgery was associated with longer hospital stays (21.8 days vs. 14.6 days, $p=0.026$) and increased complication rates (39 % vs. 21.2 %, $p=0.1$) [17, 78]. In addition, many of these patients are deemed to be not operative candidates given their associated comorbidities and limited life expectancy.

For patients presenting with a simultaneous enteral and biliary obstruction, we propose the following management algorithm (Fig. 8.9):

Complications

One of the major challenges in managing patients with a combined obstruction is stent patency due to the progressive ingrowth of tumor. One group reported a median time of duodenal stent patency was 41.5 days (range, 6–371) and that of biliary stent was 110 days (rage, 30–1054). Other groups have reported lower rates of stent occlusion. Given the limited life expectancy of 12 weeks after presenting with a combined bilioduodenal obstruction perhaps the issue of stent occlusion is less important. Additional, a high majority of patients with tumor ingrowth could be endoscopically or percutaneously managed [79]. Other complications reported include cholangitis in the setting of biliary instrumentation and biliary stent occlusion, bleeding from sphincterotomy and post ERCP pancreatitis. Stent migration is a known complication with enteral stenting; however, perhaps due to the malignant obstruction this complication is very rarely reported in this indication [13]. Of note, there have been no reported mortalities in the setting of combined enteral and biliary stenting.

As discussed earlier, performance of biliary access via EUCP has its own set of complications reported at 10.5–20 % which is higher than traditional transpapillary approach [23, 57]. These complications include pneumoperitoneum which can be managed conservatively in the majority of cases, bleeding, pancreatitis, bile leak and perforations requiring surgery. As such, EUCP should only be performed by experienced endoscopists in both EUS and ERCP. A

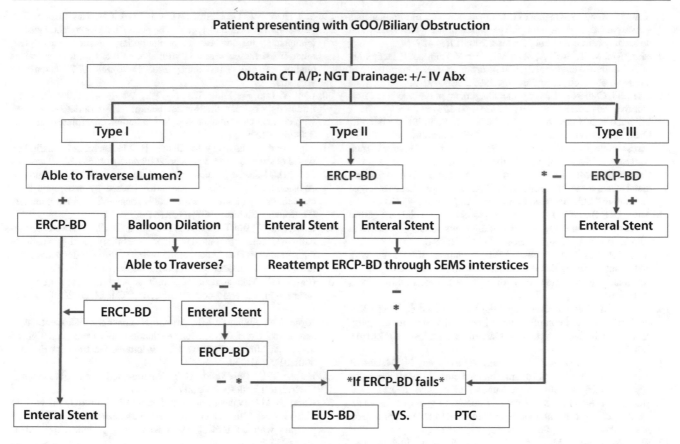

Fig. 8.9 Proposed flow diagram for endoscopic management

recent international meeting suggested that this procedure should only be attempted by endoscopists regularly performing pancreaticobiliary EUS at a high volume (200–300 EUS and ERCPs per year) with over 4 years' experience in a tertiary care environment, but this is just a suggestion [80].

Conclusion

Simultaneous biluoduodenal obstruction is a common presentation in advanced pancreaticobiliary and gastric cancers predicting a high short-term mortality. Patients will present with symptoms of nausea, vomiting, abdominal pain, jaundice, and possibly cholangitis. Endoscopic management is safe and both clinically and cost effective compared to surgical bypass. Occasionally consultation with interventional radiology assistance for PTC when ERCP fails is necessary; however, this may be increasingly rare as centers become more familiar with EUCP biliary drainage.

Video Legend
Video 8.1 Endoscopic management of combined malignant biliary obstruction and gastric outlet obstruction (MPG 182,006 kb).

References

1. Connolly MM, Dawson PJ, Michelassi F, Moossa AR, Lowenstein F. Survival in 1001 patients with carcinoma of the pancreas. Ann Surg. 1987;206(3):366–73.
2. Mosler P, Mergener KD, Brandabur JJ, Schembre DB, Kozarek RA. Palliation of gastric outlet obstruction and proximal small bowel obstruction with self-expandable metal stents: a single center series. J Clin Gastroenterol. 2005;39(2):124–8.
3. Nevitt AW, Vida F, Kozarek RA, Traverso LW, Raltz SL. Expandable metallic prostheses for malignant obstructions of gastric outlet and proximal small bowel. Gastrointest Endosc. 1998;47(3):271–6.
4. Burkill GJ, Badran M, Al-Muderis O, Meirion Thomas J, Judson IR, Fisher C, et al. Malignant gastrointestinal stromal tumor: distribution, imaging features, and pattern of metastatic spread 1. Radiology. 2003;226(2):527–32.
5. Hirano K, Tada M, Isayama H, Yagioka H, Sasaki T, Kogure H, et al. Long-term prognosis of autoimmune pancreatitis with and without corticosteroid treatment. Gut. 2007;56(12):1719–24.
6. Horton KM, Lawler LP, Fishman EK. CT findings in sclerosing mesenteritis (panniculitis): spectrum of disease 1. Radiographics. 2003;23(6):1561–7.
7. Cappell MS, Davis M. Characterization of Bouveret's syndrome: a comprehensive review of 128 cases. Am J Gastroenterol. 2006;101(9):2139–46.
8. Kim KO, Kim TN, Lee HC. Effectiveness of combined biliary and duodenal stenting in patients with malignant biliary and duodenal obstruction. Scand J Gastroenterol. 2012;47(8-9):962–7.

9. Kaw M, Singh S, Gagneja H. Clinical outcome of simultaneous self-expandable metal stents for palliation of malignant biliary and duodenal obstruction. Surg Endosc. 2003;17(3):457–61.

10. Mutignani M, Tringali A, Shah SG, Perri V, Familiari P, Iacopini F, et al. Combined endoscopic stent insertion in malignant biliary and duodenal obstruction. Endoscopy. 2007;39(5):440–7.

11. Sarr MG, Cameron JL. Surgical management of unresectable carcinoma of the pancreas. Surgery. 1982;91(2):123–33.

12. Lillemoe KD, Cameron JL, Hardacre JM, Sohn TA, Sauter PK, Coleman J, et al. Is prophylactic gastrojejunostomy indicated for unresectable periampullary cancer? A prospective randomized trial. Ann Surg. 1999;230(3):322–8. discussion 328–30.

13. Dormann A, Meisner S, Verin N, Wenk Lang A. Self-expanding metal stents for gastroduodenal malignancies: systematic review of their clinical effectiveness. Endoscopy. 2004;36(6):543–50.

14. Adler DG, Baron TH. Endoscopic palliation of malignant gastric outlet obstruction using self-expanding metal stents: experience in 36 patients. Am J Gastroenterol. 2002;97(1):72–8.

15. Holt AP, Patel M, Ahmed MM. Palliation of patients with malignant gastroduodenal obstruction with self-expanding metallic stents: the treatment of choice? Gastrointest Endosc. 2004; 60(6):1010–7.

16. Kahaleh M, Tokar J, Conaway MR, Brock A, Le T, Adams RB, et al. Efficacy and complications of covered Wallstents in malignant distal biliary obstruction. Gastrointest Endosc. 2005;61(4): 528–33.

17. Andersen JR, Sorensen SM, Kruse A, Rokkjaer M, Matzen P. Randomised trial of endoscopic endoprosthesis versus operative bypass in malignant obstructive jaundice. Gut. 1989;30(8):1132–5.

18. Siddiqui A, Spechler SJ, Huerta S. Surgical bypass versus endoscopic stenting for malignant gastroduodenal obstruction: a decision analysis. Dig Dis Sci. 2007;52(1):276–81.

19. Wong Y, Brams D, Munson L, Sanders L, Heiss F, Chase M, et al. Gastric outlet obstruction secondary to pancreatic cancer. Surg Endosc. 2002;16(2):310–2.

20. Bottger T, Menke H, Zech J, Junginger T. Risks and follow-up of choledocho-jejunostomy for nonresectable cancers of the head of the pancreas. A prospective study. Chirurg. 1992;63(5):416–20.

21. Lillemoe KD, Pitt HA. Palliation: surgical and otherwise. Cancer. 1996;78(S3):605–14.

22. Kuriansky J, Saenz A, Astudillo E, Cardona V, Fernandez-Cruz L. Simultaneous laparoscopic biliary and retrocolic gastric bypass in patients with unresectable carcinoma of the pancreas. Surg Endosc. 2000;14(2):179–81.

23. Shah JN, Marson F, Weilert F, Bhat YM, Nguyen-Tang T, Shaw RE, et al. Single-operator, single-session EUS-guided anterograde cholangiopancreatography in failed ERCP or inaccessible papilla. Gastrointest Endosc. 2012;75(1):56–64.

24. Brimhall B, Adler DG. Enteral stents for malignant gastric outlet obstruction. Gastrointest Endosc Clin N Am. 2011;21(3):389–403. vii–viii.

25. Telford JJ, Carr-Locke DL, Baron TH, Tringali A, Parsons WG, Gabbrielli A, et al. Palliation of patients with malignant gastric outlet obstruction with the enteral Wallstent: outcomes from a multicenter study. Gastrointest Endosc. 2004;60(6):916–20.

26. Singh SM, Longmire Jr WP, Reber HA. Surgical palliation for pancreatic cancer. The UCLA experience. Ann Surg. 1990;212(2): 132–9.

27. Ballinger AB, McHugh M, Catnach SM, Alstead EM, Clark ML. Symptom relief and quality of life after stenting for malignant bile duct obstruction. Gut. 1994;35(4):467–70.

28. Shepherd H, Royle G, Ross A, Diba A, Arthur M, Colin-Jones D. Endoscopic biliary endoprosthesis in the palliation of malignant obstruction of the distal common bile duct: a randomized trial. Br J Surg. 1988;75(12):1166–8.

29. Van Heek NT, De Castro SM, van Eijck CH, van Geenen RC, Hesselink EJ, Breslau PJ, et al. The need for a prophylactic gastrojejunostomy for unresectable periampullary cancer: a prospective randomized multicenter trial with special focus on assessment of quality of life. Ann Surg. 2003;238(6):894–902. discussion 902–905.

30. Lam Y, Lau JY, Fung TM, Ng EK, Wong SK, Sung JJ, et al. Endoscopic balloon dilation for benign gastric outlet obstruction with or without Helicobacter pylori infection. Gastrointest Endosc. 2004;60(2):229–33.

31. Ripamonti CI, Easson AM, Gerdes H. Management of malignant bowel obstruction. Eur J Cancer. 2008;44(8):1105–15.

32. Feretis C, Benakis P, Dimopoulos C, Manouras A, Tsimbloulis B, Apostolidis N. Duodenal obstruction caused by pancreatic head carcinoma: palliation with self-expandable endoprostheses. Gastrointest Endosc. 1997;46(2):161–5.

33. Kikuyama M, Itoi T, Sasada Y, Sofuni A, Ota Y, Itokawa F. Large-balloon technique for one-step endoscopic biliary stenting in patients with an inaccessible major papilla owing to difficult duodenal stricture (with video). Gastrointest Endosc. 2009;70(3):568–72.

34. Baron TH. Management of simultaneous biliary and duodenal obstruction: the endoscopic perspective. Gut Liver. 2010;4 Suppl 1:S50–6.

35. Joyce AM, Kochman ML, Ahmad N, Ginsberg GG. Continuous access technique for dilation, evaluation, and stent palliation of malignant luminal digestive tract strictures. Gastrointest Endosc. 2005;61(5):AB230.

36. Baron TH, Harewood GC. Enteral self-expandable stents. Gastrointest Endosc. 2003;58(3):421–33.

37. Khashab MA, Valeshabad AK, Leung W, Camilo J, Fukami N, Shieh F, et al. Multicenter experience with performance of ERCP in patients with an indwelling duodenal stent. Endoscopy. 2014; 46(3):252–5.

38. Demarquay JF, Dumas R, Peten EP, Rampal P. Argon plasma endoscopic section of biliary metallic prostheses. Endoscopy. 2001; 33(3):289–90.

39. Topazian M, Baron TH. Endoscopic fenestration of duodenal stents using argon plasma to facilitate ERCP. Gastrointest Endosc. 2009;69(1):166–9.

40. Moon JH, Choi HJ, Ko BM, Koo HC, Hong SJ, Cheon YK, et al. Combined endoscopic stent-in-stent placement for malignant biliary and duodenal obstruction by using a new duodenal metal stent (with videos). Gastrointest Endosc. 2009;70(4):772–7.

41. Kochar R, Shah N. Enteral stents: from esophagus to colon. Gastrointest Endosc. 2013;78(6):913–8.

42. Varadarajulu S, Banerjee S, Barth B, Desilets D, Kaul V, Kethu S, et al. Enteral stents. Gastrointest Endosc. 2011;74(3):455–64.

43. Simmons DT, Baron TH. Technology insight: enteral stenting and new technology. Nat Clin Pract Gastroenterol Hepatol. 2005;2(8): 365–74.

44. van der Gaag NA, Rauws EA, van Eijck CH, Bruno MJ, van der Harst E, Kubben FJ, et al. Preoperative biliary drainage for cancer of the head of the pancreas. N Engl J Med. 2010;362(2):129–37.

45. Choudari C, Sherman S, Fogel EL, Phillips S, Kochell A, Flueckiger J, et al. Success of ERCP at a referral center after a previously unsuccessful attempt. Gastrointest Endosc. 2000;52(4):478–83.

46. Carter RF, Saypol GM. Transabdominal cholangiography. JAMA. 1952;148(4):253–5.

47. Burke DR, Lewis CA, Cardella JF, Citron SJ, Drooz AT, Haskal ZJ, et al. Quality improvement guidelines for percutaneous transhepatic cholangiography and biliary drainage. J Vasc Interv Radiol. 1997;8(4):677–81.

48. Morita S, Kitanosono T, Lee D, Syed L, Butani D, Holland G, et al. Comparison of technical success and complications of percutaneous transhepatic cholangiography and biliary drainage between

patients with and without transplanted liver. Am J Roentgenol. 2012;199(5):1149–52.

49. Beissert M, Wittenberg G, Sandstede J, Beer M, Tschammler A, Burghardt W, et al. Metallic stents and plastic endoprostheses in percutaneous treatment of biliary obstruction. Z Gastroenterol. 2002;40(7):503–10.

50. Oh HC, Lee SK, Lee TY, Kwon S, Lee SS, Seo DW, et al. Analysis of percutaneous transhepatic cholangioscopy-related complications and the risk factors for those complications. Endoscopy. 2007;39(8):731–6.

51. Mendez Jr G, Russell E, Levi JU, Koolpe H, Cohen M. Percutaneous brush biopsy and internal drainage of biliary tree through endopros-thesis. AJR Am J Roentgenol. 1980;134(4):653–9.

52. Hellekant C, Jonsson K, Genell S. Percutaneous internal drainage in obstructive jaundice. AJR Am J Roentgenol. 1980;134(4): 661–4.

53. Calvo MM, Bujanda L, Heras I, Cabriada JL, Bernal A, Orive V, et al. The rendezvous technique for the treatment of choledocholi-thiasis. Gastrointest Endosc. 2001;54(4):511–3.

54. Robertson D, Hacking C, Birch S, Ayres R, Shepherd H, Wright R. Experience with a combined percutaneous and endoscopic approach to stent insertion in malignant obstructive jaundice. Lancet. 1987;330(8573):1449–52.

55. Wiersema MJ, Sandusky D, Carr R, Wiersema LM, Erdel WC, Frederick PK. Endosonography-guided cholangiopancreatography. Gastrointest Endosc. 1996;43(2):102–6.

56. Yamao K, Hara K, Mizuno N, Sawaki A, Hijioka S, Niwa Y, et al. EUS-guided biliary drainage. Gut Liver. 2010;4 Suppl 1:S67–75.

57. Shami VM, Kahaleh M. Endoscopic ultrasound-guided cholangio-pancreatography and rendezvous techniques. Dig Liver Dis. 2010;42(6):419–24.

58. Kawakubo K, Isayama H, Kato H, Itoi T, Kawakami H, Hanada K, et al. Multicenter retrospective study of endoscopic ultrasound-guided biliary drainage for malignant biliary obstruction in Japan. J Hepatobiliary Pancreat Sci. 2014;21(5):328–34.

59. Belletrutti PJ, Gerdes H, Schattner MA. Successful endoscopic ultrasound-guided transduodenal biliary drainage through a pre-existing duodenal stent. JOP. 2010;11(3):234–6.

60. Khashab MA, Fujii LL, Baron TH, Canto MI, Gostout CJ, Petersen BT, et al. EUS-guided biliary drainage for patients with malignant biliary obstruction with an indwelling duodenal stent (with videos). Gastrointest Endosc. 2012;76(1):209–13.

61. Mallery S, Matlock J, Freeman ML. EUS-guided rendezvous drain-age of obstructed biliary and pancreatic ducts: report of 6 cases. Gastrointest Endosc. 2004;59(1):100–7.

62. Lai R, Freeman ML. Endoscopic ultrasound-guided bile duct access for rendezvous ERCP drainage in the setting of intradiver-ticular papilla. Endoscopy. 2005;37(5):487–9.

63. Kahaleh M, Wang P, Shami VM, Tokar J, Yeaton P. EUS-guided transhepatic cholangiography: report of 6 cases. Gastrointest Endosc. 2005;61(2):307–13.

64. Will U, Thieme A, Fueldner F, Gerlach R, Wanzar I, Meyer F. Treatment of biliary obstruction in selected patients by endo-scopic ultrasonography (EUS)-guided transluminal biliary drain-age. Endoscopy. 2007;39(4):292–5.

65. Tarantino I, Barresi L, Repici A, Traina M. EUS-guided biliary drainage: a case series. Endoscopy. 2008;40(4):336–9.

66. Kim YS, Gupta K, Mallery S, Li R, Kinney T, Freeman ML. Endoscopic ultrasound rendezvous for bile duct access using a transduodenal approach: cumulative experience at a single center. A case series. Endoscopy. 2010;42(6):496–502.

67. Giovannini M, Moutardier V, Pesenti C, Bories E, Lelong B, Delpero JR. Endoscopic ultrasound-guided bilioduodenal anasto-mosis: a new technique for biliary drainage. Endoscopy. 2001;33(10):898–900.

68. Park DH, Koo JE, Oh J, Lee YH, Moon S, Lee SS, et al. EUS-guided biliary drainage with one-step placement of a fully covered metal stent for malignant biliary obstruction: a prospective feasibil-ity study. Am J Gastroenterol. 2009;104(9):2168–74.

69. Itoi T, Itokawa F, Sofuni A, Kurihara T, Tsuchiya T, Ishii K, et al. Endoscopic ultrasound-guided choledochoduodenostomy in patients with failed endoscopic retrograde cholangiopancreatogra-phy. World J Gastroenterol. 2008;14(39):6078–82.

70. Hara K, Yamao K, Niwa Y, Sawaki A, Mizuno N, Hijioka S, et al. Prospective clinical study of EUS-guided choledochoduodenos-tomy for malignant lower biliary tract obstruction. Am J Gastroenterol. 2011;106(7):1239–45.

71. Hanada K, Iiboshi T, Ishii Y. Endoscopic ultrasound-guided choledochoduodenostomy for palliative biliary drainage in cases with inoperable pancreas head carcinoma. Dig Endosc. 2009; 21(s1):S75–8.

72. Burmester E, Niehaus J, Leinweber T, Huetteroth T. EUS-cholangio-drainage of the bile duct: report of 4 cases. Gastrointest Endosc. 2003;57(2):246–51.

73. Park DH. Endoscopic ultrasonography-guided hepaticogastros-tomy. Gastrointest Endosc Clin N Am. 2012;22(2):271–80.

74. Bories E, Pesenti C, Caillol F, Lopes C, Giovannini M. Transgastric endoscopic ultrasonography-guided biliary drainage: results of a pilot study. Endoscopy. 2007;39(4):287–91.

75. Ramirez-Luna MA, Tellez-Avila FI, Giovannini M, Valdovinos-Andraca F, Guerrero-Hernandez I, Herrera-Esquivel J. Endoscopic ultrasound-guided biliodigestive drainage is a good alternative in patients with unresectable cancer. Endoscopy. 2011;43(9):826–30.

76. Nguyen-Tang T, Binmoeller KF, Sanchez-Yague A, Shah JN. Endoscopic ultrasound (EUS)-guided transhepatic anterograde self-expandable metal stent (SEMS) placement across malignant biliary obstruction. Endoscopy. 2010;42(3):232–6.

77. Maranki J, Hernandez AJ, Arslan B, Jaffan AA, Angle JF, Shami VM, et al. Interventional endoscopic ultrasound-guided cholangi-ography: long-term experience of an emerging alternative to percu-taneous transhepatic cholangiography. Endoscopy. 2009;41(6): 532–8.

78. Glazer ES, Hornbrook MC, Krouse RS. A meta-analysis of ran-domized trials: immediate stent placement vs. surgical bypass in the palliative management of malignant biliary obstruction. J Pain Symptom Manage. 2014;47(2):307–14.

79. Yim H, Jacobson B, Saltzman J, Johannes R, Bounds B, Lee J, et al. Clinical outcome of the use of enteral stents for palliation of patients with malignant upper GI obstruction. Gastrointest Endosc. 2001;53(3):329–32.

80. Kahaleh M, Artifon EL, Perez-Miranda M, Gupta K, Itoi T, Binmoeller KF, et al. Endoscopic ultrasonography guided biliary drainage: summary of consortium meeting, May 7th, 2011, Chicago. World J Gastroenterol. 2013;19(9):1372.

Pancreas Divisum and Minor Papilla Interventions

Jay Luther and Brenna W. Casey

Introduction

Pancreas divisum is the most common congenital anomaly of the pancreas and is frequently encountered in clinical practice. The clinical relevance of pancreas divisum is highlighted by its association with acute and chronic pancreatitis. Over the years, endoscopic and surgical therapies aimed at improving dorsal pancreatic duct drainage have been used to treat patients with idiopathic pancreatitis and pancreas divisum. In this chapter, we will provide the most updated review on the epidemiology, diagnosis, and treatment options and success rates for patients with pancreas divisum.

Epidemiology

Pancreas divisum is the most common congenital anomaly of the pancreas, with an estimated prevalence of 4.1–17.9 %. The wide range highlights the importance of method of diagnosis and population studied on the observed prevalence. Dimagno and colleagues performed the most comprehensive systematic review of the epidemiology of pancreas divisum, taking into account the aforementioned factors [1]. They examined the literature which studied the prevalence of pancreas divisum in the general population

(those without pancreatitis) and in patients with pancreatitis using either autopsy, standard magnetic resonance cholangiopancreatogram (MRCP), secretin-stimulated MRCP (s-MRCP) which allows enhanced visualization of the dorsal duct, or endoscopic retrograde cholangiopancreatography (ERCP). In the general population, ERCP studies suggested a prevalence of 4.1 %, whereas S-MRCP revealed an incidence of 17.9 %. The general prevalence of pancreas divisum in autopsy studies was found to be 7.8 %. In comparison, the prevalence of pancreas divisum in patients with pancreatitis is estimated to be 7.6 % and 8.1 %, using ERCP and S-MRCP, respectively (Table 9.1). The discrepancy in prevalence based on patient population (general population versus pancreatitis) is not fully understood and will be discussed in greater detail below (Section "Relationship to Pancreatitis"). Risk factors for the in utero development of pancreas divisum have not been thoroughly studied. There are limited data suggesting patients of Asian descent are less likely to develop divisum, with an estimated incidence of 1–2 % in this population [2, 3].

Pathogenesis

In order to appreciate the pathophysiology leading to pancreas divisum, an understanding of the normal embryonic development of the pancreas is imperative. At 4 weeks gestation the ventral and dorsal pancreas bud off from the duodenum. Over the following 3 weeks, the dorsal pancreas migrates towards the mesentery, while the ventral pancreatic bud adjoins to the common bile duct. Soon thereafter, axial rotation of the intestine leads to parenchymal and ductal fusion of the dorsal and ventral pancreas, with the ventral pancreas representing 2–20 % of the parenchymal mass. Failure of dorsal and ventral pancreatic ducts fusion leads to pancreas divisum.

Multiple variations of pancreas divisum have been reported. In the classic form, the dorsal duct of Santorini drains through the minor papilla, unconnected to the ventral duct of Wirsung,

Electronic supplementary material: The online version of this chapter (doi:10.1007/978-3-319-26854-5_9) contains supplementary material, which is available to authorized users. Videos can also be accessed at http://link.springer.com/chapter/10.1007/978-3-319-26854-5_9.

J. Luther, M.D.
Clinical and Research Fellow, Gastrointestinal Unit, Massachusetts General Hospital, Boston, MA, USA

B.W. Casey, M.D., F.A.S.G.E. (✉)
Interventional Gastroenterology, Endoscopic Training, Harvard Medical School, Blake 453D, 55 Fruit Street, Boston, MA 02114, USA
e-mail: bcasey2@partners.org

© Springer International Publishing Switzerland 2016
D.G. Adler (ed.), *Advanced Pancreaticobiliary Endoscopy*, DOI 10.1007/978-3-319-26854-5_9

135

Table 9.1 Prevalence of pancreas divisum [1]

	Autopsy	MRCP	S-MRCP	ERCP
General population	7.8 % (95 % CI=6.8–8.8)	9.3 % (95 % CI=6.8–11.8)	17.9 % (95 % CI=11.9–24.0)	4.1 % (95 % CI=3.8–4.4)
Pancreatitis	N/A	N/A	8.1 % (95 % CI=4.9–11.4)	7.6 % (95 % CI=7.0–8.3)

N/A not available, *CI* confidence interval, *MRCP* magnetic resonance cholangiopancreatography, *S-MRCP* secretin magnetic resonance cholangio-pancreatography, *ERCP* endoscopic retrograde cholangiopancreatography

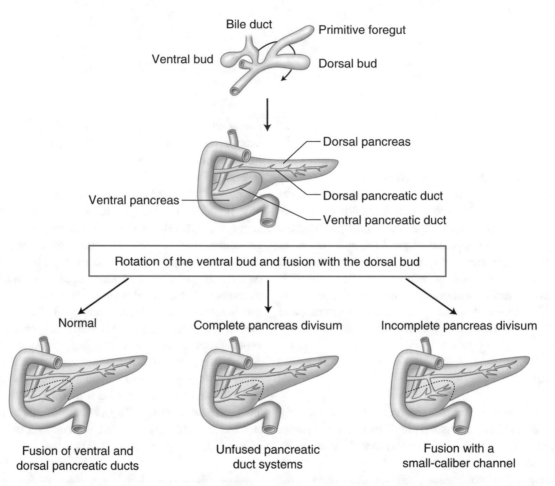

Fig. 9.1 Formation of the normal pancreas and pancreas divisum during embryological development. The schematic illustration above represents the embryological formation of the normal pancreas and abnormalities in this process that lead to the development of pancreas divisum. Reproduced with permission from Springer & Business Media. Kamisawa T. Clinical significance of the minor duodenal papilla and accessory pancreatic duct. *Journal of Gastroenterology* 2004; 39: 606

which drains through the major papilla. In the incomplete form of pancreas divisum, a small branch of the ventral duct communicates with the dorsal duct. The incomplete form represents 15 % of all pancreas divisium cases (Fig. 9.1) [4, 5]. In reverse pancreas divisum, the dorsal duct does not connect with the genu of the main duct but rather, a small segment of dorsal pancreas drains through the minor papilla, while the majority of the pancreas empties through the main pancreatic duct via the major papilla. Unlike the classic and incomplete forms of pancreas divisum, it is thought that reverse divisum has no physiological relevance [1].

Clinical Significance

Clinical Manifestations

The vast majority of patients with pancreas divisum are asymptomatic. In fact, the diagnosis is commonly made incidentally on imaging for a nonpancreatic indication. However, a small percentage of patients with pancreas divisum develop abdominal symptoms, although the causal relationship of pancreas divisum to these symptoms is debated (see section "Relationship to Pancreatitis").

Symptoms typical for acute pancreatitis, including intermittent epigastric pain or more severe pain associated with nausea, vomiting, and fevers, have been reported. Symptoms consistent with chronic pancreatitis, such as pain and diarrhea, also can be seen in patients with pancreas divisum. Chronic abdominal pain in the absence of pancreatic abnormalities has been reported in pancreas divisum patients.

Relationship to Pancreatitis

It must be emphasized that the majority of patients with pancreas divisum do not develop symptoms. However, there appears to be an increased prevalence of pancreas divisum in patients with recurrent acute idiopathic pancreatitis and chronic pancreatitis. There are three potential explanations for this observed clinical association. First, it is possible that pancreas divisum provides the physiologic setting for patients to be at increased risk for pancreatitis. Specifically, the majority of the pancreas drains through the small minor papilla, and during active secretion of enzymes there is a theoretical heightened risk for increased intraductal pressure, which may lead to pancreatitis.

A second potential explanation for the observed association between pancreas divisum and pancreatitis relates to study bias. The majority of studies illustrating an increased prevalence of pancreas divisum in patients with pancreatitis rely on ERCP as the diagnostic method. In fact, the prevalence of pancreas divisum in the general population as diagnosed by autopsy is equal to that of the prevalence in patients with pancreatitis diagnosed at ERCP [1]. This raises the possibility that endoscopists underdiagnose pancreas divisum in the general population, creating the apparent discrepancy between the prevalence rates in the general population and pancreatitis patients in ERCP studies.

Last, there are emerging data showing pancreas divisum is more prevalent in patients with another risk factor for developing pancreas, suggesting pancreas divisum on its own is not sufficient for the development of pancreatitis. For example, Bertin and colleagues studied patients with and without pancreatitis evaluating the incidence of pancreas divisum in these groups [6]. They found that 7 % of patients with either no pancreatic disease (control population) or alcohol-induced pancreatitis had evidence for pancreas divisum as diagnosed by MRCP. A smaller percentage of patients (5 %) with idiopathic pancreatitis had pancreas divisum. Last, and most interesting, 47 % of patients with a genetic mutation in *CFTR* had radiographic evidence for pancreas divisum. Additionally, patients with genetic mutations in *SPINK1* and *PRSS1* had an increased incidence of pancreas divisum than those with no pancreatic disease or with idiopathic pancreatitis. Multiple other studies found similar results, further strengthening this concept that pancreatitis in patients with pancreas divisum

Table 9.2 Conditions associated with pancreas divisum

Recurrent acute idiopathic pancreatitis
Chronic pancreatitis
Chronic abdominal pain
Annular pancreas
Sphincter of Oddi dysfunction
Partial agenesis of the dorsal pancreas

is more frequent when patients already have a genetic predisposition to pancreatitis, and that pancreas divisum itself is not the sole cause of pancreatitis [7–9]. It is possible that the abnormal duct anatomy leading to the majority of the pancreas draining through a small minor papilla, in a patient with viscous pancreatic secretions, as seen in patients with a CFTR mutation, could create the perfect scenario for pancreatitis development.

Association with Other Pancreatic Disorders

Pancreas divisum has been associated with multiple other anomalies of the pancreas (Table 9.2). Perhaps the most common association is with annular pancreas, a condition in which the pancreatic head wraps around the duodenum increasing the susceptibility to duodenal obstruction. Multiple studies have suggested that up to one-half of patients with annular pancreas have co-existing pancreas divisum [10–13]. The most recent study of 40 patients with annular pancreas conducted by Sandrasegaran and colleagues found that 37.5 % also had ERCP evidence for pancreas divisum [10]. Physiologically, this association is not surprising as both, in part, result from abnormalities of in utero rotation of the gut axis. Furthermore, there are data associating pancreas divisum with sphincter of Oddi dysfunction [14] and partial agenesis of the dorsal pancreas [15]. Importantly, there is no association between pancreas divisum and cancer.

Diagnosis

Endoscopic Methods

Endoscopic Retrograde Cholangiopancreatography (ERCP)

The gold standard test for diagnosing pancreas divisum is ERCP. Pancreas divisum is characterized by certain findings on fluoroscopy, which include (1) opacification of the ventral duct with contrast injection through the major papillary, (2) absence of a connection between the ventral and dorsal ducts, (3) absence of ductal anatomy in the body or tail with contrast injection through the major papilla, and (4) opacification of the dorsal duct with contrast injection through the minor papilla (Fig. 9.2).

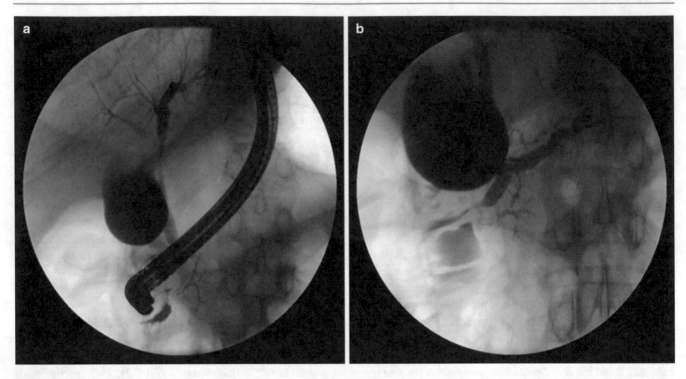

Fig. 9.2 Pancreatogram representing pancreas divisum. (**a**) Cannulation of the major papilla reveals a diminutive ventral duct, (**b**) while cannulation of the minor papilla reveals a dilated dorsal pancre-atic duct with prominence of the side branches. These findings are consistent with pancreas divisum

Cannulation of the minor papilla, required to make the diagnosis via ERCP, can be challenging even for expert endoscopists and may not be technically possible in all patients. Therefore, conditions should be optimized prior to and during endoscopy to enhance the likelihood of successful cannulation. First, the use of general anesthesia, if available, is most appropriate as these procedures tend to be lengthier than standard endoscopic procedures. Second, antispasmodics, such as glucagon, may enhance visualization of the minor papilla and should be considered for use in these procedures. Additionally, maneuvers to aid in minor papilla identification, such as secretin administration (if available) to enhance pancreatic outflow or methylene blue spray on the duodenal wall to contrast the clear pancreatic juice, may offer benefit [16].

Most commonly, the minor papilla is located proximal and anterior (to the right when viewed with a duodenoscope) of the major papilla (i.e., in the right upper quadrant) when en face with the major papilla. In some patients, the minor papilla is best visualized in the "long-scope position" (Fig. 9.3) [16]. It usually lies 2 cm cephalic and anterior to the major papilla. Establishing these landmarks prior to attempted minor papilla cannulation is critical, as the minor papilla may appear only subtly. More rarely, the minor papilla may appear bulging and have a visible orifice. In some patients, the minor papilla may not be identifiable endoscopically.

Once the minor papilla has been identified, it can be cannulated by multiple methods. A needle-tip catheter designed for minor papilla cannulation (ERCP-1-CRAMER) can be very effective; however, it does not allow for guidewire passage but instead dilates the opening of the orifice, after which a catheter with a guidewire can be used (Video 9.1). Alternatively, a 5-Fr catheter (standard or tapered) preloaded with a 0.021, 0.025, or 0.035 in. guidewire can be used to cannulate the minor papilla. Finally, direct cannulation with a 20–25 mm cutting wire pull-type sphincterotome can be very effective. When sphincterotomy is planned, the sphincterotome and guidewire technique are preferable. This approach also allows for cannulation when one is unable to achieve an en face orientation with the minor papilla, as the sphincterotome is able to bow into the correct position. Regardless of the technique used, the guidewire should be passed to the mid-dorsal duct prior to entry of the catheter or sphincterotome in hopes of avoiding trauma-related edema at the papilla.

Endoscopic methods for detecting pathological narrowing of the minor papilla are lacking. An edematous appearance around the papilla may suggest narrowing, although ultimately this provides no objective evidence. Furthermore, normalized values for the basal pressure of the minor papilla have not been established. Accordingly, papillary manometry is not useful to detect pathologic narrowing of the papilla.

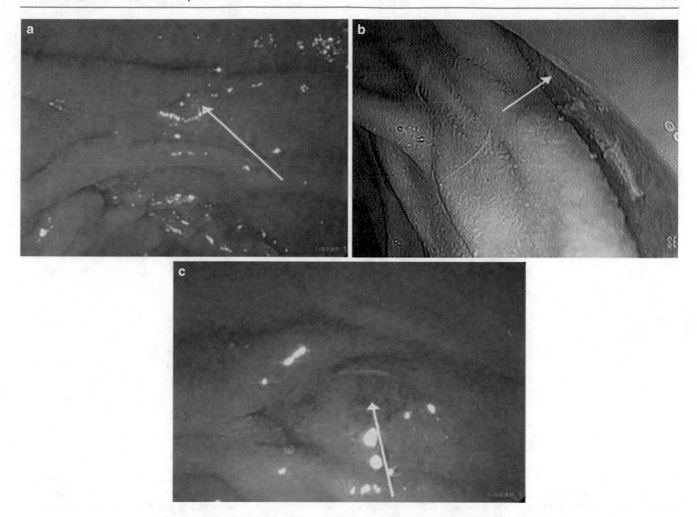

Fig. 9.3 Identification of the minor papilla. (**a**) The minor papilla may be subtle; therefore an understanding of its most common location (proximal and to the right of the major papilla when en face with the major papilla) is critical. (**b** and **c**) represent the minor papilla post-intervention (stenting and sphincterotomy, respectively). The *yellow arrow* in these photographs points to the minor papilla

Finally, some endoscopists suggest subjectively observing the resistance created by the passage of various sized catheters through the papilla may provide insight into the degree of papillary narrowing [1]. This method, however, has not been standardized, is completely subjective to operator impressions and not an actual reference standard, and therefore cannot be recommended.

Although ERCP is the gold standard diagnostic method for pancreas divisum, certain pitfalls associated with ERCP must be recognized. First, complications associated with the procedure, which can include pancreatitis, bleeding, and infection, can be substantial and must be considered. Second, the technical difficulty of accessing the minor papilla and injection of the dorsal duct may increase the risk for complications associated with ERCP. For example, Moffatt and colleagues found the rate of post-ERCP pancreatitis to be 1.2 % if dorsal duct cannulation was not attempted. Contrastingly, patients with pancreas divisum undergoing dorsal duct cannulation with or without minor papillary sphincterotomy experienced much higher rates

of pancreatitis, specifically at a rate of 8.2 % and 10.6 %, respectively [17]. Finally, there are other pancreatic disorders which may mimic pancreas divisum on pancreatography and lead to a false positive result. For example, calcifications and the presence of a fibrotic stricture in the ventral duct and obstruction of the ventral pancreatic duct to malignancy or a pancreatic pseudocyst can produce a similar pancreatogram as is seen in divisum [18, 19].

It must be emphasized that although ERCP is the gold standard diagnostic method for pancreas divisum, it should only be pursued if therapeutic intervention is also planned. Given the risks associated with the procedure, ERCP done for purely diagnostic purposes should be avoided in most cases but can be considered if other diagnostic methods are not available or not appropriate.

Endoscopic Ultrasound

Endoscopic ultrasound (EUS) has also been investigated as a diagnostic tool for pancreas divisum. Bhutani and colleagues illustrated that the absence of the "stack sign," where the bile

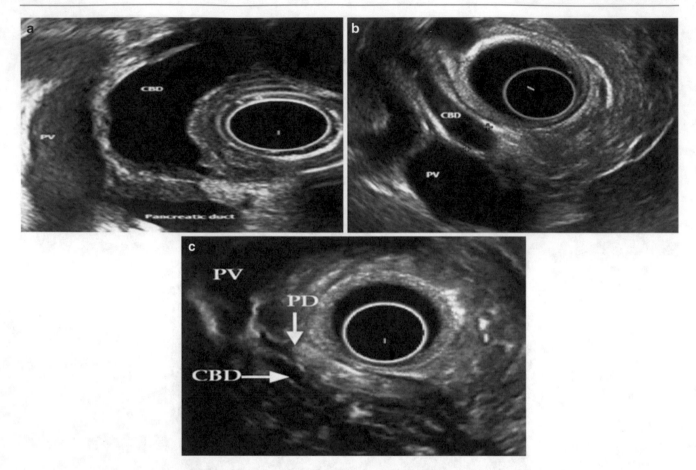

Fig. 9.4 Endoscopic ultrasound in the diagnosis of pancreas divisum. (a) The stack sign, defined by the CBD and PD running in parallel on EUS, is present in a patient with normal PD anatomy. (b) The stack sign is absent, suggesting the possibility of pancreas divisum. (c) The PD crosses the CBD towards the minor papilla, which can be seen in patients with pancreas divisum. CBD: common bile duct; EUS: endoscopic ultrasound; PD: pancreatic duct; PV: portal vein. Images obtained from: Endosc Ultrasound 2013 Jan; 2(1):7–10

duct and the pancreatic duct can be seen to run in parallel through the pancreatic head, indirectly suggests the presence of pancreas divisum [20] (Fig. 9.4). Additionally, Lai and colleagues studied 162 patients and demonstrated linear EUS to have positive and negative predictive values of 86 % and 97 %, respectively, to directly detect pancreas divisum [21]. EUS can also be an effective tool in assisting cannulation of the minor papilla in difficult cases. The main pancreatic duct can be identified and cannulated with a fine-needle aspiration catheter via a transgastric approach. Following cannulation, methylene blue or indigo carmine can be injected into the duct. The echoendoscope is then removed and the duodenoscope is passed into the duodenum. The dye will be visualized passing out of the minor papilla, greatly enhancing its identification. An alternative approach is to pass a 0.018 in. to a 0.035 in. guidewire into the pancreatic duct, using ultrasound guidance, and advance the wire anterograde into the duodenum. Leaving the wire in place, the echoendoscope can be withdrawn and the standard duodenoscope advanced into the duodenum with subsequent identification and removal of the wire. This rendezvous technique allows for passage of a catheter or sphincterotome over the guidewire.

Noninvasive Methods

MRI is the most common noninvasive technique to diagnose pancreas divisum (Fig. 9.5). Conventional MRCP and secretin-enhanced MRCP have been well studied in this clinical setting. Rustagi and colleagues performed a meta-analysis of the available literature comparing the diagnostic accuracy of MRCP to secretin-enhanced MRCP, with ERCP as the criterion standard [22]. They reviewed ten studies that included close to 1500 patients and found that secretin-enhanced MRCP to provide significantly higher diagnostic yield than conventional MRCP. The main drawback to noninvasive imaging is the high interobserver disagreement in the reading of images.

A recent study by Kushnir et al. compared the sensitivity of EUS to multi-detector computer tomography and MRCP for the diagnosis of pancreas divisum [23]. The authors found EUS to have the highest sensitivity of all the diagnostic methods studies, supporting the fact that EUS may offer the most accurate method, outside of ERCP, for the diagnosis of pancreas divisum. The authors, however, did not compare secretin-enhanced MRCP with EUS.

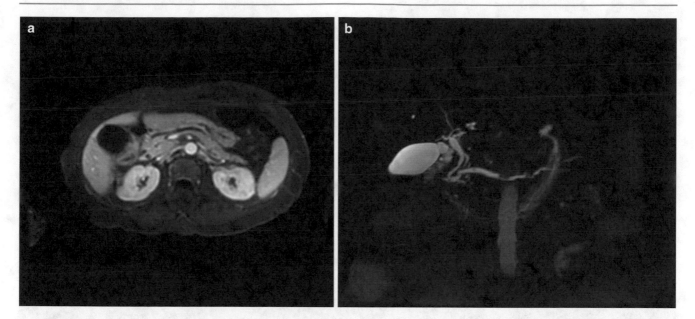

Fig. 9.5 MRI representation of pancreas divisum. (**a**) Cross-section MRI revealed a prominent dorsal duct not in communication with the ventral duct, consistent with pancreas divisum. (**b**) Three-dimensional MRI illustrating a prominent dorsal duct, suggestive of pancreas divisum

As with ERCP, there are no reliable ways to diagnose pathological narrowing of the minor papilla. Findings such as dorsal duct dilation on CT scan or ultrasound, with or without secretin stimulation, have not been rigorously studied. Accordingly, their use in the clinical management of a patient with pancreas divisum remains uncertain.

Treatment

It must be re-emphasized that most patients with pancreas divisum do not develop clinical symptoms, and in the minority that do, the symptoms are likely unrelated to their divisum. Nonetheless, in certain clinical scenarios, therapeutic endoscopic intervention may offer benefit. Therapeutic interventions in patients with symptoms believed to be related to pancreas divisum usually focus on endoscopic sphincterotomy and stenting. Although surgical interventions exist for this condition, their review falls outside the scope of this chapter.

There are multiple techniques available to perform a minor papilla sphincterotomy. One option is to use a pull-type sphincterotome over a guidewire. Once cannulation has been achieved, the sphincterotome should be advanced over the guidewire and through the papilla, with the cutting wire at 10–12 o'clock. Electrocautery settings for minor papilla sphincterotomy are not standardized. Cutting should be initiated by continuous or repeated taps on the foot pedal with the sphincterotome bowed, increasing the exposed cutting space.

Alternative approaches to minor papilla sphincterotomy include using a needle knife over a pancreatic stent and

wire-assisted needle knife. Both techniques involve the use of a needle knife cut, which allows better control of the cut and limits injury to the papillary tissue. When using a pancreatic stent, which can either be straight or with a pigtail at the duodenal end, one must be careful to ensure the pigtail is oriented inferiorly to the minor papilla, as not to interfere with cutting. Sphincterotomy with a needle knife can be performed using pure-cut current at 200 W or ENDO current at 200 W for cut and 20 W for coagulation, but, again, electrocautery settings for this maneuver are not standardized.

Although the role of endotherapy in minimizing symptoms for patients with pancreas divisum has been studied for many years, to date there is only one randomized, controlled study. Lan and colleagues randomized 19 patients with pancreas divisum and at least two episodes of unexplained acute pancreatitis to dorsal duct endotherapy or sham [17]. Specifically, patients in the treatment arm underwent papillary dilation with a graduated Soehendra catheter (4–7 Fr) and dorsal duct stenting (5 or 7 Fr). Stent changes were performed every 4 months up to 1 year. After 1 year, the stents were removed and both groups were followed for around 30 months. Compared to the sham controls, patients who received endotherapy experienced significant reductions in the frequency of pancreatitis, hospitalizations, and severity of pain.

The most common endotherapy for symptomatic pancreas divisum patients is minor papilla sphincterotomy and temporary dorsal duct stent placement (Figs. 9.6 and 9.7). Cotton and colleagues studied the outcomes of 113 patients post-minor papilla sphincterotomy who carried a diagnosis

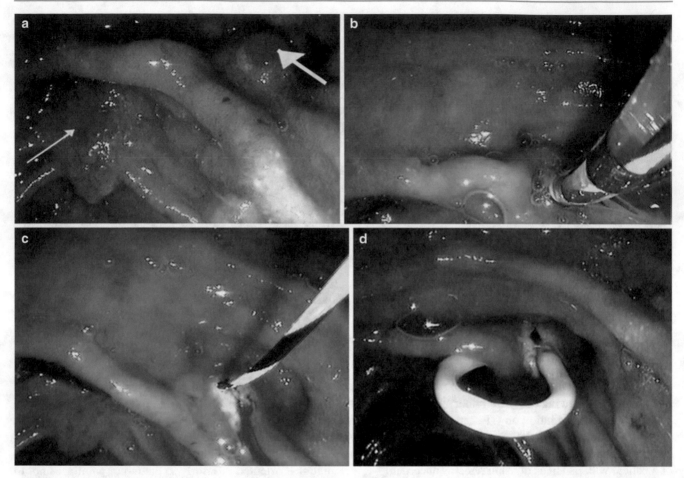

Fig. 9.6 Endoscopic therapy for pancreas divisum using sphincterotomy plus stent placement. (**a**) Major papilla (*thin arrow*); minor papilla (*thick arrow*) which is next to diverticulum. (**b**) Deep cannulation of the dorsal pancreatic duct was accomplished with the short-nosed traction sphincterotome. (**c**) A 5 mm dorsal pancreatic sphincterotomy was made with a monofilament Autotome sphincterotome using ERBE electrocautery. (**d**) One 5 Fr by 5 cm pancreatic stent with a full external pigtail and no internal flaps was placed 4 cm into the dorsal pancreatic duct

of pancreas divisum and recurrent pancreatitis, chronic pancreatitis, or chronic abdominal pain over a course of 5 years, on average [24]. The primary outcome was defined as improvement or resolution of symptoms without need for repeat ERCP or narcotic therapy. The most common endoscopic therapy was a needle-knife sphincterotomy with a temporary dorsal duct stent placement. They found that minor papilla sphincterotomy offered long-term "success" in 53.2 %, 18.2 %, and 41.4 % of patients with recurrent pancreatitis, chronic pancreatitis, and chronic pain, respectively. Complications following ERCP, however, were not trivial, as 12 patients developed pancreatitis, 2 patients had bleeding, and 1 patient suffered an anesthesia-related complication. Their results suggest endotherapy likely offers the most benefit to patients without chronic pancreatitis.

There are multiple technical approaches for sphincterotomy of the minor papilla. The two most commonly employed methods, needle knife cut over a plastic stent and standard pull-type cut using a sphincterotome, appear to be equally effective and safe. Romangnuolo and colleagues retrospec-

tively studied 133 patients who underwent needle-knife sphincterotomy and 51 patients who underwent traditional sphincterotomy and found the need for repeat endoscopic therapy, rates of papillary restenosis, and complications were similar in both groups [25]. Their results suggest both endoscopic techniques are equally effective and safe.

More recently, Yamamoto and colleagues investigated the effect of minor papilla balloon dilation on the clinical outcome of symptomatic pancreas divisum patients (Fig. 9.8) [26]. They suggest, somewhat controversially, that it is easier technically to dilate the minor papilla as opposed to performing a sphincterotomy, because a fixed endoscopic view is not needed for balloon dilation. They retrospectively studied the outcome of 16 patients undergoing balloon dilation and stent placement for symptomatic pancreas divisum and show 81 % of patients improved clinically following therapy. Information regarding the potential adverse effects of balloon dilation of the dorsal duct, including pancreatitis, is not possible given the small nature of the study. If pancreatic duct stenting is very prolonged, it

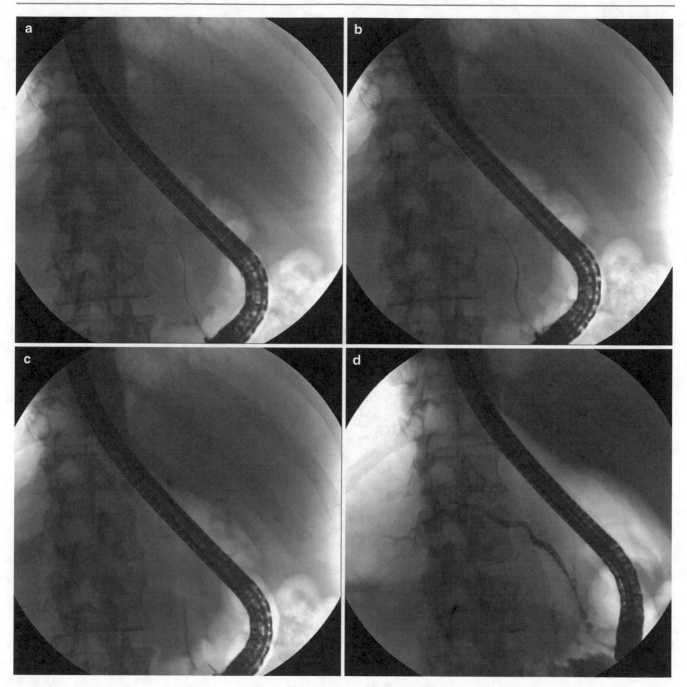

Fig. 9.7 Endoscopic therapy for pancreas divisum using sphincterotomy plus stent placement in a patient with recurrent acute pancreatitis: Endoscopic and Fluoroscopic views. (**a**) A guidewire is inserted into the pancreatic duct at the major papilla. (Image courtesy of Douglas G. Adler MD). (**b**) Injection of the duct of Wirsung at the major papilla reveals pancreas divisum (image courtesy of Douglas G. Adler MD). (**c**) A prophylactic pancreatic duct stent is placed at the major papilla (image courtesy of Douglas G. Adler MD). (**d**) Cannulation of the minor papilla confirms pancreatic divisum and shows a subtle narrow-ing of the pancreatic duct with proximal ductal dilation (image courtesy of Douglas G. Adler MD). (**e**) A minor papilla sphincterotomy is performed. Note pancreatic duct stent in major papilla as well (image courtesy of Douglas G. Adler MD). (**f**) Endoscopic view of a pancreatic duct stent after placement in the minor papilla. Note that both pancreatic duct stents can be seen in one image (image courtesy of Douglas G. Adler MD). (**g**) Final fluoroscopic view of both pancreatic duct stents in place. Note complete drainage of the entire pancreatic ductal system given stent placements (image courtesy of Douglas G. Adler MD)

may lead to a number of complications including stent occlusion or migration, pancreatitis, pancreatic duct perforation, and pseudocyst formation, although many patients tolerate long-term pancreatic duct stenting well and without

difficulty [27–29]. Larger, prospective, randomized trials are needed to confirm these results.

Endoscopic intervention studies in pancreas divisum patients are heterogeneous. The study population (acute

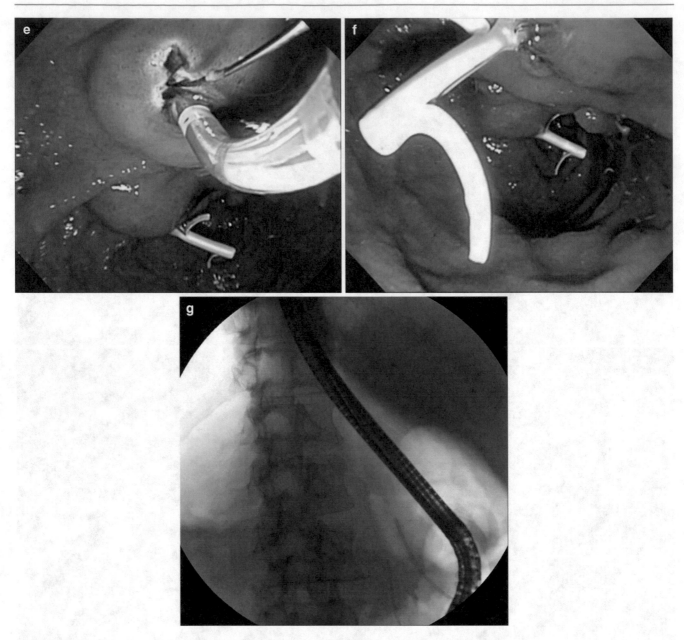

Fig. 9.7 (continued)

pancreatitis, chronic pancreatitis, chronic abdominal pain), endotherapy (duct stenting, sphincterotomy, a combination of stenting and sphincterotomy), and clinical design (retrospective versus prospective) are not uniform throughout studies, making clinical implications from these studies difficult. For example, Kanth and colleagues recently conducted a systematic review of the available literature examining the efficacy of endotherapy for patients with symptomatic pancreas divisum [30]. They included 22 studies totaling 838 patients in their analysis. Of the included studies, most were conducted in the United States and were retrospective in design. In total, 63 % of patients "responded" to endotherapy, although the definition of response varied dramatically amongst the studies. Their results also suggested that patients with acute recurrent pancreatitis were more likely to respond to endotherapy compared to pancreas divisum patients with chronic pancreatitis or chronic abdominal pain. The results of their systemic review, however, must be tempered given the heterogeneity amongst the studies.

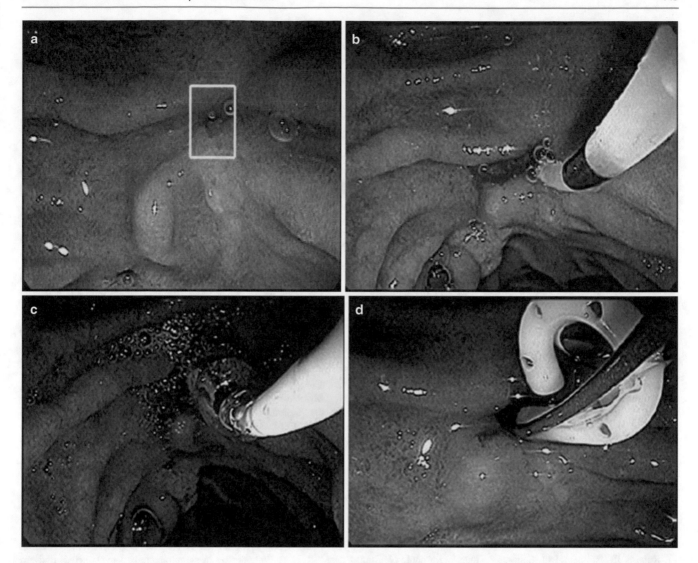

Fig. 9.8 Endoscopic therapy for pancreas divisum using balloon dilation plus stent placement. (**a**) Identification of the minor papilla (represented by the *box*), which appeared stenotic. (**b**) Cannulation of the minor papilla with a tapered catheter and 0.035 in guidewire. (**c**) A 6 mm Hurricane balloon was used to dilate the minor papilla. (**d**) Following this, a 7 Fr 7 cm Hobbs stent was placed into the dorsal pancreatic duct

Conclusion

Pancreas divisum is a common clinical finding. Patients with this finding are often asymptomatic but may have acute pancreatitis, chronic pancreatitis, or pain though to be of pancreatic origin. Taken together, the data suggest a possible benefit for endotherapy in patients with recurrent idiopathic acute pancreatitis for whom other therapies are limited. Its role in the treatment of patients with chronic pancreatitis and chronic abdominal pain, however, is much less established. A randomized, large multi-center, prospective therapeutic trial of endotherapy in symptomatic patients with pancreas divisum is much needed. For now, the risk-benefit ratio of performing ERCP with possible therapeutic intervention needs to be thoroughly reviewed with the patient and care team.

Video Legend

Video 9.1 Minor papilla intervention. A gentleman with presumed alcohol pancreatitis underwent ERCP for endoscopic intervention of a pancreatic duct stricture visualized on cross-sectional imaging. However, pancreatogram revealed the presence of pancreas divisum. Given this, minor papilla sphincterotomy and duct placement were performed (WMV 16743 kb).

References

1. Fogel EL, Toth TG, Lehman GA, et al. Does endoscopic therapy favorably affect the outcome of patients who have recurrent acute pancreatitis and pancreas divisum. Pancreas. 2007;34(1):21–45.
2. Suga T, Nagakawa T, Miyakawa H, et al. Clinical features of patients with pancreas divisum. Dig Endosc. 1994;6:80–6.

3. Aowaros V. Pancreas divisum: incidence and clinical evaluation in Thai patients. J Med Assoc Thai. 1992;75:692–6.
4. Moreira VF, Merono E, Ledo L, et al. Incomplete pancreas divisum. Gastrointest Endosc. 1991;37:104–7.
5. Ng JWD, Wong MK, Huang J, et al. Incomplete pancreas divisum associated with abnormal junction of the pancreatobiliary duct system. Gastrointest Endosc. 1992;38:105–6.
6. Bertin C, Pelletie AL, Vullierme MP, et al. Pancreas divisum is not a cause of pancreatitis by itself but acts as a partner of genetic mutations. Am J Gastroenterol. 2012;107(2):311–7.
7. Choudari CP, Imperiale TF, Sherman S, et al. Risk of pancreatitis with mutation of the cystic fibrosis gene. Am J Gastroenterol. 2004;99:1358–63.
8. Gelrud A, Sheth S, Banerjee S, et al. Analysis of cystic fibrosis gener product (CFTR) function in patients with pancreas divisum and recurrent acute pancreatitis. Am J Gastroenterol. 2004;99:1557–62.
9. Garg PK, Khajuria R, Kabra M, Shastri SS. Association of SPINK1 gene mutation and CFTR polymorphisms in patients with pancreas divisum presenting with idiopathic pancreatitis. J Clin Gastroenterol. 2009;43:848–85.
10. Sandrasegaran K, Patel A, Fogel EL, et al. Annular pancreas in adults. AJR Am J Roentgenol. 2009;193(2):455–60.
11. Lehman GA, O'Connor KW. Coexistence of annular pancreas and pancreas divisum—ERCP diagnosis. Gastrointest Endosc. 1985;31(1):25.
12. England RE, Newcomer MK, Leung JW, Cotton PB. Case report: Annular pancreas—a report of two cases and review of the literature. Br J Radiol. 1995;68(807):324.
13. Zyromoski NJ, Sandoval JA, Pitt HA, et al. Annular pancreas: dramatic difference between children and adults. J Am Coll Surg. 2008;206(5):1019.
14. Madura JA, Fiore AC, O'Connor KW, et al. Pancreas divisum. Detection and management. Am Surg. 1985;51(6):353.
15. Lehman GA, Kopecky KK, Rogge JD. Partial pancreatic agenesis combined with pancreas divisum and duodenum reflexum. Gastrointest Endosc. 1987;33(6):445.
16. Moffatt DC, Cote GA, Avula H, Watkins JL, McHenry L, Sherman S, et al. Risk factors for ERCP-related complications in patients with pancreas divisum: a retrospective study. Gastrointest Endosc. 2011;73(5):963–70.
17. Roberts JR, Romagnulo J. Endoscopic therapy for acute recurrent pancreatitis. Gastrointest Endosc Clin N Am. 2013;23:803–19.
18. Belber JP, Bill K. Fusion anomalies of the pancreatic ductal system differentiation from pathologic states. Radiology. 1977;122:637–42.
19. Warshaw AL, Cambria RP. False pancreas divisum. Acquired pancreatic duct obstruction simulating the congenital anomaly. Ann Surg. 1984;200:595–9.
20. Bhutani MS, Hoffman BJ, Hawes RH. Diagnosis of pancreas divisum by endoscopic ultrasonography. Endoscopy. 1999;31:167–9.
21. Lai R, Freeman ML, Cass OW, Mallery S. Accurate diagnosis of pancreas divisum by linear-array endoscopic ultrasonography. Endoscopy. 2004;36:705–9.
22. Rustagi T, Njei B. Magnetic resonance cholangiopancreatography in the diagnosis of pancreas divisum: a systematic review and meta-analysis. Pancreas. 2014;43:823–8.
23. Kushnir VM, Wani SB, Fowler K, Menias C, Varma R, Narra V, et al. Sensitivity of endoscopic ultrasound, multidetector computed tomography, and magnetic resonance cholangiopancreatography in the diagnosis of pancreas divisum: a tertiary center experience. Pancreas. 2013;42:436–41.
24. Borak GD, Romangnuolo J, Alsolaiman M, Holt E, Cotton PB. Long-term clinical outcomes after endoscopic minor papilla therapy in symptomatic patients with pancreas divisum. Pancreas. 2009;38(8):903–6.
25. Atwell A, Borak G, Hawes R, Cotton P, Romagnuolo J. Endoscopic pancreatic sphincterotomy for pancreas divisum by using a needle-knife or standard pull-type technique: safety and reintervention rates. Gastrointest Endosc. 2006;64(5):705–11.
26. Yamamoto N, Isayama H, Sasahira N, Tsujino T, Nakai Y, Miyabayashi K, et al. Endoscopic minor papilla balloon dilation for the treatment of symptomatic pancreas divisum. Pancreas. 2014;43(6):927–30.
27. Ikenberry SO, Sherman S, Hawes RH, Smith M, Lehman GA. The occlusion rate of pancreatic stents. Gastrointest Endosc. 1994;40(5):611.
28. Johanson JF, Schmalz MJ, Geenen JE. Incidence and risk factors for biliary and pancreatic stent migration. Gastrointest Endosc. 1992;38(3):341.
29. Johanson JF, Schmalz MJ, Geenen JE. Simple modification of a pancreatic duct stent to prevent proximal migration. Gastrointest Endosc. 1993;39(1):62.
30. Kanth R, Samji NS, Inaganti A, Komanapalli SD, Rivera R, Antillon MR, et al. Endotherapy in symptomatic patients pancreas divisum patients: a systematic review. Pancreatology. 2014;14:244–50.

Endoscopic Ampullectomy: Who, When, and How

10

Matthew E. Feurer, Eric G. Hilgenfeldt, and Peter V. Draganov

Introduction

Ampullary adenomas are dysplastic lesions of the major duodenal papilla. Although considered rare, with an estimated 3000 cases reported annually in the United States, these lesions have the potential to undergo malignant transformation to ampullary cancer following an adenoma-to-carcinoma sequence [1–5]. Ampullary adenomas are precancerous lesions, with a reported incidence of transformation to invasive or in situ carcinoma ranging from 25 to 85 % [6–8]. Therefore, removal of both premalignant and malignant ampullary lesions is to be considered in patients who are felt to be candidates for endoscopic and/or surgical resection.

Ampullary adenomas can occur sporadically or in the setting of genetic syndromes such as familial adenomatous polyposis (FAP). The prevalence of ampullary adenoma has been estimated to be 0.04–0.12 % based on autopsy series, and it is most commonly observed in patients of 50–70 years of age [9, 10]. These lesions have become increasingly more recognized due to the widespread availability of endoscopy for the evaluation of upper gastrointestinal-related issues and through screening and surveillance programs for patients with FAP. With a risk for ampullary carcinoma that is 124-fold greater than the general population, surveillance upper endoscopy plays an important role in the management of patients with FAP [11–13]. Up to 50–90 % of patients with FAP will develop duodenal adenomas, predominantly concentrated on or around the major papilla [14].

Historically, ampullary adenomas have been treated surgically. Localized resection of an ampullary lesion was first described by Halsted in 1899 using a transduodenal approach [15]. Due to a high rate of tumor recurrence associated with transduodenal ampullectomy, pancreaticoduodenectomy, or Whipple procedure, has been more traditionally performed, and remains the standard surgical approach [16, 17]. In experienced centers, pancreaticoduodenectomy offers complete removal of ampullary adenomas and is associated with relatively low mortality rates, but still carries high perioperative morbidity [18].

Endoscopic ampullectomy, first described in 1983, has evolved into an alternative first-line therapy for the evaluation and treatment of ampullary adenomas [19]. Endoscopic resection is now often considered prior to surgical intervention as it is less invasive and associated with lower morbidity than surgery [20]. The technique is often described in literature as endoscopic papillectomy, with the term ampullectomy traditionally referring to a surgical approach, although many centers still use the term endoscopic ampullectomy. These two terms, however, are often used interchangeably and we generally refer to endoscopic resection as ampullectomy throughout this text.

Adverse events tend to be more commonly encountered when treating ampullary lesions endoscopically as compared to other endoscopic procedures (highlighting the relatively high-risk nature of endoscopic ampullectomy), with improved outcomes based on the practitioner's experience. With significant advances in our ability and means to perform endoscopic ampullectomy, the endoscopic approach is being performed with increasing frequency. This chapter examines the role of imaging and endoscopy in evaluating ampullary adenomas and provides an overview of the various endoscopic techniques available for resection. Potential adverse events and their avoidance and management, as well as long-term surveillance for recurrence following resection, are also discussed.

Electronic supplementary material: The online version of this chapter (doi:10.1007/978-3-319-26854-5_10) contains supplementary material, which is available to authorized users. Videos can also be accessed at http://link.springer.com/chapter/10.1007/978-3-319-26854-5_10.

M.E. Feurer, M.D., M.S. • E.G. Hilgenfeldt, M.D.
P.V. Draganov, M.D. (✉)
Division of Gastroenterology, Hepatology, and Nutrition,
University of Florida College of Medicine,
1329 SW 16th Street, Room 5251, Gainesville, FL 32608, USA
e-mail: Peter.Draganov@medicine.ufl.edu

Clinical Presentation and Diagnosis

Presentation

Many ampullary adenomas are asymptomatic and are discovered incidentally on upper endoscopy performed for unrelated reasons. For those who develop symptoms, obstructive jaundice tends to be the most common presentation [21]. Nonspecific findings such as progressive weight loss and abdominal and back pain can be observed as well. With increasing lesion size, nausea and vomiting can be seen in the setting of gastric outlet obstruction. Recurrent acute pancreatitis can also occur from pancreatic duct obstruction, which may be intermittent [22]. In conjunction with pancreatic duct obstruction, diarrhea may occur due to the absence of lipase within the gut lumen. Significant weight loss may indicate a more invasive process; however, ampullary malignancies tend to manifest at an early stage due to biliary outflow obstruction (as opposed to pancreatic adenocarcinoma that is often advanced at the time of diagnosis).

Diagnosis

It may be difficult to differentiate ampullary adenomas from ampullary carcinomas or nonadenomatous polyps based on endoscopic appearance alone. Nevertheless, there are certain endoscopic features which may suggest a benign lesion including regular margins, soft consistency, lack of ulceration or friability, and no spontaneous bleeding [23]. A side-viewing endoscope is necessary for a complete endoscopic evaluation. In order to confirm the presence of an adenoma or carcinoma however, a tissue diagnosis of the lesion is typically required.

Although forceps biopsy of an ampullary lesion can be carried out readily, the accuracy of this technique for diagnosing adenocarcinoma is reported as 62–85 % [24–26]. This demonstrates that forceps biopsy does not sufficiently detect infiltrating carcinomas. It has been argued that deeper biopsy after sphincterotomy may provide a more accurate diagnosis, but sensitivity in determining adenocarcinoma was shown to increase from only 21 to 37 % before and after sphincterotomy [27]. Given the high false negative rates associated with forceps biopsy, endoscopic ampullectomy can be recommended also as a diagnostic tool to provide sufficient tissue for histological examination, recognizing that some patients initially thought to have ampullary adenomas may be found to have ampullary cancers [28].

Staging

Use of Imaging

Following biopsy, further management decisions regarding high-risk lesions or confirmed ampullary adenocarcinoma are guided by adjunctive staging modalities that may include transabdominal ultrasound (US), computed tomography (CT), magnetic resonance cholangiopancreatography (MRCP), endoscopic retrograde cholangiopancreatography (ERCP), endoscopic ultrasound (EUS), and intraductal ultrasound (IDUS).

Transabdominal ultrasound is an inexpensive and readily available noninvasive procedure that can identify dilated biliary ducts and liver metastasis. CT can also provide useful information regarding invasion or compression of vasculature and adjacent organs, as well as identification of lymphadenopathy and distant metastatic lesions. Both US and CT, however, fail to provide adequate visualization of the ampullary area for the local staging of ampullary lesions. MRCP may not prove useful for staging purposes unless there are specific bile duct abnormalities previously identified on CT or US that need further clarification prior to more invasive investigative studies, and the ampulla itself is often poorly seen on MRI/MRCP. Nevertheless, MRCP is frequently used in patients with obstructive jaundice in an attempt to identify the level and cause of obstruction. If used, MRCP may provide evidence of intraductal extension and anatomical variants such as pancreas divisum. Although there are no formal studies that have reported the benefits of MRCP prior to ampullectomy, additional information obtained from this imaging modality may help guide management decisions and avoid potential adverse events. Knowledge of anatomic conditions such as pancreas divisum may help to prevent difficulties in pancreatic duct stenting, which is generally performed during ampullectomy. One can forgo pancreatic duct stenting at the time of endoscopic ampullectomy if pancreas divisum is detected ahead of time, although in practice this discovery is often made during the ampullectomy procedure itself.

Role of Endoscopic Ultrasound

Endoscopic ultrasonography (EUS) can provide specific information regarding the depth of invasion of an ampullary lesion and the extent of any metastasis to adjacent lymph nodes. EUS can also be used to obtain tissue samples in cases where the diagnosis remains unclear. EUS has been demonstrated to be superior to CT, MRCP, or transabdominal US for tumor staging; it has emerged as the staging modality of choice in the evaluation of ampullary carcinoma [29–31]. EUS, most often performed at a frequency of 7.5–10 MHz, is capable of identifying tumors significantly smaller than 1 cm in size and has an accuracy of 97 % for diagnosing adenomas and pTis tumors [32]. The ability of EUS to correctly stage carcinomas was reported to be between 67 and 92 % [27, 29, 30, 33–35].

There have been several staging systems applied to ampullary adenomas that are used to dictate appropriate therapy. With the TNM staging classification system, tumor staging for ampullary adenomas is based on the extent of invasion into surrounding tissues (see Table 10.1). The symbol "p" is based on gross and microscopic examination and indicates resection of the primary tumor or biopsy adequate

Table 10.1 TNM classification system for carcinoma of the Ampulla of Vater

TNM descriptors for carcinoma of the ampulla of Vater	
pT0	No evidence of primary tumor
pTis	Carcinoma in situ
pT1	Tumor limited to ampulla of Vater or sphincter of Oddi
pT2	Tumor invades duodenal wall
pT3	Tumor invades pancreas
pT4	Tumor invades peripancreatic soft tissues or other adjacent organs or structures other than pancreas

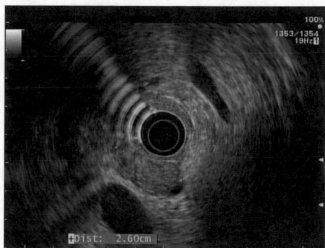

Fig. 10.2 EUS demonstrates a well-defined 25 mm hypoechoic mass in the ampulla visible from 6 to 7 ô'clock

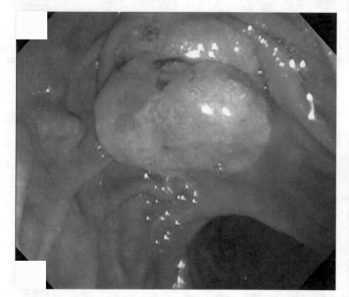

Fig. 10.1 Ampullary adenoma

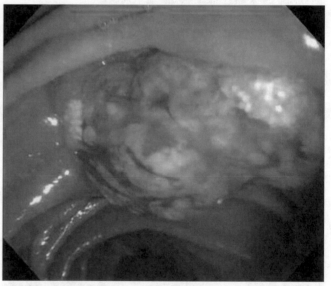

Fig. 10.3 Ampullary mass with ulceration

for evaluation. For ampullary carcinomas, the term "carcinoma in situ" (pTis) describes cancer cells confined within the glandular basement membrane and includes noninvasive ampullary carcinomas. An alternative system, the Vienna classification of histologic grading for gastrointestinal epithelial neoplasms, categorizes ampullary lesions into low- or high-grade dysplasia, noninvasive carcinoma (carcinoma in situ), and invasive carcinoma.

Figures 10.1 and 10.2 show an ampullary lesion that was diagnosed as adenoma based on biopsy. EUS was used (Fig. 10.2) to further define a 25 mm mass without definitive extension into the pancreatic duct or biliary duct.

An ulcerated ampullary mass determined to be adenocarcinoma is highlighted in Figs. 10.3, 10.4, 10.5, and 10.6. EUS staging was T2N0. Dilation and thickening of the common bile duct was observed without obvious extension.

IDUS, operating at higher frequencies (20–30 MHz), can provide higher-resolution images than EUS at the expense of decreased depth penetration. These small diameter probes (from 1.1 to 2.6 mm) can be passed directly into the bile duct over a biliary guidewire and allow visualization of tumors at and above the sphincter of Oddi. IDUS has been reported to have greater accuracy in the staging of ampullary lesions when compared to EUS, with rates up to 100 % [27, 35].

Despite the improved rates of accuracy, IDUS is not routinely used in the staging of ampullary adenomas and carcinomas due to its limited availability, cost, need for a second EUS processor, and the fragility of the probes themselves.

To date, there has been no general consensus on the use of EUS prior to treatment of ampullary adenomas. Several experts have recommended that patients with ampullary adenomas that exhibit any high-risk features including size >1 cm, high-grade dysplasia, or signs of malignancy on endoscopic exam (ulceration, irregular margins, spontaneous bleeding, or firmness) undergo EUS for staging [36, 37]. It is reasonable to consider the use of EUS prior to endoscopic or surgical resection of an ampullary adenoma when it is available given the degree of detail it can provide regarding the lesion although its role has not been firmly established [38]. It has recently been reported that EUS is comparable to ERCP and surgical pathology for evaluating the extent of

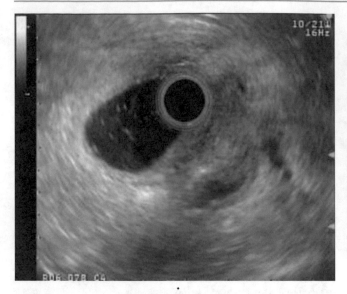

Fig. 10.4 An ampullary mass is shown inferior with thickened bile duct at 5 o'clock and pancreatic duct at 4 o'clock

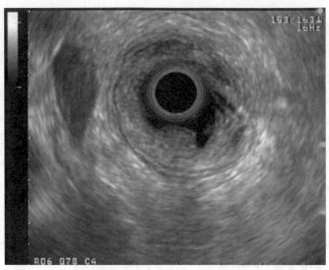

Fig. 10.6 The ampullary mass is visualized on EUS in 6 o'clock position

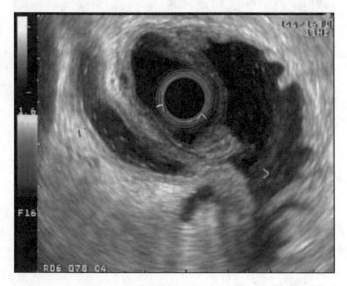

Fig. 10.5 The bile duct and pancreatic ducts are clearly visualized

intraductal extension of an ampullary lesion with a specificity and accuracy of 97 % and 90 % respectively [39]. This implies that patients that demonstrate significant intraductal extension on EUS (≥1 cm) may be referred directly for surgical resection, thus avoiding potential adverse effects and incomplete resection associated with ERCP and endoscopic ampullectomy [40]. In our institution, EUS is routinely performed for adenomatous lesions greater than 2 cm and for all ampullary carcinomas.

Role of ERCP

ERCP with both biliary and pancreatic duct evaluation is performed immediately prior to possible endoscopic therapeutic intervention [41]. ERCP can also be performed before ampullectomy if EUS is unavailable or the findings on EUS

are equivocal. ERCP is utilized primarily to detect possible extension of the ampullary lesion into the biliary or pancreatic duct and to remove any obstruction that may be present at the time. Evidence of intraductal extension as detected by ERCP is generally accepted as criteria for surgical referral; however, successful endoscopic resection and ablation of benign intraductal lesions with less than 1 cm of extension into the common bile or pancreatic duct, although not commonly performed, have been demonstrated following biliary sphincterotomy [42–45].

Indication for Resection

The indications for endoscopic ampullectomy are not firmly established due in part to the continued advances in endoscopic therapy. Generally accepted criteria for endoscopic resection include adenomas confined to the ampullary region without evidence of malignancy on endoscopy or biopsy, absence of extension into the biliary or pancreatic ducts, lack of invasion of the muscularis propria of the duodenum, and size less than 4 cm [11, 36, 46–49]. Although there have been reports of focal or unanticipated ampullary adenocarcinoma being endoscopically removed, surgical resection remains the general recommendation [50–54].

Special consideration is given when a newly diagnosed ampullary adenoma is detected in the setting of FAP. Multiple duodenal polyps are often observed in these patients, which are assigned a stage 0–IV according to the Spigelman classification system based on number of polyps, size, histology, and dysplasia [55]. Patients with Spigelman stage 0–III have traditionally been followed with close endoscopic surveillance. Those FAP patients who progress to Spigelman stage IV carry a cumulative cancer risk between 30 and 40 %, prompting more aggressive therapies including endoscopic resection of nonampullary duodenal adenomas or pancreaticoduodenectomy [13]. In patients with FAP who have a normal appearing ampulla, biopsies will almost universally reveal adenoma. In general, adenomatous tissue in the ampulla of a FAP patient with a normal appearing ampulla is not considered an indication for ampullectomy. Given that many of the duodenal malignancies that arise in FAP are nonampullary, endoscopic ampullectomy has not been shown to reduce the need for eventual pancreaticoduodenectomy [56, 57].

Endoscopic Versus Surgical Resection: How to Decide?

There are currently no consensus guidelines regarding which lesions are amendable to either surgery or endoscopic resection. Each case should be addressed on an individual basis due to variability in patient populations and lesions encountered. A proposed algorithm based on previous recommendations for the management of a newly diagnosed ampullary adenoma is depicted in Fig. 10.7 [8, 37].

Previous consensus advocated that all ampullary lesions demonstrating adenocarcinoma be treated surgically. It has been reported, however, that high-grade dysplasia (HGD) and focal T1 ampullary adenocarcinoma can be treated endoscopically without evidence of residual tumor on follow-up

[58]. Endoscopic resection has been deemed appropriate management for ampullary adenomas with HGD in instances where the lesion is extraductal only [59]. Other studies have observed that HGD has been associated with high rates of recurrence [60]. Despite the lack of universally agreed upon management strategies, endoscopic therapy is accepted as a first-line approach for ampullary adenomas (with or without HGD) with surgery generally indicated for ampullary carcinomas. The availability of local expertise also plays an important role in management as ampullary adenomas/carcinomas are relatively rare and the endoscopic and/or surgical techniques for their resection can be technically and resource demanding. It is reasonable to refer patients to tertiary care centers with proven experience in both endoscopic and surgical treatment of ampullary lesions.

Endoscopic Resection Techniques

Endoscopic Ampullectomy

Since Binmoeller et al. first reported curative endoscopic resection of an ampullary adenoma, the techniques associated with endoscopic ampullectomy have continued to evolve [46]. Although it shares many of the basic principles of colonic polypectomy, a variety of new techniques have been deployed due to the unique anatomy and known adverse events associated with endoscopy ampullectomy. Some of these techniques include differing methods of resection,

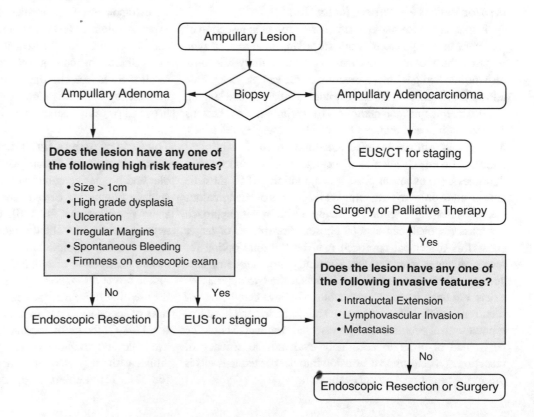

Fig. 10.7 Management of ampullary lesion

ablative therapy, and prophylactic measures to avert post-procedural adverse events. The paragraphs that follow will highlight these measures in detail.

Submucosal Injection Versus No Injection

The purported benefit of submucosal injection of a lesion prior to ampullectomy is to aid in removal by lifting the lesion and to protect the duodenal muscularis propria from thermal injury. The most commonly used fluid for injection remains either normal saline or a mixture of epinephrine diluted with normal saline to reduce bleeding following resection [50, 61]. The need for submucosal injection is disputed but may increase the visibility of and prognosticate the lesion [45, 47, 54]. The presence of a "lift sign" in which the adenoma elevates off of the mucosa is said to predict a favorable pathology and less chance of malignancy. The absence of a "lift sign" (suggesting deeper involvement and/or malignancy) can in some cases be an indication for cessation of endoscopic ampullectomy. Injection of methylene blue is stated to similarly reflect a likelihood of malignancy depending on its pattern of uptake in the tissue [62].

Submucosal injection, although commonly performed, is not required per se prior to endoscopic resection and may carry potential deleterious effects [63–65]. The lifting of the mucosa may alter the anatomy of the lesion, thus decreasing the chance of successful *en bloc* resection [37, 66]. Furthermore, the usefulness of the "lift sign" has been questioned because even superficial lesions may not always lift due to the bile and pancreatic duct "anchoring" the lesion.

En Bloc Versus Piecemeal Resection

As is inherent in the name itself, *en bloc* refers to resection of the mass in one piece. It is not surprising then that *en bloc* remains the recommended method of ampullary adenoma resection, when possible. Resection of the sample as a whole allows for the most accurate histological analysis and staging of both lateral and deep margins. This technique also shortens procedure time and requires less electrocautery. Often times, despite best efforts, *en bloc* resection is not feasible and additional methods such as piecemeal removal and thermal therapies such as argon plasma coagulation (APC) must be employed in order to treat remnant fragments of adenomatous tissue. Piecemeal resection, utilizing a bite-by-bite approach for mass removal, can also be chosen. For masses of larger sizes, this piecemeal approach may be the only option for resection other than surgery. Currently, no long-term data comparing the recurrence rates between the two approaches exists, although it seems reasonable to believe that the rate of recurrence with *en bloc* resection should be lower. Close histopathological evaluation of all resected segments should be performed in order to accurately evaluate the efficacy of resection and determine if invasion into deeper tissue levels is present, warranting surgical evaluation.

Endoscopic Snares

Endoscopic ampullectomy for an ampullary adenoma, similar to a colorectal polypectomy, utilizes an endoscopic snare with electrocautery. Both monofilament and braided snares have been utilized with similar success [11, 42, 43, 47]. After the decision is made to excise the ampullary tumor, it is snared at its base. This can prove difficult depending on the size and flatness of the lesion, leading to novel methods [67]. Ghidirim et al. noted one such method of resection for sessile adenomas utilizing an intraductal balloon catheter. Once placed within the duct, the balloon is inflated and withdrawn lifting the lesion, thus exposing a larger portion of the ampullary mass for snaring. Once snared, constant tension is applied as the lesion is transected. Following transection of the lesion, efforts to retrieve all of the resected tissue are made in order to ensure careful pathological evaluation. The step can be completed using suction, a retrieval snare or retrieval net. The use of intravenous glucagon may decrease the risk of losing the specimen due to downstream migration from peristaltic contractions but this approach has not been formally evaluated.

Electrocautery

No standardization exists regarding the type of current or the power settings used for electrocautery. Blended, endocut, and pure-cut curre nt have all been shown to be effective [43, 68, 69]. A specific mode of electrocautery should not only be measured on its effectiveness of transection and coagulation, but also on its effect to the surrounding structures and histopathological analysis of the transected lesion. Since no studies have addressed the optimal electrocautery mode, one can only rely on extrapolation from studies on colonic polypectomy and expert opinion. In our institution we favor the use of endocut current based on the theoretical considerations. Endocut provides alternating cutting and coagulating currents and as a result there is less charring of the ampullectomy base which may facilitate identification of the biliary and pancreatic orifices and possibly decrease the risk of post-ERCP pancreatitis.

The Role of Adjunctive Tissue Ablation

Argon plasma coagulation (APC), laser therapy, and monopolar and bipolar coagulation are adjunctive methods used to achieve fulguration of remnant tissue following endoscopic snare resection [11, 42, 46]. Complete *en bloc* resection negates the need for ablative techniques. More often than not, *en bloc* is not possible and ablative methods are utilized to ensure destruction of remaining suspicious tissue. For large tumor resection where a piecemeal technique is employed, the use of ablative methods has been found to achieve similar rates of success and recurrence as compared to surgical resection [70]. Of the modalities, APC tends to be the most widely available and frequently used form of adjunctive ablation. Ablative therapy has been attempted as primary treatment [68, 71, 72]. Leinert et al. conducted a study in which endoscopic snare resection with adjuvant ablation was compared to APC treatment alone for treatment of duodenal adenomas [71]. In addition to the higher rate of recurrence identified in this patient cohort, barriers to APC as primary treatment were identified which included the need for multiple treatment sessions and the inability to histologically examine each lesion. Given the reported 20 % of occult carcinoma identified in ampullary adenomas, some advise against its use, although it is still widely performed [41, 62, 73].

Pancreatic or Biliary Sphincterotomy

Adjunctive biliary sphincterotomy is commonly performed either prior to or after snaring of the ampullary lesion. When performed prior to snaring of the lesion, this technique can be useful in preserving the ampullary opening following resection of small lesions [8]. Mixing radiopaque contrast with methylene blue and injecting the bile and pancreatic ducts prior to snare resection has also been reported to improve visualization of the biliary and pancreatic orifices following ampullectomy [67]. Additionally, contrast injection may allow detection of intraductal growth of the lesion [64]. Some authors have advocated sphincterotomy prior to resection; however, post-ampullectomy sphincterotomy with pancreatic stent placement is generally performed to maximize the possibility of *en bloc* resection [37, 47, 50]. The issue remains controversial and no uniform consensus exists on the timing of the biliary sphincterotomy. Nevertheless, biliary sphincterotomy is typically recommended before or after the ampullectomy. Although pancreatic stenting after ampullectomy is generally performed to decrease the risk of post-ERCP pancreatitis following procedure, the addition of pancreatic sphincterotomy is debatable. Some centers universally perform pancreatic sphincterotomy during ampullectomy and others use it in a limited manner or not at all. The advantage of performing a pancreatic sphincterotomy is that it may facilitate access to the pancreatic duct following ampullectomy for pancreatic stent placement. Downsides include the potential increased risk of bleeding and/or pancreatitis.

Pancreatic or Biliary Stenting

Ampullectomy can lead to both pancreatitis and papillary stenosis. In patients for whom stenting was not performed, adverse events were five times more likely to occur [11, 42, 43, 74]. Several studies have looked at the effectiveness of using post-ampullectomy pancreatic duct stenting in order to limit post-procedural pancreatitis [43, 47, 63, 75–78]. Current data supports routine use following ampullectomy, although again this practice is not universally applied. Preprocedural pancreatic duct stenting has also been evaluated; however the

data is not as conclusive. Moon et al. looked at using wire-guided endoscopic snare ampullectomy during tumor resection involving the major papilla. It was found that utilization of a guidewire improved the ability to traverse the recently snared ampulla. This was in part due to the resulting edema from ampullectomy that can make it difficult to visualize the ampullary lumen. Utilization of a guidewire allowed for constant awareness of the pancreatic duct [79]. Biliary stenting remains a case-by-case decision and is done when suspicion exists for poor biliary drainage [11, 37, 46, 47, 67].

Figures 10.8, 10.9, 10.10, and 10.11 illustrate an ampullary adenoma that was resected *en bloc* using snare and electrocautery. A temporary pancreatic stent was also placed for pancreatitis prophylaxis.

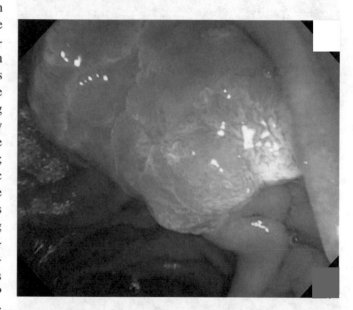

Fig. 10.8 Ampullary adenoma visualized through side-viewer scope

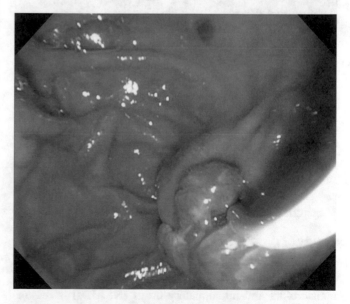

Fig. 10.9 ERCP cannulation prior to ampullectomy

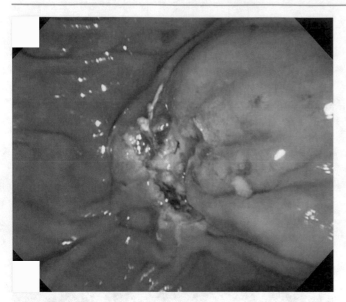

Fig. 10.10 Endoscopic ampullectomy performed with snare and electrocautery

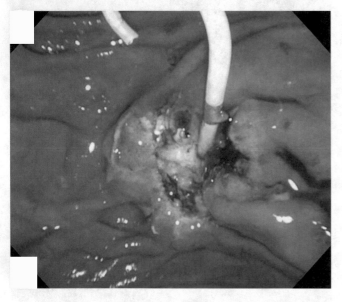

Fig. 10.11 Placement of pancreatic duct stent following ampullectomy

Video 10.1 demonstrates an endoscopic ampullectomy of an ampullary adenoma using an *en bloc* snare technique with biliary sphincterotomy and post-ampullectomy pancreatic stenting.

Medical Prophylaxis for Post-ERCP Pancreatitis

No study has directly addressed the benefit from medical prophylaxis for post-ERCP pancreatitis in the setting of endoscopic ampullectomy. We believe that prophylaxis with nonsteroidal anti-inflammatory drugs (NSAIDs) is reasonable in all ampullectomy patients. These patients are at high

risk for post-ERCP pancreatitis and a single dose of NSAIDs has been shown to have an excellent safety profile [80]. The most commonly used NSAID in North America is rectally administered indomethacin.

Results of Endoscopic Therapy

Outcomes

The most recent results of endoscopic ampullectomy reported in the literature are summarized in Table 10.2. In the vast majority of available literature, the reported outcomes are the result of data analyzed from small to medium cohorts of patients. Patient demographics, techniques, and the methods of post-procedural monitoring all vary, thus leading to a heterogeneous group. The lack of large, prospective, randomized trials limit the generalizability of treatment and thus case-by-case considerations must be considered prior to pursuing endoscopic resection. It should be observed that the rarity of cases, as well as the significant difference in the treatment between both surgical and endoscopic approaches, would make it difficult to design and conduct a randomized and prospective trial.

When evaluating the use of endoscopic ampullectomy for treatment of ampullary adenomas, successful resection is difficult to completely define. Success should be considered to represent an absence of histological residual adenoma during regular short-term (<6 months) follow-up. Best estimates for the reported success approaches 80 %; however, this is highly variable and depends on a multitude of factors which include but are not limited to the experience of the endoscopist, lesion size, lesion location, comorbid conditions, and the ability to perform surveillance follow-up. Overall analysis of the current trials has shown that the rate of recurrence varies between 0 and 26 % and is similar to previous meta-analysis [81]. It can be confidently concluded that the use of pancreatic stenting, as noted by previous guidelines, should be universally practiced in an effort to minimize potential morbidity [38].

Adverse Events

Endoscopic ampullectomy has reported adverse event rates between 10 and 30 % and depends on a multitude of factors related to both the lesion characteristics and the experience of the endoscopist. Mortality following endoscopic resection is extremely rare. In comparison, surgical ampullectomy is associated with a morbidity upwards of 40 % with a small but slightly higher chance of mortality [70]. Additionally, given the high percentage of false positives noted on forceps biopsy, pursuit of the least invasive approach possible should be undertaken [81].

Table 10.2 Outcomes of endoscopic ampullectomy of ampullary adenomas

Author, year	n	Median/mean f/u (in months)	Injection/ medium used	Pancreatic stenting	Success rate	Recurrence rate	Morbidity	Mortality	Need for surgery
Binmoeller et al., 1993	25	37	No	No	23/25 (95 %)	6/23 (26 %)	5	0	3
Desilets et al., 2001	13	NR	Yes/epi	Yes	12/13 (92 %)	0/12 (0 %)	1	0	1
Catalano et al., 2004	103	36	No	Yes	83/103 (80 %)	20/103 (19 %)	10	0	16
Cheng et al., 2004	55	30	No	Yes	39/55 (71 %)	9/55 (16 %)	12	0	4
Bohnacker et al., 2005	87	43	No	Yes	74/87 (85 %)	15/87 (17 %)	29	0	17
Han et al., 2006	33	9	Yes/saline or epi	Yes	20/33 (61 %)	2/33 (6 %)	11	0	2
Jung et al., 2009	22	5	NR	Yes	17/22 (77 %)	2/12 (17 %)	5	0	6
Yamao et al., 2010	36	14	No	Yes	29/36 (81 %)	1/36 (3 %)	6	0	1
Hopper et al., 2010	23	12	Yes/saline	Yes	21/23 (91 %)	4/23 (17 %)	6	0	2
Heinzow et al., 2012	21	64	Yes/saline	Yes	21/21 (100 %)	3/18 (17 %)	7	0	3
Ceppa et al., 2013	68	NR	No	Yes	48/68 (71 %)	0/68 (0 %)	12	0	NR
Overall	486	–	–	–	387/486 (79 %)	62/470 (13 %)	104	0	–

Similar to colonic polypectomy, bleeding and perforation are possible and typically controlled with conservative or local measures such as clips or epinephrine injection. Additionally, both pancreatitis and cholangitis have been described but can be minimized by periprocedural pancreatic duct stent placement. When pancreatitis does develop, it tends to be mild to moderate and resolves with conservative therapy. Later stage adverse events are rare and include the development of pancreatic or biliary duct stenosis. This is often treated with sphincterotomy in conjunction with further stenting or dilation [20, 82].

Surveillance for Residual Tissue or Recurrence

With the rate of recurrence for ampullary adenomas reported up to 33 %, endoscopic surveillance is required. There is currently no standardized method of surveillance monitoring following initial endoscopic resection of an ampullary adenoma. Aside from the recommendations of expert consensus in patients with FAP, initial follow-up following endoscopic resection is performed at 1–3 months. Surveillance is continued at 3–6 month intervals until biopsy demonstrates no residual adenoma. If no further adenoma is identified, routine surveillance is performed at 6–12 month intervals for the next 2 years followed by less frequent intervals [11, 37, 43, 47, 74, 83, 84]. The reported mean duration of recurrence is approximately 26 months [81].

Conclusions

The role of endoscopy in the diagnosis and treatment of ampullary adenomas continues to expand due to improvements in resection techniques and increased availability of staging modalities such as EUS. Appropriate staging,

awareness of high-risk features, and consideration for special circumstances such as adenoma in the setting of FAP can help guide the clinician in making the appropriate management decisions. Although surgery remains the treatment of choice for ampullary adenocarcinoma, endoscopic therapy has now become the preferred treatment for ampullary adenomas without extensive intraductal involvement. Pancreatic stent placement is highly recommended to prevent post-procedure pancreatitis. Endoscopic surveillance is an important aspect of ongoing care to ensure complete resection and monitoring for the possibility of recurrence.

Video Legend

Video 10.1 Endoscopic ampullectomy (MOV 130921 kb).

References

1. Brandt LJ. Clinical practice of gastroenterology. Philadelphia: Current Medicine; 1999.
2. Baczako K, Büchler M, Beger HG, Kirkpatrick CJ, Haferkamp O. Morphogenesis and possible precursor lesions of invasive carcinoma of the papilla of Vater: epithelial dysplasia and adenoma. Hum Pathol. 1985;16(3):305–10.
3. Yamaguchi K, Enjoji M. Carcinoma of the ampulla of vater. A clinicopathologic study and pathologic staging of 109 cases of carcinoma and 5 cases of adenoma. Cancer. 1987;59(3):506–15.
4. Stolte M, Pscherer C. Adenoma-carcinoma sequence in the papilla of Vater. Scand J Gastroenterol. 1996;31(4):376–82.
5. Fischer HP, Zhou H. Pathogenesis of carcinoma of the papilla of Vater. J Hepatobiliary Pancreat Surg. 2004;11(5):301–9.
6. Takashima M, Ueki T, Nagai E, Yao T, Yamaguchi K, Tanaka M, et al. Carcinoma of the ampulla of Vater associated with or without adenoma: a clinicopathologic analysis of 198 cases with reference to p53 and Ki-67 immunohistochemical expressions. Mod Pathol. 2000;13(12):1300–7.
7. Seifert E, Schulte F, Stolte M. Adenoma and carcinoma of the duodenum and papilla of Vater: a clinicopathologic study. Am J Gastroenterol. 1992;87(1):37–42.

8. Patel R, Varadarajulu S, Wilcox CM. Endoscopic ampullectomy: techniques and outcomes. J Clin Gastroenterol. 2012;46(1):8–15.

9. Baker HL, Caldwell DW. Lesions of the ampulla of Vater. Surgery. 1947;21(4):523–31.

10. Sato T, Konishi K, Kimura H, Maeda K, Yabushita K, Tsuji M, et al. Adenoma and tiny carcinoma in adenoma of the papilla of Vater—p53 and PCNA. Hepatogastroenterology. 1999;46(27):1959–62.

11. Cheng CL, Sherman S, Fogel EL, McHenry L, Watkins JL, Fukushima T, et al. Endoscopic snare papillectomy for tumors of the duodenal papillae. Gastrointest Endosc. 2004;60(5):757–64.

12. Yao T, Ida M, Ohsato K, Watanabe H, Omae T. Duodenal lesions in familial polyposis of the colon. Gastroenterology. 1977;73(5):1086–92.

13. Offerhaus GJ, Giardiello FM, Krush AJ, Booker SV, Tersmette AC, Kelley NC, et al. The risk of upper gastrointestinal cancer in familial adenomatous polyposis. Gastroenterology. 1992;102(6):1980–2.

14. Griffioen G, Bus PJ, Vasen HF, Verspaget HW, Lamers CB. Extracolonic manifestations of familial adenomatous polyposis: desmoid tumours, and upper gastrointestinal adenomas and carcinomas. Scand J Gastroenterol Suppl. 1998;225:85–91.

15. Halsted W. Contributions to the surgery of the bile passages, especially of the common bile duct. Boston Med Surg J. 1899;141:645–54.

16. Bohra AK, McKie L, Diamond T. Transduodenal excision of ampullary tumours. Ulster Med J. 2002;71(2):121–7.

17. Di Giorgio A, Alfieri S, Rotondi F, Prete F, Di Miceli D, Ridolfini MP, et al. Pancreatoduodenectomy for tumors of Vater's ampulla: report on 94 consecutive patients. World J Surg. 2005;29(4):513–8.

18. Grobmyer SR, Pieracci FM, Allen PJ, Brennan MF, Jaques DP. Defining morbidity after pancreaticoduodenectomy: use of a prospective complication grading system. J Am Coll Surg. 2007;204(3):356–64.

19. Suzuki K, Kantou U, Murakami Y. Two cases with ampullary cancer who underwent endoscopic excision. Prog Digest Endosc. 1983;23:236–9.

20. Han J, Lee SK, Park DH, Choi JS, Lee SS, Seo DW, et al. Treatment outcome after endoscopic papillectomy of tumors of the major duodenal papilla. Korean J Gastroenterol. 2005;46(2):110–9.

21. Talamini MA, Moesinger RC, Pitt HA, Sohn TA, Hruban RH, Lillemoe KD, et al. Adenocarcinoma of the ampulla of Vater. A 28-year experience. Ann Surg. 1997;225(5):590–9. discussion 599–600.

22. Guzzardo G, Kleinman MS, Krackov JH, Schwartz SI. Recurrent acute pancreatitis caused by ampullary villous adenoma. J Clin Gastroenterol. 1990;12(2):200–2.

23. Schwarz M, Pauls S, Sokiranski R, Brambs HJ, Glasbrenner B, Adler G, et al. Is a preoperative multidiagnostic approach to predict surgical resectability of periampullary tumors still effective? Am J Surg. 2001;182(3):243–9.

24. Elek G, Györi S, Tóth B, Pap A. Histological evaluation of preoperative biopsies from ampulla vateri. Pathol Oncol Res. 2003;9(1):32–41.

25. Blackman E, Nash SV. Diagnosis of duodenal and ampullary epithelial neoplasms by endoscopic biopsy: a clinicopathologic and immunohistochemical study. Hum Pathol. 1985;16(9):901–10.

26. Grobmyer SR, Stasik CN, Draganov P, Hemming AW, Dixon LR, Vogel SB, et al. Contemporary results with ampullectomy for 29 "benign" neoplasms of the ampulla. J Am Coll Surg. 2008;206(3):466–71.

27. Menzel J, Hoepffner N, Sulkowski U, Reimer P, Heinecke A, Poremba C, et al. Polypoid tumors of the major duodenal papilla: preoperative staging with intraductal US, EUS, and CT—a prospective, histopathologically controlled study. Gastrointest Endosc. 1999;49(3 Pt 1):349–57.

28. Ogawa T, Ito K, Fujita N, Noda Y, Kobayashi G, Horaguchi J, et al. Endoscopic papillectomy as a method of total biopsy for possible early ampullary cancer. Dig Endosc. 2012;24(4):291.

29. Skordilis P, Mouzas IA, Dimoulios PD, Alexandrakis G, Moschandrea J, Kouroumalis E. Is endosonography an effective method for detection and local staging of the ampullary carcinoma? A prospective study. BMC Surg. 2002;2:1.

30. Chen CH, Tseng LJ, Yang CC, Yeh YH, Mo LR. The accuracy of endoscopic ultrasound, endoscopic retrograde cholangiopancreatography, computed tomography, and transabdominal ultrasound in the detection and staging of primary ampullary tumors. Hepatogastroenterology. 2001;48(42):1750–3.

31. Cannon ME, Carpenter SL, Elta GH, Nostrant TT, Kochman ML, Ginsberg GG, et al. EUS compared with CT, magnetic resonance imaging, and angiography and the influence of biliary stenting on staging accuracy of ampullary neoplasms. Gastrointest Endosc. 1999;50(1):27–33.

32. Okano N, Igarashi Y, Hara S, Takuma K, Kamata I, Kishimoto Y, et al. Endosonographic preoperative evaluation for tumors of the ampulla of Vater using endoscopic ultrasonography and intraductal ultrasonography. Clin Endosc. 2014;47(2):174–7.

33. Artifon EL, Couto D, Sakai P, da Silveira EB. Prospective evaluation of EUS versus CT scan for staging of ampullary cancer. Gastrointest Endosc. 2009;70(2):290–6.

34. Kubo H, Chijiiwa Y, Akahoshi K, Hamada S, Matsui N, Nawata H. Pre-operative staging of ampullary tumours by endoscopic ultrasound. Br J Radiol. 1999;72(857):443–7.

35. Ito K, Fujita N, Noda Y, Kobayashi G, Horaguchi J, Takasawa O, et al. Preoperative evaluation of ampullary neoplasm with EUS and transpapillary intraductal US: a prospective and histopathologically controlled study. Gastrointest Endosc. 2007;66(4):740–7.

36. Baillie J. Endoscopic ampullectomy: does pancreatic stent placement make it safer? Gastrointest Endosc. 2005;62(3):371–3.

37. Chini P, Draganov PV. Diagnosis and management of ampullary adenoma: the expanding role of endoscopy. World J Gastrointest Endosc. 2011;3(12):241–7.

38. Adler DG, Qureshi W, Davila R, Gan SI, Lichtenstein D, Rajan E, et al. The role of endoscopy in ampullary and duodenal adenomas. Gastrointest Endosc. 2006;64(6):849–54.

39. Ridtitid W, Schmidt SE, Al-Haddad MA, LeBlanc J, DeWitt JM, McHenry L, et al. Performance characteristics of EUS for locoregional evaluation of ampullary lesions. Gastrointest Endosc. 2015;81(2):380–8.

40. Gaspar J, Shami VM. The role of EUS in ampullary lesions: is the answer black and white? Gastrointest Endosc. 2015;81(2):389–90.

41. Hopper AD, Bourke MJ, Williams SJ, Swan MP. Giant laterally spreading tumors of the papilla: endoscopic features, resection technique, and outcome (with videos). Gastrointest Endosc. 2010;71(6):967–75.

42. Norton ID, Gostout CJ, Baron TH, Geller A, Petersen BT, Wiersema MJ. Safety and outcome of endoscopic snare excision of the major duodenal papilla. Gastrointest Endosc. 2002;56(2):239–43.

43. Catalano MF, Linder JD, Chak A, Sivak Jr MV, Raijman I, Geenen JE, et al. Endoscopic management of adenoma of the major duodenal papilla. Gastrointest Endosc. 2004;59(2):225–32.

44. Kim JH, Moon JH, Choi HJ, Lee HS, Kim HK, Cheon YK, et al. Endoscopic snare papillectomy by using a balloon catheter for an unexposed ampullary adenoma with intraductal extension (with videos). Gastrointest Endosc. 2009;69(7):1404–6.

45. Bohnacker S, Seitz U, Nguyen D, Thonke F, Seewald S, deWeerth A, et al. Endoscopic resection of benign tumors of the duodenal papilla without and with intraductal growth. Gastrointest Endosc. 2005;62(4):551–60.

46. Binmoeller KF, Boaventura S, Ramsperger K, Soehendra N. Endoscopic snare excision of benign adenomas of the papilla of Vater. Gastrointest Endosc. 1993;39(2):127–31.

47. Desilets DJ, Dy RM, Ku PM, Hanson BL, Elton E, Mattia A, et al. Endoscopic management of tumors of the major duodenal papilla: refined techniques to improve outcome and avoid complications. Gastrointest Endosc. 2001;54(2):202–8.

48. Silvis SE. Endoscopic snare papillectomy. Gastrointest Endosc. 1993;39(2):205–7.
49. El Hajj II, Coté GA. Endoscopic diagnosis and management of ampullary lesions. Gastrointest Endosc Clin N Am. 2013;23(1):95–109.
50. Eswaran SL, Sanders M, Bernadino KP, Ansari A, Lawrence C, Stefan A, et al. Success and complications of endoscopic removal of giant duodenal and ampullary polyps: a comparative series. Gastrointest Endosc. 2006;64(6):925–32.
51. Jung MK, Cho CM, Park SY, Jeon SW, Tak WY, Kweon YO, et al. Endoscopic resection of ampullary neoplasms: a single-center experience. Surg Endosc. 2009;23(11):2568–74.
52. Ito K, Fujita N, Noda Y. Endoscopic diagnosis and treatment of ampullary neoplasm (with video). Dig Endosc. 2011;23(2):113–7.
53. Small AJ, Baron TH. Successful endoscopic resection of ampullary adenoma with intraductal extension and invasive carcinoma (with video). Gastrointest Endosc. 2006;64(1):148–51.
54. Fukushima H, Yamamoto H, Nakano H, Nakazawa K, Sunada K, Wada S, et al. Complete en bloc resection of a large ampullary adenoma with a focal adenocarcinoma by using endoscopic submucosal dissection (with video). Gastrointest Endosc. 2009;70(3):592–5.
55. Spigelman AD, Williams CB, Talbot IC, Domizio P, Phillips RK. Upper gastrointestinal cancer in patients with familial adenomatous polyposis. Lancet. 1989;2(8666):783–5.
56. Baron TH. Ampullary adenoma. Curr Treat Options Gastroenterol. 2008;11(2):96–102.
57. Björk J, Akerbrant H, Iselius L, Bergman A, Engwall Y, Wahlström J, et al. Periampullary adenomas and adenocarcinomas in familial adenomatous polyposis: cumulative risks and APC gene mutations. Gastroenterology. 2001;121(5):1127–35.
58. Yoon SM, Kim MH, Kim MJ, Jang SJ, Lee TY, Kwon S, et al. Focal early stage cancer in ampullary adenoma: surgery or endoscopic papillectomy? Gastrointest Endosc. 2007;66(4):701–7.
59. Seewald S, Omar S, Soehendra N. Endoscopic resection of tumors of the ampulla of Vater: how far up and how deep down can we go? Gastrointest Endosc. 2006;63(6):789–91.
60. Kim JH, Han JH, Yoo BM, Kim MW, Kim WH. Is endoscopic papillectomy safe for ampullary adenomas with high-grade dysplasia? Ann Surg Oncol. 2009;16(9):2547–54.
61. Pandolfi M, Martino M, Gabbrielli A. Endoscopic treatment of ampullary adenomas. JOP. 2008;9(1):1–8.
62. Kim MH, Lee SK, Seo DW, Won SY, Lee SS, Min YI. Tumors of the major duodenal papilla. Gastrointest Endosc. 2001;54(5):609–20.
63. Yamao T, Isomoto H, Kohno S, Mizuta Y, Yamakawa M, Nakao K, et al. Endoscopic snare papillectomy with biliary and pancreatic stent placement for tumors of the major duodenal papilla. Surg Endosc. 2010;24(1):119–24.
64. Boix J, Lorenzo-Zúñiga V, Moreno de Vega V, Domènech E, Gassull MA. Endoscopic resection of ampullary tumors: 12-year review of 21 cases. Surg Endosc. 2009;23(1):45–9.
65. Irani S, Arai A, Ayub K, Biehl T, Brandabur JJ, Dorer R, et al. Papillectomy for ampullary neoplasm: results of a single referral center over a 10-year period. Gastrointest Endosc. 2009;70(5):923–32.
66. Wong RF, DiSario JA. Approaches to endoscopic ampullectomy. Curr Opin Gastroenterol. 2004;20(5):460–7.
67. Ghidirim G, Mişin I, Istrate V, Cazacu S. Endoscopic papillectomy into the treatment of neoplastic lesions of Vater papilla. Curr Health Sci J. 2009;35(2):92–7.
68. Saurin JC, Chavaillon A, Napoléon B, Descos F, Bory R, Berger F, et al. Long-term follow-up of patients with endoscopic treatment of sporadic adenomas of the papilla of Vater. Endoscopy. 2003;35(5):402–6.
69. Norton ID, Geller A, Petersen BT, Sorbi D, Gostout CJ. Endoscopic surveillance and ablative therapy for periampullary adenomas. Am J Gastroenterol. 2001;96(1):101–6.
70. Ceppa EP, Burbridge RA, Rialon KL, Omotosho PA, Emick D, Jowell PS, et al. Endoscopic versus surgical ampullectomy: an algorithm to treat disease of the ampulla of Vater. Ann Surg. 2013;257(2):315–22.
71. Lienert A, Bagshaw PF. Treatment of duodenal adenomas with endoscopic argon plasma coagulation. ANZ J Surg. 2007;77(5):371–3.
72. Ghilain JM, Dive C. Endoscopic laser therapy for small villous adenomas of the duodenum. Endoscopy. 1994;26(3):308–10.
73. Farnell MB, Sakorafas GH, Sarr MG, Rowland CM, Tsiotos GG, Farley DR, et al. Villous tumors of the duodenum: reappraisal of local vs. extended resection. J Gastrointest Surg. 2000;4(1):13–21. discussion 2–3.
74. Zádorová Z, Dvořák M, Hajer J. Endoscopic therapy of benign tumors of the papilla of Vater. Endoscopy. 2001;33(4):345–7.
75. Chacko A, Dutta AK. Endoscopic resection of ampullary adenomas: novel technique to reduce post procedure pancreatitis. J Gastroenterol Hepatol. 2010;25(8):1338–9.
76. Fazel A, Quadri A, Catalano MF, Meyerson SM, Geenen JE. Does a pancreatic duct stent prevent post-ERCP pancreatitis? A prospective randomized study. Gastrointest Endosc. 2003;57(3):291–4.
77. Tarnasky PR, Palesch YY, Cunningham JT, Mauldin PD, Cotton PB, Hawes RH. Pancreatic stenting prevents pancreatitis after biliary sphincterotomy in patients with sphincter of Oddi dysfunction. Gastroenterology. 1998;115(6):1518–24.
78. Harewood GC, Pochron NL, Gostout CJ. Prospective, randomized, controlled trial of prophylactic pancreatic stent placement for endoscopic snare excision of the duodenal ampulla. Gastrointest Endosc. 2005;62(3):367–70.
79. Moon JH, Cha SW, Cho YD, Ryu CB, Cheon YK, Kwon KW, et al. Wire-guided endoscopic snare papillectomy for tumors of the major duodenal papilla. Gastrointest Endosc. 2005;61(3):461–6.
80. Kubiliun NM, Adams MA, Akshintala VS, Conte ML, Cote GA, Cotton PB, et al. Evaluation of pharmacologic prevention of pancreatitis after endoscopic retrograde cholangiopancreatography: a systematic review. Clin Gastroenterol Hepatol. 2015;13(7):1231–9.
81. Heinzow HS, Lenz P, Lenze F, Domagk D, Domschke W, Meister T. Feasibility of snare papillectomy in ampulla of Vater tumors: meta-analysis and study results from a tertiary referral center. Hepatogastroenterology. 2012;59(114):332–5.
82. De Palma GD. Endoscopic papillectomy: indications, techniques, and results. World J Gastroenterol. 2014;20(6):1537–43.
83. Charton JP, Deinert K, Schumacher B, Neuhaus H. Endoscopic resection for neoplastic diseases of the papilla of Vater. J Hepatobiliary Pancreat Surg. 2004;11(4):245–51.
84. Vogt M, Jakobs R, Benz C, Arnold JC, Adamek HE, Riemann JF. Endoscopic therapy of adenomas of the papilla of Vater. A retrospective analysis with long-term follow-up. Dig Liver Dis. 2000;32(4):339–45.

ERCP in Children, Pregnant Patients, and the Elderly

Mohamed O. Othman and Waqar A. Qureshi

ERCP in Children

Although once only rarely performed, the use of ERCP in the pediatric population is on the increase. This is mainly due to an increase in gallstone complications amongst children and young adolescents. Obesity and metabolic syndrome are recognized risk factors for gallstone formation [1]. It is estimated that as many as 16.9 % of children and adolescents are obese [2]. The surge in ERCP in this particular group of children and young adolescents focuses on managing complications of gallstone disease such as choledoholithiasis, ascending cholangitis, impacted common bile duct (CBD)s stone, and recurrent acute pancreatitis.

In the United States today, there are not many pediatric gastroenterologists who are adequately trained to perform ERCP in pediatric patients. Most ERCP procedures performed in children are carried out by gastroenterologists who are also advanced endoscopists and who received their training primarily in treating adult patients [3].

Procedure Indications

Most indications for ERCP in pediatrics are for benign disease given the low prevalence of pancreaticobiliary cancer in this age group, although occasionally young patients can develop primary pancreaticobiliary malignancy or biliary obstruction as a consequence of portal or hepatic metastases or malignant adenopathy.

Chronic pancreatitis and the management of complications of gallstones disease are the most common indications for ERCP in children and account for more than two-thirds of the procedures performed [4–6]. Other indications include management of choledochal cysts [4, 7, 8], preoperative evaluation in pancreaticobiliary maljunction [9], management of CBD strictures after liver transplant [10], management of postcholecystectomy leaks or biliary ductal injuries from surgery [11], acute or recurrent pancreatitis [4], pancreatic divisum [12], or pancreatic duct disruption from trauma [4, 12]. On rare occasions, ERCP is indicated for CBD obstruction from malignant tumors [13].

Safety

The safety of ERCP in children is comparable to that seen in the adult population. One of the largest retrospective studies in the pediatric population found that post-ERCP complications occurred in 11 out of 231 procedures (4.7 %) while pancreatitis occurred in 7 patients (3 %) [5]. In a case control study which matched 116 pediatric patients who underwent ERCP to a 116 adult patients who underwent ERCP found no difference in post-ERCP complications between pediatric and adult patients (3.5 % versus 2.5 %) [14]. Although post-ERCP pancreatitis in the pediatric population was comparable to the adult population, post-ERCP pancreatitis (PEP) was as high as 6–10 % in some case series [4, 15]. As in adults, pancreatic duct injection and pancreatic sphincterotomy were the most common risk factors for PEP in pediatric patients [16]. In one study, prophylactic pancreatic duct stenting was associated with higher rates of PEP in a retrospective series of 432 ERCP performed in pediatric patients in a large referral center for pediatric ERCP in the United States [15]. The reasons for this result in this study are unknown and prophylactic pancreatic duct stenting is not considered a violation of the standard of care in these patients.

Electronic supplementary material: The online version of this chapter (doi:10.1007/978-3-319-26854-5_11) contains supplementary material, which is available to authorized users. Videos can also be accessed at http://link.springer.com/chapter/10.1007/978-3-319-26854-5_11.

M.O. Othman, M.B.Bch • W.A. Qureshi, M.D. (✉)
Gastroenterology and Hepatology Section, Department of Internal Medicine, Baylor College of Medicine, Houston, TX 77030, USA
e-mail: wqureshi@bcm.edu

Rectal nonsteroidal anti-inflammatory drugs (NSAIDs), primarily indomethacin and diclofenac, have been proven to decrease the incidence of PEP in adult patients [17]. Currently, there is no data in pediatric literature discussing the role of rectal NSAIDs in preventing PEP, although it is likely the benefits of these agents extend to children as well.

Technical Considerations

There are two main technical issues when performing ERCP in the pediatric population: the type of anesthesia to be selected and the patient's size [14].

General anesthesia was the most common form of sedation in published series of ERCP in children [5, 8, 13, 14, 16]. The increased airflow resistance in children, in addition to the reduced ventilation from the semi-prone position, favors general anesthesia for ERCP performed in infants and young children [3]. Recently, emerging data suggest that Propofol-based sedation is also safe in pediatric patients undergoing endoscopy in general but no specific data comparing general anesthesia with Propofol-based sedation for ERCP in children has been published to date [18, 19].

Most ERCPs performed in pediatric patients utilize a standard adult duodenoscope (outer diameter of 11 mm and accessory channel of 3.2 mm) [14]. Therapeutic duodenoscopes (outer diameter of 12.5 mm and accessory channel of 4.2 mm) were used in some series for young adolescents (age 12–18 years) [13]. The use of pediatric duodenoscopes (outer diameter of 7.5 mm and an accessory channel diameter of 2.0 mm) is reserved for children under 2 years of age or children who weigh less than 10 kg [3]. The 2 mm diameter of the accessory channel limits the therapeutic uses of this pediatric duodenoscope and therefore is mainly used in infants. In addition, the pediatric duodenoscope has been produced in only limited numbers, and many institutions will not have access to one of these devices. As a general rule of thumb, children over 3 years of age can undergo ERCP with adult instruments (Fig. 11.1). Adolescents can almost always undergo ERCP with adult instruments.

The use of the tapered-tip catheter or tapered-tip sphincterotomes for CBD cannulation has been recommended in

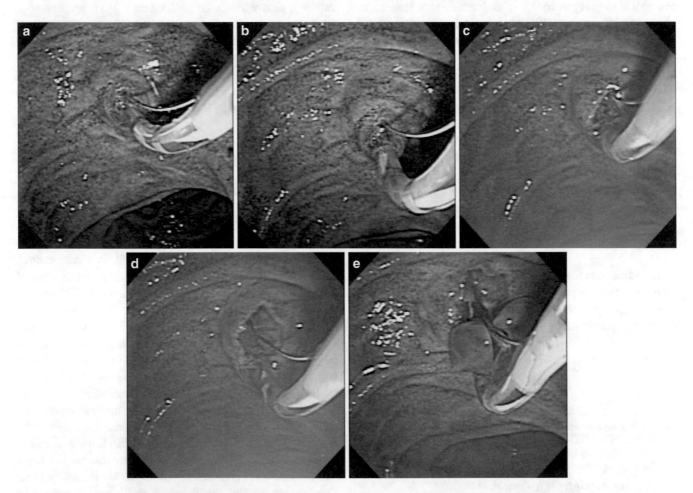

Fig. 11.1 Five image series showing ERCP performed with adult duodenoscope in a 9-year-old boy with choledocholithiasis. Sphincterotomy was performed with a tapered-tip sphincterotome and several stones passed spontaneously into the duodenum thereafter. The remainder of the stones were cleared with an occlusion balloon. (**a–e** courtesy of Douglas G. Adler MD)

younger patients with a smaller ampulla, although many endoscopists use standard adult sphincterotomes for these procedures without difficulty or increased risk [13, 14]. Different therapeutic maneuvers such as stricture dilation, stent placement, or sphincteroplasty can be performed in the pediatric population without any modification of standard technique [6, 13, 16].

The technical success of ERCP in children is comparable to that seen in adults undergoing ERCP in the hands of trained endoscopists. CBD cannulation was achieved in more than 95 % of cases in several recently published case series [15, 16]. Due to the paucity of trained pediatric gastroenterologists in ERCP, the majority of ERCP in children are done by advanced endoscopists whose training and practice specializes in adults.

Halvorson et al. reported the outcomes of 70 ERCPs performed in children by an adult gastroenterologist with no formal training in pediatric ERCP. In this study, the cannulation success rate was 98 % and the complication rate was 7 % without any major complications [20]. A similar success rate and complications rate were also noted in a smaller case series of 26 pediatric ERCPs performed by a general surgeon with fellowship training in ERCP in a community practice setting [21]. Although limited, these data support the common and widespread practice of gastroenterologists that practice on adult patients performing ERCP in pediatric patients.

Advanced endoscopists with expertise in adult patients should be familiar with fluoroscopic findings of certain congenital anomalies and conditions which are seen in pediatric patients before embarking on performing ERCPs in children. The endoscopist should be able to differentiate subtypes of choledochal cysts [22], evaluate pancreaticobiliary maljunction [23], diagnose pancreatic divisum [24], recognize annular pancreas endoscopically and via pancreatogram, as well as other rare anomalies which may be seen in the pediatric population such as wirsungocele [25] or Santorinicele [26].

Overall, ERCP in children can be safely performed with similar technical success as adult populations in the hands of advanced endoscopists trained in this procedure.

ERCP in the Elderly

The use of ERCP in the elderly is increasing as a result of increasing life expectancy, especially in developed countries. It is expected that people aged 60 years or older will represent 22 % of the population in the next four decades (a jump from the current 8–10 %) [27]. Physiological changes associated with aging, in addition to increased comorbidities in the elderly, may increase the risk of invasive procedures such as ERCP. In this part of the chapter, we discuss the indication, safety, and technical consideration of ERCP in the elderly.

Procedure Indications

Common bile duct stones and CBD obstruction due to pancreatic head malignancy are the two most common indications for ERCP in the elderly [28]. Cholangitis is the main presentation leading to ERCP in up to one-third of procedures performed in patients 80 years old or older [28, 29] (Fig. 11.2).

Safety

It was noted in one prospective series that hypotension and prolonged sedation are more frequently seen in very elderly patients (80 years or older) compared to patients younger

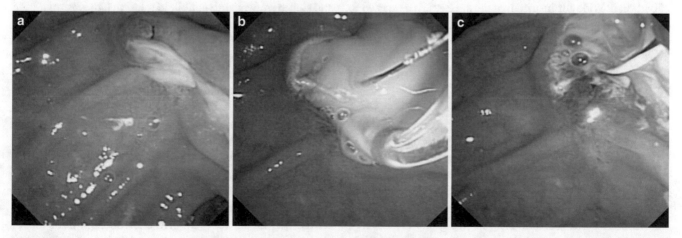

Fig. 11.2 Three image series showing ascending cholangitis in an 87-year-old man. (**a**) Shows spontaneous passage of a small amount of pus prior to cannulation. (**b**) Shows copious pus draining to the duodenum after biliary sphincterotomy. (**c**) Shows some spontaneous passage of stone fragments into the duodenum. A balloon was used to sweep out the remaining stones and stone fragments. (**a–c** courtesy of Douglas G. Adler MD)

than 80 years old. However, there was no difference with regard to other post-ERCP complications such as pancreatitis or perforation in elderly patients compared to younger patients [30]. Post-ERCP pancreatitis was significantly less frequently encountered in patients 90 years or older compared to younger patients in a recently published case control study (0 with 13 [10 %], respectively; $p=0.004$) [31]. The exact reasons for this lower rate of PEP were unclear. A possibility for this lower rate of PEP may be the fact that as people age some atrophy of the pancreas can be normal, and perhaps an atrophic pancreas is more resistant to PEP than a normal one.

Caution should be exercised when performing ERCP in the elderly with coexisting cardiopulmonary diseases. Transient ischemia and different types of arrhythmia have been noted on electrocardiography of elderly patients during ERCP procedures, although these findings can be seen in non-elderly patients as well [32]. In a prospective series of 130 ERCPs, elevated cardiac troponin was noted in 6 out of 53 (11 %) patients 65 years or older. Myocardial injury and hypoxia were risk factors for post-ERCP pancreatitis in this study [33].

The type of anesthesia used in ERCP is changing. Older studies showed a significant number of ERCP were performed with the use of moderate sedation (generally a narcotic/benzodiazepine combination). Most recently published series utilized general anesthesia or propofol sedation for ERCP. Propofol sedation was administered safely in elderly patients undergoing ERCP with a low rate of complications. In a prospective study of 150 consecutive patients aged 80 years or older who underwent ERCP with either propofol sedation or moderate anesthesia, hypoxic events were significantly lower in the propofol sedation group compared to the moderate sedation group (12 % versus 26 %). Of note, recovery time was also significantly shorter in the propofol group [34]. Although not directly related to sedation, the use of carbon dioxide for insufflation during ERCP has shown to decrease post-procedure abdominal distension and nausea in patients 75 years or older [35].

Technical Considerations

Managing CBD stones in the elderly is occasionally challenging. Due to advanced age and delayed presentation, some stones in elderly patients are too large or too difficult to capture and crush to be removed with conventional methods of balloon sweep or basket extraction. Endoscopic large balloon dilation of the papilla combined with biliary sphincterotomy can facilitate stone extraction in this age group (Video 1.1). The success rate of large balloon dilation of the ampulla in extracting stones larger than 1 cm in one session is reported to be higher than 80 % [36, 37]. Large balloon dilation of the

papilla (up to 15 or 18 mm) was not associated with an increased risk of post-ERCP pancreatitis in a published series of 341 patients [38].

Long-term CBD stent placement has been suggested as an alternative treatment for multiple or very large, irretrievable CBD stones. The concept behind this idea is that some of these patients may not tolerate prolonged sedation or anesthesia or aggressive attempts to remove large stones and that long-term stenting provides relief from jaundice and biliary obstruction. Some authors also feel that long-term plastic biliary stenting can help fragment large stones by mechanical forces within the CBD, but this is not universally agreed upon.

Plastic biliary stent placement was associated with a 6 mm decrease in stone diameter after 4 months of insertion in a single center retrospective study of 52 patients, suggesting at least some validity to the idea that a stent could help to break up a stone [39]. The combination of choleretic agents such as Ursodeoxycholic acid and terpene along with common bile duct stenting was suggested in elderly patients to further enhance the decrease of the CBD stone diameter [40]. However, there was no statistically significant difference in the reduction of the CBD stone diameter in a randomized trial which compared common bile duct stenting alone versus common bile duct stenting in addition to choleretic agents in elderly patients with irretrievable CBD stones [41]. This technique, however, is limited by the need to change plastic stents every few months to prevent cholangitis [42]. Furthermore, even with appropriately scheduled stent changes some patients will still develop ascending cholangitis and require more frequent ERCP.

Another issue which arises in elderly patients with choledocholithiasis and cholelithiasis is the frequently associated need for laparoscopic cholecystectomy. Many patients with choledocholithiasis and/or cholangitis develop simultaneous cholecystitis. ERCP with endoscopic sphincterotomy and stone removal with gallbladder left in situ was suggested as an alternative to cholecystectomy in high-risk surgical patients or the elderly, although this approach does not remove the risk of cholecystitis [43].

The rates of biliary complications after endoscopic treatment in patients with the gallbladder left in situ vary in several cohort studies. In a trial of 186 patients with choledocholithiasis who were considered to be at high risk for surgery and who underwent endoscopic therapy alone, subsequent cholecystectomy was required due to biliary complications in 9.6 % of the patients, during a median follow-up period of 36 months [44]. In another cohort of 461 patients who underwent endoscopic therapy with the gallbladder left in situ for presumed choledocholithiasis and/or cholelithiasis, a CBD stone was seen in 19 % of patients and acute cholecystitis developed in 13 % of patients over a median follow-up period of 79 months [45].

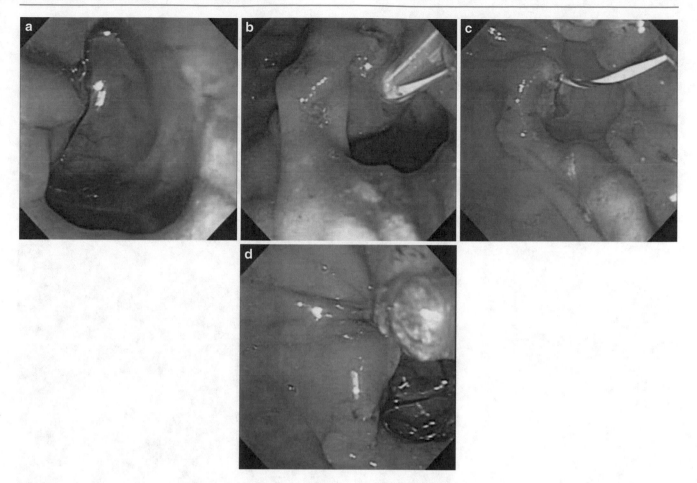

Fig. 11.3 Four image series showing an ERCP in a 92-year-old woman with a large periampullary diverticulum and a common bile duct stone and jaundice. (**a**) A large duodenal diverticula with the major papilla inside the diverticula itself. (**b**) Cannulation of the common bile duct allows the ampullary orifice to be everted, improving visualization. (**c**) Appearance of major papilla inside diverticula after biliary sphincterotomy. (**d**) The stone is visible in the duodenum after balloon extraction. (**a–d** courtesy of Douglas G. Adler MD)

On the other hand, there is accumulating evidence from the surgical literature which advocates for cholecystectomy in this subset of patients given the excellent safety profile of laparoscopic cholecystectomy in the elderly [46]. A Cochrane meta-analysis which included five randomized trials comparing endoscopic treatment alone with prophylactic cholecystectomy recommended prophylactic cholecystectomy after ERCP with CBD clearance given the high recurrence rate of cholangitis and retained CBD stones [47]. In an attempt to decrease morbidity and increase cost-effectiveness, laparoscopic cholecystectomy with ERCP can be performed in the same session in the elderly with common bile duct stone without any increase in morbidity, although this requires a high degree of coordination between surgeons and endoscopists and is not always feasible or realistic [48]. Usually, these two procedures can be performed within a few days of each other to the same effect with fewer logistical difficulties.

Another technical issue which may complicate ERCP performance in the elderly is the presence of periampullary diverticulum (Fig. 11.3). The prevalence of periampullary diverticula is increasing with advanced age and is rarely found in patients younger than 40 years old [49]. Traction on the duodenal wall at the level of the ampulla by the common bile duct may lead to diverticulum formation. The presence of the ampulla within a diverticulum may impact the success of CBD cannulation, although this is still usually successful. The utilization of advanced techniques to facilitate cannulation in this scenario may be necessary. Needle knife sphincterotomy [50] (Video 11.4), double wire technique (Video 11.2), pancreatic duct stenting [51], cap-assisted ERCP [52], clip placement over the diverticulum to help evert the major papilla [53], and EUS-guided ERCP have all previously been used to overcome difficulties in cannulation that arose due to periampullary diverticulum. With the exception of increased fluoroscopy time, ERCP outcomes in patients with periampullary diverticulum (Video 11.3) are similar to patients without periampullary diverticula [54]. Patients with periampullary diverticula may develop a very generous common bile duct diameter and may form large stones that require

Fig. 11.4 A 73-year-old man
with a duodenal diverticula
and a common bile duct
stricture. (**a**) Cholangiogram
shows many large stones
above a distal CBD stricture.
(**b**) Digital cholangioscopy
shows a benign appearing
stenosis. This was confirmed
by brushing and biopsy. (**c**)
Laser lithotripsy is used to
break up the stones above the
stenosis so they could be
removed endoscopically

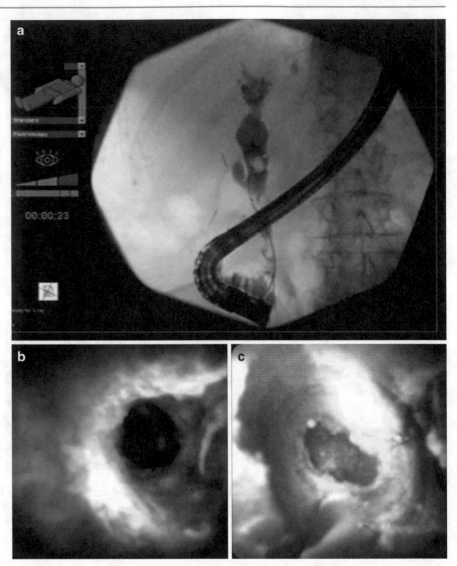

aggressive endoscopic treatments (Fig. 11.4). Cholangioscopy (Video 11.5) may be performed to allow direct vision of the duct lumen if a tumor is suspected in the bile duct or laser- or hydro-lithotripsy is planned.

ERCP in Pregnant Patients

Pregnancy poses an increased risk for developing pancreatic and biliary disease. Increased estrogen and progesterone predisposes patients for the development of gallstone formation that can be further complicated by cholecystitis, choledocholithiasis, and pancreatitis [55]. The major effect of estrogen on the biliary system is to increase cholesterol secretion into bile resulting in increased saturation of cholesterol in bile, favoring stone formation ("lithogenic bile") [56]. Progesterone slows gallbladder contractility and emptying, promoting stasis of bile [57]. These factors all increase the risk of stone

formation during pregnancy. The risk is further increased with subsequent pregnancies, especially in women who have preexisting cholelithiasis or biliary colic. Multiparous women are nine times more likely to have gallstones than nulliparous women [58]. In a study of 980 pregnant women, cholelithiasis was seen on transabdominal ultrasounds in 12 % of the patients in the postpartum period [58].

Symptomatic common bile duct stones during pregnancy may require ERCP with various interventions such as biliary sphincterotomy, biliary stone extraction, and/or stent placement. ERCP infrequently could be complicated with post-ERCP pancreatitis, hemorrhage, or perforation, which could pose a danger to the mother, the fetus, and the overall clinical arc of the pregnancy itself [59]. In addition, radiation exposure during fluoroscopy can be hazardous to the fetus, primarily in the first trimester [60].

The safety, use, and outcomes of ERCP during pregnancy have not been studied comprehensively in published literature as it has frequently been difficult to identify enough pregnant patients at a single center to study. The rate of complications following ERCP to mother and fetus is an important measure to guide the use of this procedure. In this section we discuss the indications, safety of ERCP during pregnancy, and various ERCP techniques to minimize harm and increase safety of ERCP in pregnancy.

Indications

Choledocholithiasis and acute biliary pancreatitis were the main indications of ERCP in pregnancy in many large published series [61–63]. Other indications include biliary colic, cholangitis [64], and chronic pancreatitis [65]. Diagnostic ERCP is rarely performed in pregnant patients and should be substituted with magnetic resonance cholangio-pancreaticography (MRCP) if possible [66] (Fig. 11.5). MRCP is generally felt to be safe in pregnancy and can be used to "screen" a patient who may have passed a stone before committing the patient to an ERCP.

Safety of ERCP in Pregnancy

ERCP in pregnancy is safe and the risk of maternal and fetal complications is low [62]. In some published series, post-ERCP pancreatitis was seen in up to 10 % in pregnant patients who underwent ERCP. This is slightly higher than what has been

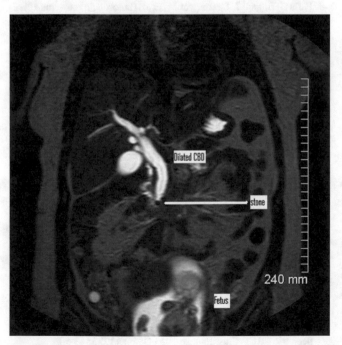

Fig. 11.5 MRCP showing choledocholithiasis and the fetus in a pregnant woman

reported in other populations. However, pancreatitis in these patients was generally mild and was managed with conservative measures alone in most cases [61]. The majority of pregnancies ended in full-term deliveries of healthy newborns. One study followed subjects over 7 years following ERCP in pregnancy and no association was established between radiation exposure time and long-term complications. Premature delivery was reported to be around 3 % in published literature and does not appear to be more common among patients who undergo ERCP compared to those who did not [61, 67].

Fetal outcomes were uncomplicated in the majority of pregnancies. Fetal complications were reported in 5 % of patients who underwent ERPC in pregnancy. This included abortions [68], low birth weight [61, 69], intrauterine growth retardation [67], and fetal death [70]. ERCP with cholangioscopy has been shown to be safe in management of choledocholithiasis in pregnancy [71].

Technical Considerations

Timing of ERCP in pregnancy and preventing harm to the fetus are important considerations in pregnancy.

Generally, avoiding ERCP in the first trimester is advised if possible, but this may not always be possible. Patients with significant symptoms of choledocholithiasis, ascending cholangitis, or other severe problems may have to undergo ERCP in the first trimester. The risk of congenital malformations, low birth weight, abortion, and cancer increases with exposure to ionizing radiation in the first trimester [72]. The second trimester and early third trimester are in the perfect window for performing ERCP as most true development has already taken place and at this stage the fetus and the gravid uterus are still not at their final size. The gravid uterus in the late third trimester may interfere with prone positioning for the procedure. There is also the possibility of compression of the aorta and/or the inferior vena cava by the gravid uterus if the patient is placed in supine position [73].

Many physicians will try to avoid ERCP in pregnant patients, if possible, out of a concern for causing harm to the mother, fetus, or both. In some cases, especially if the patient is near the end of her pregnancy, conservative treatment until after delivery (at which time an ERCP is performed) can be sufficient. Still, conservative treatment of CBD stones and its complications in pregnancy and delaying ERCP until after labor is associated with frequent emergency room visits, recurrent symptoms, and increased hospitalization [74]. Given the safety profile of ERCP in pregnancy, therapeutic ERCP should, in general, not be deferred until the postpartum period if it can be accomplished in a reasonable and safe manner and especially if the patient presents with CBD stone complications early in pregnancy. Often, delaying the procedure until the second trimester is a reasonable option. As above, some pregnant patients will require urgent or emergent ERCP regardless of their trimester.

Limiting fluoroscopy use and placing an external shield (underneath the patient) to cover the pelvic area is recommended to minimize fetal radiation [73]. Fluoroscopy can also be limited by reducing the frame rate, using X-rays only when strictly needed, and limiting or avoiding the use of "hard shots" and only using "spot fluoroscopy" during the procedure. Performing a radiation-free ERCP in pregnancy is gaining popularity, although in most cases at least some exposure to radiation will be required and is likely of little clinical consequence. Endoscopic ultrasound (EUS), which utilizes no radiation, prior to ERCP can aid in identifying the location and number of stones in the CBD and measure the length of the CBD to allow balloon sweep up to the bifurcation without fluoroscopy guidance [75]. In addition, starting with EUS prior to ERCP may help in avoiding the performance of unnecessary ERCP when the EUS shows no CBD stones [76].

Consulting with the obstetric service regarding fetal monitoring during the ERCP procedure is often helpful but is not mandatory [73].

Conclusion

ERCP in the children, the elderly, and pregnant patients is often required. In general, these special patient subsets can undergo ERCP safely and with complication rates comparable to that seen in most patients. Endoscopists performing ERCP in these settings should be aware of the anatomic, physiologic, and procedural differences in these patient subsets and plan accordingly to ensure good clinical outcomes.

Video Legends

Video 11.1 This clip shows the removal of multiple large stones with balloon extraction following endoscopic sphincterotomy and balloon dilation of the sphincter of Oddi (MP4 13528 kb).

Video 11.2 Double wire method to access the CBD in a case of difficult cannulation. The firstl wire kept going into the PD so is left in place and a second wire aids in both selecting the access of the CBD and blocking re-entry into the PD (MP4 11457 kb).

Video 11.3 Here the ampulla os is inside a diverticulum and difficult to cannulate with a standard 0.035 wire. A loop tip wire enables entry into the CBD and an endoscopic sphincterotomy and plastic stent placement are then performed (MP4 11523 kb).

Video 11.4 A precut sphincterotomy is performed here with small upward cuts from the os along the axis of the CBD fol-

lowing frequent attempts to advance the wire. Once access is gained, dye is injected to confirm entry into the CBD and then an ES is completed (MP4 13393 kb).

Video 11.5 In this video clip, an endoscopic sphincterotomy is performed over a wire and then the spyglass cholangioscope is advanced into the biliary tree. Some blood is seen over an ulcerated mass. Towards the end of the video, a forceps is introduced to biopsy this area (MP4 16757 kb).

References

1. Stinton LM, Myers RP, Shaffer EA. Epidemiology of gallstones. Gastroenterol Clin North Am. 2010;39:157–69. vii.
2. Ogden CL, Carroll MD, Kit BK, et al. Prevalence of childhood and adult obesity in the United States, 2011–2012. JAMA. 2014;311:806–14.
3. ASGE Standards of Practice Committee, Lightdale JR, Acosta R, et al. Modifications in endoscopic practice for pediatric patients. Gastrointest Endosc. 2014;79:699–710.
4. Jang JY, Yoon CH, Kim KM. Endoscopic retrograde cholangiopancreatography in pancreatic and biliary tract disease in Korean children. World J Gastroenterol. 2010;16:490–5.
5. Otto AK, Neal MD, Slivka AN, et al. An appraisal of endoscopic retrograde cholangiopancreatography (ERCP) for pancreaticobiliary disease in children: our institutional experience in 231 cases. Surg Endosc. 2011;25:2536–40.
6. Durakbasa CU, Balik E, Yamaner S, et al. Diagnostic and therapeutic endoscopic retrograde cholangiopancreatography (ERCP) in children and adolescents: experience in a single institution. Eur J Pediatr Surg. 2008;18:241–4.
7. Hukkinen M, Koivusalo A, Lindahl H, et al. Increasing occurrence of choledochal malformations in children: a single-center 37-year experience from Finland. Scand J Gastroenterol. 2014;49:1255–60.
8. Paris C, Bejjani J, Beaunoyer M, et al. Endoscopic retrograde cholangiopancreatography is useful and safe in children. J Pediatr Surg. 2010;45:938–42.
9. Hiramatsu T, Itoh A, Kawashima H, et al. Usefulness and safety of endoscopic retrograde cholangiopancreatography in children with pancreaticobiliary maljunction. J Pediatr Surg. 2015;50:377–81.
10. Otto AK, Neal MD, Mazariegos GV, et al. Endoscopic retrograde cholangiopancreatography is safe and effective for the diagnosis and treatment of pancreaticobiliary disease following abdominal organ transplant in children. Pediatr Transplant. 2012;16:829–34.
11. Issa H, Al-Haddad A, Al-Salem AH. Diagnostic and therapeutic ERCP in the pediatric age group. Pediatr Surg Int. 2007;23:111–6.
12. Poddar U, Thapa BR, Bhasin DK, et al. Endoscopic retrograde cholangiopancreatography in the management of pancreaticobiliary disorders in children. J Gastroenterol Hepatol. 2001;16:927–31.
13. Cheng CL, Fogel EL, Sherman S, et al. Diagnostic and therapeutic endoscopic retrograde cholangiopancreatography in children: a large series report. J Pediatr Gastroenterol Nutr. 2005;41:445–53.
14. Varadarajulu S, Wilcox CM, Hawes RH, et al. Technical outcomes and complications of ERCP in children. Gastrointest Endosc. 2004;60:367–71.
15. Troendle DM, Abraham O, Huang R, et al. Factors associated with post-ERCP pancreatitis and the effect of pancreatic duct stenting in a pediatric population. Gastrointest Endosc. 2015;81(6):1408–16.
16. Giefer MJ, Kozarek RA. Technical outcomes and complications of pediatric ERCP. Surg Endosc 2015.Dec;29(12):3543-50.
17. Sun HL, Han B, Zhai HP, et al. Rectal NSAIDs for the prevention of post-ERCP pancreatitis: a meta-analysis of randomized controlled trials. Surgeon. 2014;12:141–7.

18. Kaddu R, Bhattacharya D, Metriyakool K, et al. Propofol compared with general anesthesia for pediatric GI endoscopy: is propofol better? Gastrointest Endosc. 2002;55:27–32.

19. Dar AQ, Shah ZA. Anesthesia and sedation in pediatric gastrointestinal endoscopic procedures: a review. World J Gastrointest Endosc. 2010;2:257–62.

20. Halvorson L, Halsey K, Darwin P, et al. The safety and efficacy of therapeutic ERCP in the pediatric population performed by adult gastroenterologists. Dig Dis Sci. 2013;58:3611–9.

21. Green JA, Scheeres DE, Conrad HA, et al. Pediatric ERCP in a multidisciplinary community setting: experience with a fellowship-trained general surgeon. Surg Endosc. 2007;21:2187–92.

22. Kieling CO, Hallal C, Spessato CO, et al. Changing pattern of indications of endoscopic retrograde cholangiopancreatography in children and adolescents: a twelve-year experience. World J Pediatr. 2014;11:154–9.

23. Kim Y, Hyun JJ, Lee JM, et al. Anomalous union of the pancreaticobiliary duct without choledochal cyst: is cholecystectomy alone sufficient? Langenbecks Arch Surg. 2014;399:1071–6.

24. Terui K, Hishiki T, Saito T, et al. Pancreas divisum in pancreaticobiliary maljunction in children. Pediatr Surg Int. 2010;26:419–22.

25. Coelho DE, Ardengh JC, Lima-Filho ER, et al. Different clinical aspects of Wirsungocele: case series of three patients and review of literature. Acta Gastroenterol Latinoam. 2011;41:230–3.

26. Lutzak GD, Gluck M, Ross AS, et al. Endoscopic minor papilla sphincterotomy in patients with santoriniceles reduces pain and improves quality of life. Dig Dis Sci. 2013;58:2075–81.

27. Bloom DE, Chatterji S, Kowal P, et al. Macroeconomic implications of population ageing and selected policy responses. Lancet. 2015;385:649–57.

28. Fritz E, Kirchgatterer A, Hubner D, et al. ERCP is safe and effective in patients 80 years of age and older compared with younger patients. Gastrointest Endosc. 2006;64:899–905.

29. Katsinelos P, Paroutoglou G, Kountouras J, et al. Efficacy and safety of therapeutic ERCP in patients 90 years of age and older. Gastrointest Endosc. 2006;63:417–23.

30. Katsinelos P, Kountouras J, Chatzimavroudis G, et al. Outpatient therapeutic endoscopic retrograde cholangiopancreatography is safe in patients aged 80 years and older. Endoscopy. 2011;43:128–33.

31. Yun DY, Han J, Oh JS, et al. Is endoscopic retrograde cholangiopancreatography safe in patients 90 years of age and older? Gut Liver. 2014;8:552–6.

32. Kounis NG, Zavras GM, Papadaki PJ, et al. Electrocardiographic changes in elderly patients during endoscopic retrograde cholangiopancreatography. Can J Gastroenterol. 2003;17:539–44.

33. Fisher L, Fisher A, Thomson A. Cardiopulmonary complications of ERCP in older patients. Gastrointest Endosc. 2006;63:948–55.

34. Riphaus A, Stergiou N, Wehrmann T. Sedation with propofol for routine ERCP in high-risk octogenarians: a randomized, controlled study. Am J Gastroenterol. 2005;100:1957–63.

35. Nakamura K, Yamaguchi Y, Hasue T, et al. The usefulness and safety of carbon dioxide insufflation during endoscopic retrograde cholangiopancreatography in elderly patients: a prospective, double-blind, randomized, controlled trial. Hepatogastroenterology. 2014;61:2191–5.

36. Oh MJ, Kim TN. Prospective comparative study of endoscopic papillary large balloon dilation and endoscopic sphincterotomy for removal of large bile duct stones in patients above 45 years of age. Scand J Gastroenterol. 2012;47:1071–7.

37. Jin PP, Cheng JF, Liu D, et al. Endoscopic papillary large balloon dilation vs endoscopic sphincterotomy for retrieval of common bile duct stones: a meta-analysis. World J Gastroenterol. 2014; 20:5548–56.

38. Park JS, Kim TN, Kim KH. Endoscopic papillary large balloon dilation for treatment of large bile duct stones does not increase the risk of post-procedure pancreatitis. Dig Dis Sci. 2014;59: 3092–8.

39. Hong WD, Zhu QH, Huang QK. Endoscopic sphincterotomy plus endoprostheses in the treatment of large or multiple common bile duct stones. Dig Endosc. 2011;23:240–3.

40. Han J, Moon JH, Koo HC, et al. Effect of biliary stenting combined with ursodeoxycholic acid and terpene treatment on retained common bile duct stones in elderly patients: a multicenter study. Am J Gastroenterol. 2009;104:2418–21.

41. Lee TH, Han JH, Kim HJ, et al. Is the addition of choleretic agents in multiple double-pigtail biliary stents effective for difficult common bile duct stones in elderly patients? A prospective, multicenter study. Gastrointest Endosc. 2011;74:96–102.

42. Di Giorgio P, Manes G, Grimaldi E, et al. Endoscopic plastic stenting for bile duct stones: stent changing on demand or every 3 months. A prospective comparison study. Endoscopy. 2013;45:1014–7.

43. Kwon SK, Lee BS, Kim NJ, et al. Is cholecystectomy necessary after ERCP for bile duct stones in patients with gallbladder in situ? Korean J Intern Med. 2001;16:254–9.

44. Ingoldby CJ, el-Saadi J, Hall RI, et al. Late results of endoscopic sphincterotomy for bile duct stones in elderly patients with gall bladders in situ. Gut. 1989;30:1129–31.

45. Cui ML, Cho JH, Kim TN. Long-term follow-up study of gallbladder in situ after endoscopic common duct stone removal in Korean patients. Surg Endosc. 2013;27:1711–6.

46. Weber DM. Laparoscopic surgery: an excellent approach in elderly patients. Arch Surg. 2003;138:1083–8.

47. McAlister VC, Davenport E, Renouf E. Cholecystectomy deferral in patients with endoscopic sphincterotomy. Cochrane Database Syst Rev 2007:CD006233.

48. Di Mauro D, Faraci R, Mariani L, et al. Rendezvous technique for cholecystocholedochal lithiasis in octogenarians: is it as effective as in younger patients, or should endoscopic sphincterotomy followed by laparoscopic cholecystectomy be preferred? J Laparoendosc Adv Surg Tech A. 2014;24:13–21.

49. Zippi M, Traversa G, Pica R, et al. Efficacy and safety of endoscopic retrograde cholangiopancreatography (ERCP) performed in patients with Periampullary duodenal diverticula (PAD). Clin Ter. 2014;165:e291–4.

50. Tyagi P, Sharma P, Sharma BC, et al. Periampullary diverticula and technical success of endoscopic retrograde cholangiopancreatography. Surg Endosc. 2009;23:1342–5.

51. Fogel EL, Sherman S, Lehman GA. Increased selective biliary cannulation rates in the setting of periampullary diverticula: main pancreatic duct stent placement followed by pre-cut biliary sphincterotomy. Gastrointest Endosc. 1998;47:396–400.

52. Myung DS, Park CH, Koh HR, et al. Cap-assisted ERCP in patients with difficult cannulation due to periampullary diverticulum. Endoscopy. 2014;46:352–5.

53. Ustundag Y, Karakaya K, Aydemir S. Biliary cannulation facilitated by endoscopic clip assistance in the setting of intra-diverticular papilla. Turk J Gastroenterol. 2009;20:279–81.

54. Katsinelos P, Chatzimavroudis G, Tziomalos K, et al. Impact of periampullary diverticula on the outcome and fluoroscopy time in endoscopic retrograde cholangiopancreatography. Hepatobiliary Pancreat Dis Int. 2013;12:408–14.

55. Ko CW, Beresford SA, Schulte SJ, et al. Incidence, natural history, and risk factors for biliary sludge and stones during pregnancy. Hepatology. 2005;41:359–65.

56. Wang HH, Afdhal NH, Wang DQ. Estrogen receptor alpha, but not beta, plays a major role in 17beta-estradiol-induced murine cholesterol gallstones. Gastroenterology. 2004;127:239–49.

57. Abu-Hayyeh S, Papacleovoulou G, Lovgren-Sandblom A, et al. Intrahepatic cholestasis of pregnancy levels of sulfated progesterone metabolites inhibit farnesoid X receptor resulting in a cholestatic phenotype. Hepatology. 2013;57:716–26.

58. Valdivieso V, Covarrubias C, Siegel F, et al. Pregnancy and cholelithiasis: pathogenesis and natural course of gallstones diagnosed in early puerperium. Hepatology. 1993;17:1–4.

59. Freeman ML. Adverse outcomes of endoscopic retrograde cholan-giopancreatography: avoidance and management. Gastrointest Endosc Clin N Am. 2003;13:775–98. xi.

60. Lowe SA. Diagnostic radiography in pregnancy: risks and reality. Aust N Z J Obstet Gynaecol. 2004;44:191–6.

61. Tang SJ, Mayo MJ, Rodriguez-Frias E, et al. Safety and utility of ERCP during pregnancy. Gastrointest Endosc. 2009;69:453–61.

62. Fine S, Beirne J, Delgi-Esposti S, et al. Continued evidence for safety of endoscopic retrograde cholangiopancreatography during pregnancy. World J Gastrointest Endosc. 2014;6:352–8.

63. Yang J, Zhang X, Zhang X. Therapeutic efficacy of endoscopic retrograde cholangiopancreatography among pregnant women with severe acute biliary pancreatitis. J Laparoendosc Adv Surg Tech A. 2013;23:437–40.

64. Gupta R, Tandan M, Lakhtakia S, et al. Safety of therapeutic ERCP in pregnancy—an Indian experience. Indian J Gastroenterol. 2005;24:161–3.

65. Tham TC, Vandervoort J, Wong RC, et al. Safety of ERCP during pregnancy. Am J Gastroenterol. 2003;98:308–11.

66. Oto A, Ernst R, Ghulmiyyah L, et al. The role of MR cholangiopan-creatography in the evaluation of pregnant patients with acute pan-creaticobiliary disease. Br J Radiol. 2009;82:279–85.

67. Simmons DC, Tarnasky PR, Rivera-Alsina ME, et al. Endoscopic retrograde cholangiopancreatography (ERCP) in pregnancy with-out the use of radiation. Am J Obstet Gynecol. 2004;190:1467–9.

68. Daas AY, Agha A, Pinkas H, et al. ERCP in pregnancy: is it safe? Gastroenterol Hepatol (N Y). 2009;5:851–5.

69. Shelton J, Linder JD, Rivera-Alsina ME, et al. Commitment, con-firmation, and clearance: new techniques for nonradiation ERCP during pregnancy (with videos). Gastrointest Endosc. 2008;67:364–8.

70. Chong VH, Jalihal A. Endoscopic management of biliary disor-ders during pregnancy. Hepatobiliary Pancreat Dis Int. 2010;9:180–5.

71. Uradomo L, Pandolfe F, Aragon G, et al. SpyGlass cholangioscopy for management of choledocholithiasis during pregnancy. Hepatobiliary Pancreat Dis Int. 2011;10:107.

72. Brent RL. Counseling patients exposed to ionizing radiation during pregnancy. Rev Panam Salud Publica. 2006;20:198–204.

73. ASGE Standards of Practice Committee, Shergill AK, Ben-Menachem T, et al. Guidelines for endoscopy in pregnant and lac-tating women. Gastrointest Endosc. 2012;76:18–24.

74. Othman MO, Stone E, Hashimi M, et al. Conservative management of cholelithiasis and its complications in pregnancy is associated with recurrent symptoms and more emergency department visits. Gastrointest Endosc. 2012;76:564–9.

75. Sethi S, Thosani N, Banerjee S. Radiation-free ERCP in pregnancy: a "sound" approach to leaving no stone unturned. Dig Dis Sci. 2015;60:2604–7.

76. Vohra S, Holt EW, Bhat YM, et al. Successful single-session endosonography-based endoscopic retrograde cholangiopancrea-tography without fluoroscopy in pregnant patients with suspected choledocholithiasis: a case series. J Hepatobiliary Pancreat Sci. 2014;21:93–7.

Mariano Gonzalez-Haba and Uzma D. Siddiqui

Introduction

Endoscopic retrograde cholangiopancreatography (ERCP) is one of the most technically demanding and high-risk procedures performed by gastrointestinal (GI) endoscopists. Amongst all the currently performed endoscopic procedures it carries the highest complication rate, including pancreatitis, bleeding, cholangitis, and perforation. Of these complications, post-ERCP pancreatitis (PEP) is the most frequent and can be the most severe.

Since it was first reported in 1968 [1], ERCP has evolved from a diagnostic procedure to an almost exclusively therapeutic procedure. Although the increasing use of less invasive modalities to image the pancreaticobiliary system such as magnetic resonance cholangiopancreatography (MRCP) and endoscopic ultrasound (EUS) has led to a 16 % decline in total volume since 2000, there is still an estimated 700,000 ERCPs performed annually in the United States [2].

The rate of PEP can vary widely depending on a variety of factors, but the typical rate of post-ERCP pancreatitis is generally between 1 and 10 % for average-risk patients [3–5]. In a recent systematic review of the control groups (placebo or no pancreatic duct stent arms) of 108 randomized controlled trials, which included 13,296 patients undergoing both diagnostic and therapeutic ERCP, the overall rate of PEP was found to be 9.7 %, with a mortality rate of 0.7 % and an incidence of severe PEP of 0.5 %. In this study, the incidence of severe PEP and mortality caused by PEP was similar among patients in non-risk stratified (8.5 %) and high-risk (14.7 %)

randomized control trials (RCTs) [6]. Interestingly the incidence of PEP was reported to be higher in North American RCTs compared with European and Asian RCTs (13 % vs. 9.9 % vs. 8.4 % respectively). The incidence of PEP was higher on ERCPs conducted after the year 2000 than before it (10 % and 7.7 % respectively) likely due a trend towards more therapeutic indications for ERCP [6].

Although the specialty of gastroenterology may be thought of as low risk for medical malpractice lawsuits, a recent study has shown that gastroenterology ranks 6 out of 25 specialties, before obstetrics and gynecology, in terms of proportion of physicians facing malpractice claims [7]. Total claim payments for colonoscopy and ERCP have increased over time [8]. In an interesting analysis performed by Cotton on 59 cases in which ERCP malpractice was alleged, the most common allegation (54 % of cases) was that the ERCP, or the therapeutic procedure, was not indicated [9].

The risk of PEP can be influenced by multiple factors, both patient related and procedure related, and needs to be taken into account when planning for the procedure and obtaining informed consent [10]. Identification of these factors is warranted for risk stratification of patients and therefore implementation of appropriate measures to reduce the incidence and severity of PEP, particularly in high-risk groups. As will be discussed in further detail to follow, this high-risk group would include young to middle-aged women with recurrent abdominal pain, normal bilirubin, and no biliary obstructive pathology [11].

Definition of PEP

Early recognition of PEP is essential, especially when performed on an outpatient basis. The diagnosis of PEP is often difficult as mild pancreatic enzyme elevation and postprocedure abdominal discomfort are common following ERCP procedures. However, a proposed consensus definition of PEP would be: new or worsened abdominal pain after ERCP requiring or prolonging hospitalization and associated elevation of serum amylase >3 times upper limit of normal,

Electronic supplementary material: The online version of this chapter (doi:10.1007/978-3-319-26854-5_12) contains supplementary material, which is available to authorized users. Videos can also be accessed at http://link.springer.com/chapter/10.1007/978-3-319-26854-5_12.

M. Gonzalez-Haba, M.D. • U.D. Siddiqui, M.D., F.A.S.G.E. (✉)
Center for Endoscopic Research and Therapeutics (CERT),
University of Chicago Medicine, 5700 S. Maryland Avenue,
MC 8043, Chicago, IL 60637, USA
e-mail: usiddiqui@medicine.bsd.uchicago.edu

D.G. Adler (ed.), *Advanced Pancreaticobiliary Endoscopy*, DOI 10.1007/978-3-319-26854-5_12

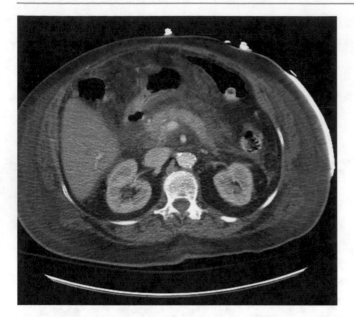

Fig. 12.1 CT scan showing changes of post-ERCP pancreatitis (PEP). Mesenteric and pancreatic edema noted, with thickening of renal fascia bilaterally and free fluid within the abdomen and pelvis. No definite evidence of pancreatic necrosis. ERCP with dilation-assisted sphincterotomy (dilation to 12 mm) and balloon sweep for large common bile stones was performed. Rectal Indomethacin and aggressive fluid hydration were administered during ERCP as part of routine practice. The pancreatic duct was cannulated once with a guidewire but not injected during the ERCP

Table 12.1 Most recognized risk factors for post-ERCP pancreatitis

Patient-related factors
• Younger age (<60 years)
• Female gender
• Prior post-ERCP pancreatitis
• Suspected sphincter of Oddi dysfunction
• Normal serum bilirubin
• Absence of chronic pancreatitis
Procedure-related factors
• Difficult cannulation
• Pancreatic duct trauma (multiple pancreatic injections/guidewire placement)
• Pancreatic sphincterotomy
• Pancreatic tissue sampling
• Balloon dilation of intact biliary sphincter
• Endoscopic papillectomy/ampullectomy
Endoscopist factors
• Endoscopist's adequate training
• Hospital volume
• Trainee participation

measured more than 24 h after the procedure [12]. This definition and cut-off value have been used in most but not all recent studies. Some studies have used higher cut-off levels in amylase levels or used lipase elevation solely, which may be more sensitive than amylase for predicting pancreatitis [13–16]. Amylase and lipase >1.5 and 4 times the upper normal limit obtained at 2–4 h after ERCP have a very high negative predictive value for PEP and can be useful when there is concern in patients with post-procedural pain [17–20].

PEP may be confused with post-procedural pain due to a perforation. ERCP-related perforation is significantly less frequent than PEP, with rates ranging from 0.1 to 0.6 % [21]. Depending on the location and type, this may be associated with more severe abdominal distension, tenderness, tachycardia, fever, and leukocytosis, although delayed and more unspecific symptomatology is not infrequent. Abdominal imaging (i.e., CT scan) may help to differentiate findings of PEP (pancreatic inflammation and edema, fat stranding, fluid collections) (Fig. 12.1) from perforation (free air). A surgical consultation should be obtained if perforation is suspected.

Pathogenesis

Several mechanisms of injury to the pancreas during ERCP have been postulated in the pathogenesis of PEP [22, 23]. Among these, the most recognized are (a) mechanical injury

from instrumentation of the papilla and pancreatic duct with subsequent obstruction to the outflow of pancreatic secretions, (b) hydrostatic injury from increased pressure following injection of contrast medium into the pancreatic duct or during sphincter of Oddi manometry, and (c) thermal injury resulting from application of electrosurgical current during biliary or pancreatic sphincterotomy. Once one or several of these "trigger events" have initiated PEP, the cascade of inflammatory activation is comparable to acute pancreatitis from other etiologies [24]. This fact is important, as the prevention of post-ERCP pancreatitis should also be focused in the early interruption of this cascade.

Risk Factors for PEP

Multiple risk factors have been demonstrated to increase the risk of post-ERCP pancreatitis. These factors can be further divided into factors related to the patient, procedure, and operator (Table 12.1). Identification and knowledge of these risk factors is critical for preventing or minimizing PEP.

Patient Related

Patient-related risk factors for PEP have been studied in multiple large, prospective studies. The patient-specific independent risk factors that have been most frequently associated with higher rates of PEP on multivariate analyses include younger age (<60 years), female gender, history of previous PEP, nondilated ducts, normal bilirubin level, and suspected sphincter of Oddi dysfunction (SOD) [3, 11, 14, 25–28]. A review of some of the larger studies is summarized below.

In a prospective multicenter study published by Freeman et al. in 2001 examining 1963 consecutive ERCP procedures, multivariate risk factors for PEP with adjusted odds ratios (OR) were prior ERCP-induced pancreatitis (5.4), biliary sphincter balloon dilation (4.5), difficult cannulation (3.4), pancreatic sphincterotomy (3.1), one or more injections of contrast into the pancreatic duct (2.7), suspected sphincter of Oddi dysfunction (2.6), female gender (2.5), normal serum bilirubin (1.9), and absence of chronic pancreatitis (1.9). In this study, small bile duct diameter, sphincter of Oddi manometry, biliary sphincterotomy, and lower ERCP case volume were not multivariate risk factors for pancreatitis [11]. One of the most remarkable findings in this study was the additive effect of these risk factors. A combination of factors like female gender, normal serum bilirubin level, and suspected sphincter of Oddi dysfunction (SOD) by the absence of stones and with a difficult cannulation would have the highest risk of PEP (42 %) as opposed to a reference rate of pancreatitis of 1.1 % for a typical low-risk patient [11]. In a more recent 2006 multicenter study enrolling 1115 patients undergoing diagnostic (48.1 %) and therapeutic (51.9 %) ERCP (suspected SOD was the indication in 33.9 %), significant risk factors for PEP in the multivariate risk model with adjusted odds ratios (OR) were minor papilla sphincterotomy (3.8), suspected SOD (2.6), history of PEP (2.0), age <60 years (1.6), ≥2 contrast injections into the pancreatic duct (1.5), and trainee involvement (1.5). In this study, female gender, history of recurrent idiopathic pancreatitis, pancreas divisum, SOM, difficult cannulation, and major papilla sphincterotomy (either biliary or pancreatic) were not multivariate risk factors for post-ERCP pancreatitis [25]. Cotton et al. reported in 2009 their experience on a total of 11,497 ERCP, with a 2.6 % rate of PEP (304 patients). Variables that were independent predictors of pancreatitis included performance of a pancreatogram at the major papilla (OR 1.70 [95 % CI, 1.17–2.41]) or at the minor papilla (OR 1.54 [95 % CI, 1.06–2.24]) and suspected SOD [3]. In a 2003 meta-analysis by Masci et al., when patient-related risk factors were analyzed, the relative risk for suspected sphincter of Oddi dysfunction was 4.09 (95 % CI 3.37–4.96; $P < 0.001$); for female gender, 2.23 (95 % CI 1.75–2.84, $P < 0.001$); and for previous pancreatitis, 2.46 (95 % CI 1.93–3.12, $P < 0.001$) [28].

These data highlight the importance of careful patient selection, as most of these additive risk factors are often associated with a weaker indication of ERCP. Therefore, less invasive tests such as MRCP and EUS should be considered first for solely diagnostic purposes [29].

Operator Related

Operator-related risk factors, such as trainee participation and the case volume and experience of the endoscopist, have been suggested to independently contribute to the risk of PEP, but with inconsistent results [30, 31].

Freeman et al. did not find lower ERCP case volume in their multivariate analysis to be a risk factor for PEP, although endoscopists performing on average more than two ERCPs per week had significantly greater success at bile duct cannulation (96.5 % vs. 91.5 %) for low-volume endoscopists performing <2 ERCPs per week, $P = 0.0001$ [11]. Several multivariate analyses have also failed to prove a relationship between annual hospital volume of ERCPs and PEP [26, 32, 33]. But these results may be biased by the higher proportion of high-risk patients and complex ERCP performed in high-volume centers that would therefore raise the incidence of complications. Trainee participation has also been postulated as an independent risk factor for PEP, as shown by Cheng et al. [25], but this factor was not significant on other large multicenter studies [11, 27]. Nevertheless, there is a high consensus among experts in the fact that ERCP must be performed by individuals who are trained and competent in order to provide safe and effective quality examinations, given the higher complexity of the procedure and rate of potential severe adverse events [10, 34].

Procedure Related

Cannulation Technique

Cannulation techniques are recognized to play an important role in the risk of PEP. Injection of contrast into the pancreatic duct may lead to both chemical and hydrostatic injuries of the pancreas. The use of guidewire-assisted cannulation (GW) instead of contrast injection cannulation (CC) has been shown in some studies to decrease PEP [35–39], as first demonstrated by Lella et al. in a RCT of 400 patients in 2004 [35]. This technique is based on the use of a hydrophilic wire as the primary cannulation device, either by pushing the wire directly into the papilla or by inserting the catheter into the papilla and then advancing the guidewire towards the desired duct.

In a systematic review and meta-analysis by Cheung on seven RCT and 2128 patients, there was significant reduction in PEP when using GW (3.2 %) compared with CC (8.7 %) (relative risk [RR] 0.38; 95 % CI, 0.19–0.76) [39]. In a more recent meta-analysis by Tse et al. that included 12 RCTs (3450 patients), the risk of PEP was significantly reduced with GW when compared with CC (risk ratio [RR] 0.51, 95 % confidence interval [CI] 0.32–0.82). Furthermore, GW technique was associated with greater primary cannulation success (RR 1.07, 95 % CI 1.00–1.15), fewer precut

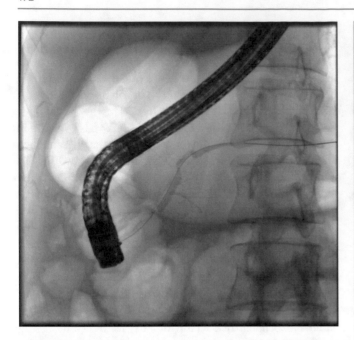

Fig. 12.2 Pancreatic duct (PD) injection. Inadvertent contrast injection of the PD during attempt at biliary cannulation is associated with higher rates of PEP. Unintentional guidewire cannulation of the PD has also been associated with an increased risk of PEP

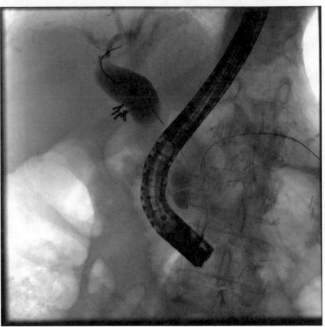

Fig. 12.3 Double-wire technique to aid biliary cannulation. Guidewire placement in the PD can help aid in subsequent cannulation of the common bile duct (CBD) and can then be used for PD stent placement to prevent PEP

sphincterotomies (RR 0.75, 95 % CI 0.60–0.95), and no increase in other ERCP-related complications [40]. A noteworthy point raised was that this risk reduction was not significant in any of the publications when analyzing only crossover trials. In addition, multiple other studies have failed to prove this reduction of risk [41–43].

Although guidewire-assisted cannulation has shown to decrease the rate of PEP in some studies, unintentional guidewire cannulation into the pancreatic duct has also been associated with an increased risk of PEP [44]. In the large meta-analysis performed by Masci et al., pancreatic duct injection was found to be an independent predictor of PEP (RR 2.2; 95 % CI 1.60–3.01) [28]. The risk of developing PEP might be directly proportional to the extent of pancreatic ductal opacification [45]. This highlights the concept to avoid any undesired PD manipulation during ERCP if possible, whether it is guidewire insertion or contrast injection (Fig. 12.2).

Difficult Cannulation

Mechanical injury to the papilla and pancreatic duct from repeated cannulation attempts may lead to edema and obstruction of pancreatic ductal flow. The term "difficult cannulation" is nonspecific, but frequently refers to failure to obtain deep biliary access despite multiple attempts at cannulation or the unintentional cannulation of the undesired duct [17]. Difficult cannulation, when defined as >5 attempts on papilla before cannulation of desired ducts, has shown to be an independent risk factor for a PEP [11, 46, 47].

For difficult cannulation, commonly used options include pancreatic guidewire placement (with biliary cannulation attempted either using a guidewire, the so-called double guidewire (DGW) technique, or using contrast medium injection), precut of various types, repeat attempts at ERCP 24–48 h later, or patient referral to another endoscopist. In the DGW technique, first described by Dumonceau et al. in 1998 [48], a guidewire is left in the pancreatic duct to aid wire cannulation of the common bile duct by straightening the papillary anatomy (Fig. 12.3). The DGW has shown disparate results in RCT [44, 49–51]. If this method is used, a pancreatic stent should be placed for PEP prophylaxis, as failed pancreatic stenting is also an independent predictor of PEP [44, 51–53].

Precut refers to the action of performing sphincterotomy before biliary access is achieved, and it has been reported to be associated with an increased risk of complications including PEP, bleeding, and perforation [5, 15, 28, 54–58]. However, it is still debated whether the risk of PEP is due to the precut itself or to the prior prolonged failed attempts at biliary cannulation [56]. A meta-analysis from six RCTs including 966 patients comparing early precut implementation vs. persistent cannulation attempts and showed a reduced risk of PEP when the former was performed (2.5 % vs. 5.3 %; OR 0.47, 95 % CI 0.24–0.91) with similar overall cannulation and complication rates in both groups [55]. A more recent meta-analysis including seven RCTs and seven non-RCTs showed a decrease in PEP with precut usage, but this was not statistically significant (OR of PEP with early precut sphincterotomy=0.58; 95 % CI: 0.32–1.05; P=0.07) [57]. Among precut techniques, the fistulotomy technique may present a lower incidence of PEP than standard needle knife or transpancreatic sphincterotomy [58].

Balloon Dilatation

Balloon dilatation of the ampulla using a small caliber balloon may be utilized over endoscopic sphincterotomy in certain circumstances, by decreasing clinically significant bleeding in patients with coagulopathy, for preserving sphincter of Oddi function in younger patients [59] and in patients with altered anatomy (Billroth II) where sphincterotomy is technically difficult [60]. The limited use of this technique in a select group of patients is due to the markedly increased risk of PEP [61, 62] when performed in an intact papilla.

A large randomized, controlled multicenter study comparing endoscopic balloon dilation to sphincterotomy for extraction of bile duct stones had to be terminated at the first interim analysis due to a significant increased rate of PEP, short-term morbidity rates, and death due to pancreatitis in the balloon dilation group [61]. The higher incidence of PEP was confirmed later by two meta-analyses [63, 64], although there was statistically significant lower rates of bleeding than biliary sphincterotomy. A more recent meta-analysis that included 12 RCTs (1649 patients) examined the risk of PEP to the duration of the balloon dilation, with no increased risk noted when there is a prolonged dilation balloon inflation time (>1 min) (OR 1.14; 95 % CI 0.56–2.35) [65]. According to the available data, balloon dilation of the sphincter of Oddi for routine stone extraction should be avoided [17, 62].

Conversely, dilation-assisted biliary sphincterotomy using larger diameter balloons (>10 mm) to facilitate removal of large biliary stones has been shown to have a lower overall rate of complications and similar PEP rates when compared to sphincterotomy alone (Fig. 12.4). However, most of the published data comes from retrospective studies [66, 67].

Sphincter of Oddi Manometry

It has been well documented that patients undergoing ERCP for known or suspected sphincter of Oddi dysfunction (SOD) carry a higher risk of PEP, but as opposed to the widely spread belief, sphincter of Oddi manometry (SOM) by itself does not appear to increase the risk of PEP, especially with the widespread use of aspiration instead of perfusion manometry catheters, which reduces the risk of hydrostatic injury and PEP [68]. In the aforementioned analysis of 11,497 ERCPs performed by Cotton et al., neither pancreatic (OR 1.43, 95 % CI 0.99–2.08) nor biliary manometry (1.16, 95 % CI 0.83–1.62) was found to be a statistically significant risk factor for PEP [3]. Nevertheless, these results should not interfere with the fact that patients with SOD are at high risk of PEP as stated earlier and preventive measures of PEP should always be taken in these cases regardless of whether SOM is performed or not.

Self-Expandable Metal Stents (SEMS)

Self-expandable metal stents (SEMS) are used worldwide for management of biliary strictures, more frequently in malignancy. The compression of the pancreatic duct by the tensile forces of larger caliber (8–10 mm) SEMS has been postulated as a risk factor for PEP. Cote et al. demonstrated

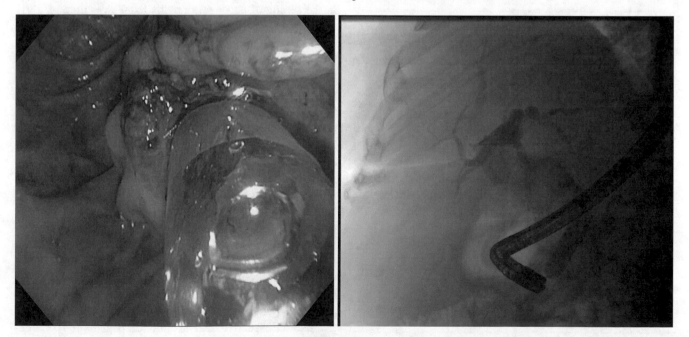

Fig. 12.4 Ampullary dilation can facilitate large stone removal and has been shown to have similar rates of PEP compared to biliary sphincterotomy alone. In order to prevent PEP, prior biliary sphincterotomy should be performed

this in a retrospective cohort of 544 patients undergoing ERCP with either SEMS or plastic stent (PS) first time biliary stent placement for malignant biliary obstruction. They observed a significantly higher frequency of PEP in the SEMS group (7.3 %) vs. the PS group (1.3 %) (OR 5.7 [95 % CI, 1.9–17.1]) with no difference between covered and uncovered SEMS [38]. Kawakubo et al. reviewed 370 consecutive patients who underwent initial transpapillary SEMS placement for biliary decompression and found that SEMSs with high axial force (odds ratio [OR], 3.69; $P=0.022$) and nonpancreatic cancer (OR, 5.52; $P<0.001$) to be significant risk factors for pancreatitis in these patients [69]. Biliary sphincterotomy was not associated with a decreased risk.

Maneuvers That Have NOT Been Shown to Influence the Risk of PEP

There is no evidence that the risk of PEP is influenced by patient position during ERCP [70, 71]. Carbon dioxide is recommended for insufflation, and might be particularly useful for outpatient ERCPs, to reduce post-procedural abdominal pain from overdistention and to avoid confusion with PEP [72, 73]. The type of electrosurgical current used has also been studied, pure-cut current produces less edema than blended current [74], and it was hypothesized that it might reduce the incidence of PEP after biliary sphincterotomy. A meta-analysis of four RCTs that included 804 patients found no significant difference in the incidence of PEP following the use of pure vs. blended current [75]. However, the incidence of bleeding was significantly higher when pure-cut current was used.

Prevention of Post-ERCP Pancreatitis

Preventive strategies to reduce the risk or minimize the severity of PEP are listed in Table 12.2.

Appropriate ERCP Indication

The first and probably the more important preventive strategy for PEP is careful patient selection. Now that safer alternative radiologic and endoscopic modalities are

Table 12.2 Most accepted methods to reduce the incidence of PEP

• Adequate indication for ERCP (careful patient selection)
• Recognize high-risk patients and maneuvers
• Minimize ampullary trauma
• Guidewire cannulation technique
• Early precut (access) sphincterotomy when difficult cannulation
• Aggressive hydration
• Chemoprophylaxis (i.e., rectal NSAIDs)
• Pancreatic duct stenting, particularly in high-risk cases

becoming increasingly available, the role of diagnostic ERCP has been reexamined. MRCP, intraoperative laparoscopic cholangiography in patients undergoing cholecystectomy, and EUS all have accuracy rates rivaling that of ERCP for diagnostic purposes and are widely available [76–79]. These techniques are preferable to ERCP for patients with equivocal evidence of biliary obstruction or during initial workup, especially those who are at high risk for post-ERCP pancreatitis.

According to current evidence [10], ERCP is generally not indicated in patients with abdominal pain without objective evidence of pancreaticobiliary or routinely before cholecystectomy in the absence of cholangitis, biliary obstruction, or confirmed or highly suspected bile duct stones. In patients with malignant distal pancreaticobiliary tumors who are potentially resectable and can undergo surgery immediately, the role of preoperative biliary decompression has not been shown to improve postoperative outcomes and can potentially jeopardize or worsen the surgical outcomes [80]. Furthermore, with regard to SOD patients, there is recent evidence to suggest that ERCP is not warranted in this high-risk PEP population. Cotton et al. presented their data in 2014 from a multicenter, prospective, sham-controlled randomized trial demonstrating that endoscopic sphincterotomy did not reduce disability due to pain in patients presenting with abdominal pain (suspected SOD, type III) after cholecystectomy [81].

Intravenous Fluid Hydration

In the setting of acute pancreatitis from any etiology, early aggressive intravenous hydration, during the first 12–24 h, with close monitoring is of paramount importance [82]. Early aggressive intravenous fluid resuscitation provides micro- and macrocirculatory support to prevent serious complications such as pancreatic necrosis [83–85]. In this setting, Lactated Ringer's (LR) solution is the preferred isotonic crystalloid replacement as it may be less likely to induce metabolic acidosis and the lactate component may stimulate an anti-inflammatory response [86, 87].

This same conclusion was reached from a pilot study in which aggressive intravenous hydration with LR solution appeared to reduce the development of PEP in patients undergoing first ERCP when compared with standard hydration (0–16 % ($P=0.016$)). Reduced length of hospitalization and rate of readmission were also seen in a retrospective study in patients with greater IV hydration during the first 24 h after ERCP [88]. Larger fluid volume during the ERCP procedure was also associated with less severe PEP in a multivariate retrospective analysis in 6505 patients [89]. Large-scale RCTs to establish an evidence-based approach to intensive hydration are needed.

Fig. 12.5 Pancreatic duct
stent placement has been
shown to reduce the risk of
PEP

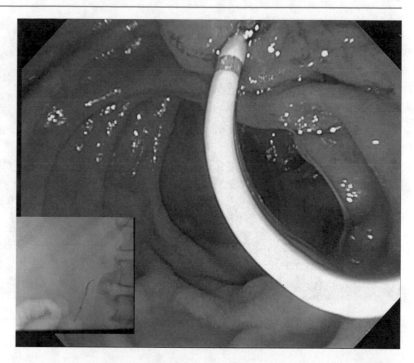

Pancreatic Stent Placement (PSP)

Endoscopic placement of a pancreatic duct stent mechanically facilitates pancreatic duct drainage by relieving the increased pressure across the pancreatic sphincter that might have developed as a result of transient procedure-induced blockage of the pancreatic orifice (Fig. 12.5). Pancreatic stent placement (PSP) has been widely studied for more than 20 years as a prophylactic measure for the prevention of PEP and has been demonstrated to be effective in high-risk patients [90, 91]. In the most recent meta-analysis, published by Matzaki et al. and including 14 studies and 1541 patients, PSP was associated with a statistically significant reduction of PEP (RR 0.39; 95 % CI 0.29–0.53; $P < 0.001$). Subgroup analysis of those with PEP showed that a pancreatic stent was beneficial in patients with mild to moderate PEP (RR 0.45; 95 % CI 0.32–0.62; $P < 0.001$) and in patients with severe PEP (RR 0.26; 95 % CI 0.09–0.76; $P = 0.01$) [92]. In addition, subgroup analysis demonstrated that PSP was effective for both high-risk and mixed-case groups [93].

PSP is currently considered the standard of care in high-risk circumstances such as patients with a difficult cannulation (including when double-wire cannulation has been performed), precut sphincterotomy (Fig. 12.6 and Video 12.1), pancreatic sphincterotomy (major or minor) (Fig. 12.7), pancreatic endotherapy, diagnostic or therapeutic ERCP for suspected or confirmed SOD, past history of PEP, balloon dilation of an intact biliary sphincter, and endoscopic ampullectomy [94–98].

The ideal stent features and its optimal duration for preventing PEP prophylaxis have not yet been defined. The ideal

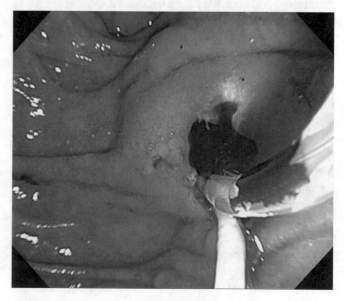

Fig. 12.6 Precut sphincterotomy using a needle knife over a PD stent. Early precut sphincterotomy can prevent excessive manipulation of the ampulla and facilitate cannulation

pancreatic duct stent would be easy to place, stay in position for at least a few days, and then fall out spontaneously without inducing any duct changes. There has been discussion comparing various pancreatic stent features such as: length (short 2–3 cm vs. long 8–12 cm), caliber (3 Fr requiring smaller caliber 0.018–0.21 guidewires vs. 4–5 Fr), having an internal flange vs. none, and type (single pigtail vs. straight). There is a general consensus to avoid medium length stents that can end in the genu and induce duct damage leading to

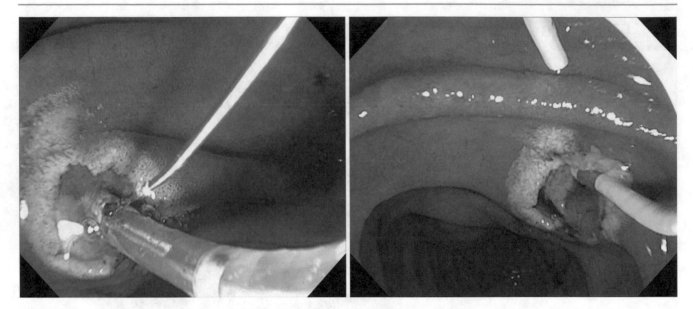

Fig. 12.7 Minor papilla sphincterotomy is associated with a higher risk of PEP and thus prophylactic pancreatic duct stent placement is recommended

stricturing. A recent 2014 meta-analysis including six RCTs and 561 patients demonstrated that larger stent caliber may be the most important factor in preventing PEP [99]. This study demonstrated that 5 Fr single pigtail, unflanged pancreatic stents and 5 Fr straight, flanged pancreatic stents performed similarly and both were superior to 3 Fr stents. Our practice is to use pancreatic duct stents that are typically short (3 cm), 5 Fr, single pigtail, and without an internal flange. Passage of the stent from the pancreatic duct must be documented and should be evaluated within 10–14 days of placement with an abdominal X-ray. Retained stents should be promptly removed endoscopically so as not to induce pancreatic duct damage if left in long term.

Despite the undoubtful efficacy of PSP for clearly reducing PEP risk, it can be technically challenging, time-consuming, and requires follow-up with either abdominal X-ray or another endoscopy to ensure passage or removal. This technique has some major drawbacks, like potential long-term stent-related duct injury, unsuccessful stent placement (e.g., inability to advance a wire into PD, or inability to place a stent after wire placement), or inadvertent duct injury during stent placement that may substantially increase the risk of PEP by adding further trauma to the pancreatic duct without providing ductal decompression [100, 101]. In a recent secondary analysis of a multicenter RCT of rectal indomethacin vs. placebo for preventing PEP from Elmunzer et al. [102], Choksi et al. analyzed the incidence of PEP among patients in the placebo group who experienced failed pancreatic stenting, and it was significantly higher than was for those who underwent successful stent placement and in those without a stent attempt (34.7 % vs. 16.4 % vs. 12.1 %) [103].

The major issue raised with the use of pancreatic stents is variable expertise and familiarity with their placement. PD stent placement alone may therefore not be the whole answer, especially in less-specialized hands, but this data highlight that proper training and experience that endoscopists performing ERCP should have to achieve the documented risk reduction demonstrated by PD stent placement.

Chemoprophylaxis

PEP is an unavoidable complication even in the hands of expert endoscopists. With this premise, pharmacologic prophylaxis of PEP has been extensively researched in an attempt to prevent or reduce the severity of PEP. Some of the main targets for chemoprevention include prevention of intra-acinar trypsinogen activation (protease inhibitors such as gabexate, ulinastatin, nafamostat mesylate) [104–106]; reduction of pancreatic enzyme secretion (somatostatin and octreotide) [107, 108]; reduction of sphincter of Oddi pressure (nitroglycerin, nifedipine, phosphodiesterase-5 inhibitors) [109–112]; and interruption of the inflammatory cascade (nonsteroidal anti-inflammatory drugs [NSAIDs], interleukin-10, corticosteroids, allopurinol, heparin, N-acetylcysteine) [113–120].

In 2012, Elmunzer et al. published a multicenter, randomized, placebo-controlled, double blind clinical trial with 602 patients at elevated risk for post-ERCP (82 % had a clinical suspicion of sphincter of Oddi dysfunction) in the *New England Journal of Medicine*. This study showed a significantly reduced rate of PEP in patients randomized to a single dose of rectal indomethacin (100 mg) after ERCP than in the placebo group (27/295 9.2 % vs. 52/307 16.9 % (P=0.005)).

Moderate-to-severe pancreatitis developed in 13 patients (4.4 %) in the indomethacin group and in 27 patients (8.8 %) in the placebo group ($P=0.03$) [102].

Since then, there have been several meta-analyses published comparing NSAIDs vs. placebo administration for prevention of PEP, and all of them concordantly showed the benefit of NSAIDs in preventing either mild or moderate/severe PEP. The number needed to treat (NNT) figures, reported in the majority of these studies, has varied from 11 to 34 [102, 106, 121–128]. Furthermore, in their most recent guidelines, the European Society of Gastrointestinal Endoscopy (ESGE) recommends routine use of rectally administered NSAIDS to prevent post-ERCP pancreatitis (e.g., 100 mg of diclofenac or indomethacin rectally immediately before or after every ERCP) in all patients, not only high-risk ones [17]. Our group supports this practice as well given the excellent safety profile and low cost of this strategy.

Combining NSAIDs with other pharmacologic agents has also been studied in an attempt to achieve higher prophylactic efficacy from synergistic action. In a recent randomized trial by Sotoudehmanesh et al., the combination of rectal indomethacin and sublingual nitrate given before ERCP was significantly more likely to reduce the incidence of PEP than indomethacin suppository alone. Absolute risk reduction, relative risk reduction, and NNT for the prevention of PEP were 8.6 % (95 % CI: 4.7–14.5), 56.2 % (95 % CI: 50.6–60.8), and 12 (95 % CI: 7–22), respectively [129].

There are scarce data directly comparing NSAIDs with PSP. In a post hoc analysis of an RCT of NSAIDs vs. placebo for PEP prophylaxis, administration of rectal NSAIDs alone was more effective and less costly than prophylactic PSP alone or combined with rectal NSAIDs [116]. NSAIDs were also superior to placebo in preventing post-ERCP pancreatitis. Rectal NSAIDs alone were again demonstrated to be superior to PSP alone in preventing PEP in a recent network meta-analysis (odds ratio, 0.48; 95 % confidence interval, 0.26–0.87) with no superiority shown by the combination of rectal NSAIDs with PSP to either approach alone [130].

Rectal NSAID administration also proved to be the most cost-effective prophylactic strategy used to prevent PEP in a recent cost-effectiveness decision analysis when compared to PSP plus rectal indomethacin, and no prophylaxis [131]. However, these results must be carefully interpreted, the hypothesis of obviating the need of PD stent placement by the administration of NSAIDs is still under debate, and results from randomized trials comparing both strategies are awaited before a consensus is reached.

Discussion

Post-ERCP pancreatitis (PEP) is the most common and feared complication of ERCP given its potential for causing prolonged hospitalization, major morbidity, and even death. PEP is still an unavoidable complication even in the hands of expert endoscopists, but every effort to minimize this risk should be undertaken. The first and *MOST* important preventive strategy for PEP is a careful selection of patients and adherence to the current evidence-based indications. Diagnostic ERCP should generally be avoided, and the use of noninvasive techniques such as MRCP or EUS are preferred in the setting.

Our knowledge and understanding of PEP has grown significantly over the past decades with numerous studies examining this complication and identifying high-risk patients and methods to prevent or minimize it. Several post-ERCP pancreatitis risk factors have been identified and are associated with patient characteristics, procedure techniques, and operator expertise. When a patient at high risk for post-ERCP pancreatitis is recognized, prophylactic measures like aggressive intravenous hydration during the ERCP, rectal NSAIDs, and/or prophylactic pancreatic stent placement should all be considered since they have been shown to decrease the risk and severity of PEP. Research on PEP continues to grow with our overall ERCP experience and further evidence is awaited to demonstrate the most effective and safest approaches to minimize, if not eliminate, the risk of this dreaded complication.

Acknowledgement *Conflicts of interest*: None
   Financial disclosures: None
   Funding/Grant Support: None
   Writing Assistance: None
   Author(s) have nothing to disclose. All author(s) disclose that there are NO potential conflicts (financial, professional, or personal) that are relevant to the manuscript.

Video Legend

Video 12.1 In this video demonstration, a prophylactive pancreatic duct (PD) stent (5 Fr diameter, 3 cm length, single pigtail without any internal flange) is placed to assist with a difficult biliary cannulation and to prevent post-ERCP pancreatitis (PEP). Once the PD stent has been deployed, a needle knife is used to perform a precut to gain access to the bile duct and then the biliary sphincterotomy is completed using a standard sphincterotome. Finally, a biliary stent is placed with good drainage of bile coming through it at the end of the procedure. (MP4 372069 kb).

References

1. McCune WS, Shorb PE, Moscovitz H. Endoscopic cannulation of the ampulla of Vater: a preliminary report. Ann Surg. 1968; 167(5):752–6.
2. Peery AF, Dellon ES, Lund J, Crockett SD, McGowan CE, Bulsiewicz WJ, et al. Burden of gastrointestinal disease in the United States: 2012 update. Gastroenterology. 2012;143(5):1179–87 e1–3.
3. Cotton PB, Garrow DA, Gallagher J, Romagnuolo J. Risk factors for complications after ERCP: a multivariate analysis of 11,497 procedures over 12 years. Gastrointest Endosc. 2009;70(1):80–8.

4. Freeman ML. Adverse outcomes of ERCP. Gastrointest Endosc. 2002;56(6 Suppl):S273–82.
5. Freeman ML, Nelson DB, Sherman S, Haber GB, Herman ME, Dorsher PJ, et al. Complications of endoscopic biliary sphincterotomy. N Engl J Med. 1996;335(13):909–18.
6. Kochar B, Akshintala VS, Afghani E, Elmunzer BJ, Kim KJ, Lennon AM, et al. Incidence, severity, and mortality of post-ERCP pancreatitis: a systematic review by using randomized, controlled trials. Gastrointest Endosc. 2015;81(1):143–9. e9.
7. Jena AB, Seabury S, Lakdawalla D, Chandra A. Malpractice risk according to physician specialty. N Engl J Med. 2011;365(7):629–36.
8. Hernandez LV, Klyve D, Regenbogen SE. Malpractice claims for endoscopy. World J Gastrointest Endosc. 2013;5(4):169–73.
9. Cotton PB. Analysis of 59 ERCP lawsuits; mainly about indications. Gastrointest Endosc. 2006;63(3):378–82. quiz 464.
10. Adler DG, Lieb II JG, Cohen J, Pike IM, Park WG, Rizk MK, et al. Quality indicators for ERCP. Gastrointest Endosc. 2015;81(1):54–66.
11. Freeman ML, DiSario JA, Nelson DB, Fennerty MB, Lee JG, Bjorkman DJ, et al. Risk factors for post-ERCP pancreatitis: a prospective, multicenter study. Gastrointest Endosc. 2001; 54(4):425–34.
12. Cotton PB, Lehman G, Vennes J, Geenen JE, Russell RC, Meyers WC, et al. Endoscopic sphincterotomy complications and their management: an attempt at consensus. Gastrointest Endosc. 1991;37(3):383–93.
13. Gottlieb K, Sherman S. ERCP and biliary endoscopic sphincterotomy-induced pancreatitis. Gastrointest Endosc Clin N Am. 1998;8(1):87–114.
14. Christoforidis E, Goulimaris I, Kanellos I, Tsalis K, Demetriades C, Betsis D. Post-ERCP pancreatitis and hyperamylasemia: patient-related and operative risk factors. Endoscopy. 2002;34(4):286–92.
15. Masci E, Toti G, Mariani A, Curioni S, Lomazzi A, Dinelli M, et al. Complications of diagnostic and therapeutic ERCP: a prospective multicenter study. Am J Gastroenterol. 2001;96(2):417–23.
16. Sutton VR, Hong MK, Thomas PR. Using the 4-hour Post-ERCP amylase level to predict post-ERCP pancreatitis. JOP. 2011;12(4):372–6.
17. Dumonceau JM, Andriulli A, Elmunzer BJ, Mariani A, Meister T, Deviere J, et al. Prophylaxis of post-ERCP pancreatitis: European Society of Gastrointestinal Endoscopy (ESGE) Guideline—updated June 2014. Endoscopy. 2014;46(9):799–815.
18. Artifon EL, Chu A, Freeman M, Sakai P, Usmani A, Kumar A. A comparison of the consensus and clinical definitions of pancreatitis with a proposal to redefine post-endoscopic retrograde cholangiopancreatography pancreatitis. Pancreas. 2010;39(4):530–5.
19. Sultan S, Baillie J. What are the predictors of post-ERCP pancreatitis, and how useful are they? JOP. 2002;3(6):188–94.
20. Thomas PR, Sengupta S. Prediction of pancreatitis following endoscopic retrograde cholangiopancreatography by the 4-h post procedure amylase level. J Gastroenterol Hepatol. 2001;16(8):923–6.
21. Anderson MA, Fisher L, Jain R, Evans JA, Appalaneni V, Ben-Menachem T, et al. Complications of ERCP. Gastrointest Endosc. 2012;75(3):467–73.
22. Freeman ML, Guda NM. Prevention of post-ERCP pancreatitis: a comprehensive review. Gastrointest Endosc. 2004;59(7):845–64.
23. Pezzilli R, Romboli E, Campana D, Corinaldesi R. Mechanisms involved in the onset of post-ERCP pancreatitis. JOP. 2002;3(6):162–8.
24. Sinha A, Cader R, Akshintala VS, Hutfless SM, Zaheer A, Khan VN, et al. Systemic inflammatory response syndrome between 24 and 48 h after ERCP predicts prolonged length of stay in patients with post-ERCP pancreatitis: a retrospective study. Pancreatology. 2015;15:105–10.
25. Cheng CL, Sherman S, Watkins JL, Barnett J, Freeman M, Geenen J, et al. Risk factors for post-ERCP pancreatitis: a prospective multicenter study. Am J Gastroenterol. 2006;101(1):139–47.
26. Testoni PA, Mariani A, Giussani A, Vailati C, Masci E, Macarri G, et al. Risk factors for post-ERCP pancreatitis in high- and low-volume centers and among expert and non-expert operators: a prospective multicenter study. Am J Gastroenterol. 2010; 105(8):1753–61.
27. Vandervoort J, Soetikno RM, Tham TC, Wong RC, Ferrari Jr AP, Montes H, et al. Risk factors for complications after performance of ERCP. Gastrointest Endosc. 2002;56(5):652–6.
28. Masci E, Mariani A, Curioni S, Testoni PA. Risk factors for pancreatitis following endoscopic retrograde cholangiopancreatography: a meta-analysis. Endoscopy. 2003;35(10):830–4.
29. Cotton PB. ERCP is most dangerous for people who need it least. Gastrointest Endosc. 2001;54(4):535–6.
30. Kapral C, Duller C, Wewalka F, Kerstan E, Vogel W, Schreiber F. Case volume and outcome of endoscopic retrograde cholangiopancreatography: results of a nationwide Austrian benchmarking project. Endoscopy. 2008;40(8):625–30.
31. Williams EJ, Taylor S, Fairclough P, Hamlyn A, Logan RF, Martin D, et al. Risk factors for complication following ERCP; results of a large-scale, prospective multicenter study. Endoscopy. 2007;39(9):793–801.
32. Swahn F, Nilsson M, Arnelo U, Lohr M, Persson G, Enochsson L. Rendezvous cannulation technique reduces post-ERCP pancreatitis: a prospective nationwide study of 12,718 ERCP procedures. Am J Gastroenterol. 2013;108(4):552–9.
33. Colton JB, Curran CC. Quality indicators, including complications, of ERCP in a community setting: a prospective study. Gastrointest Endosc. 2009;70(3):457–67.
34. Chutkan RK, Ahmad AS, Cohen J, Cruz-Correa MR, Desilets DJ, Dominitz JA, et al. ERCP core curriculum. Gastrointest Endosc. 2006;63(3):361–76.
35. Lella F, Bagnolo F, Colombo E, Bonassi U. A simple way of avoiding post-ERCP pancreatitis. Gastrointest Endosc. 2004; 59(7):830–4.
36. Artifon EL, Sakai P, Cunha JE, Halwan B, Ishioka S, Kumar A. Guidewire cannulation reduces risk of post-ERCP pancreatitis and facilitates bile duct cannulation. Am J Gastroenterol. 2007;102(10):2147–53.
37. Lee TH, Parkdo H, Park JY, Kim EO, Lee YS, Park JH, et al. Can wire-guided cannulation prevent post-ERCP pancreatitis? A prospective randomized trial. Gastrointest Endosc. 2009;69(3 Pt 1):444–9.
38. Cote GA, Ansstas M, Pawa R, Edmundowicz SA, Jonnalagadda SS, Pleskow DK, et al. Difficult biliary cannulation: use of physician-controlled wire-guided cannulation over a pancreatic duct stent to reduce the rate of precut sphincterotomy (with video). Gastrointest Endosc. 2010;71(2):275–9.
39. Cheung J, Tsoi KK, Quan WL, Lau JY, Sung JJ. Guidewire versus conventional contrast cannulation of the common bile duct for the prevention of post-ERCP pancreatitis: a systematic review and meta-analysis. Gastrointest Endosc. 2009;70(6):1211–9.
40. Tse F, Yuan Y, Moayyedi P, Leontiadis GI. Guide wire-assisted cannulation for the prevention of post-ERCP pancreatitis: a systematic review and meta-analysis. Endoscopy. 2013;45(8):605–18.
41. Bailey AA, Bourke MJ, Williams SJ, Walsh PR, Murray MA, Lee EY, et al. A prospective randomized trial of cannulation technique in ERCP: effects on technical success and post-ERCP pancreatitis. Endoscopy. 2008;40(4):296–301.
42. Mariani A, Giussani A, Di Leo M, Testoni S, Testoni PA. Guidewire biliary cannulation does not reduce post-ERCP pancreatitis com-

pared with the contrast injection technique in low-risk and high-risk patients. Gastrointest Endosc. 2012;75(2):339–46.

43. Kobayashi G, Fujita N, Imaizumi K, Irisawa A, Suzuki M, Murakami A, et al. Wire-guided biliary cannulation technique does not reduce the risk of post-ERCP pancreatitis: multicenter randomized controlled trial. Dig Endosc. 2013;25(3):295–302.

44. Tsujino T, Komatsu Y, Isayama H, Hirano K, Sasahira N, Yamamoto N, et al. Ulinastatin for pancreatitis after endoscopic retrograde cholangiopancreatography: a randomized, controlled trial. Clin Gastroenterol Hepatol. 2005;3(4):376–83.

45. Cheon YK, Cho KB, Watkins JL, McHenry L, Fogel EL, Sherman S, et al. Frequency and severity of post-ERCP pancreatitis correlated with extent of pancreatic ductal opacification. Gastrointest Endosc. 2007;65(3):385–93.

46. Wang P, Li ZS, Liu F, Ren X, Lu NH, Fan ZN, et al. Risk factors for ERCP-related complications: a prospective multicenter study. Am J Gastroenterol. 2009;104(1):31–40.

47. Halttunen J, Meisner S, Aabakken L, Arnelo U, Gronroos J, Hauge T, et al. Difficult cannulation as defined by a prospective study of the Scandinavian Association for Digestive Endoscopy (SADE) in 907 ERCPs. Scand J Gastroenterol. 2014;49(6):752–8.

48. Dumonceau JM, Deviere J, Cremer M. A new method of achieving deep cannulation of the common bile duct during endoscopic retrograde cholangiopancreatography. Endoscopy. 1998;30(7):S80.

49. Maeda S, Hayashi H, Hosokawa O, Dohden K, Hattori M, Morita M, et al. Prospective randomized pilot trial of selective biliary cannulation using pancreatic guide-wire placement. Endoscopy. 2003;35(9):721–4.

50. Herreros de Tejada A, Calleja JL, Diaz G, Pertejo V, Espinel J, Cacho G, et al. Double-guidewire technique for difficult bile duct cannulation: a multicenter randomized, controlled trial. Gastrointest Endosc. 2009;70(4):700–9.

51. Ito K, Horaguchi J, Fujita N, Noda Y, Kobayashi G, Koshita S, et al. Clinical usefulness of double-guidewire technique for difficult biliary cannulation in endoscopic retrograde cholangiopancreatography. Dig Endosc. 2014;26(3):442–9.

52. Ito K, Fujita N, Noda Y, Kobayashi G, Obana T, Horaguchi J, et al. Can pancreatic duct stenting prevent post-ERCP pancreatitis in patients who undergo pancreatic duct guidewire placement for achieving selective biliary cannulation? A prospective randomized controlled trial. J Gastroenterol. 2010;45(11):1183–91.

53. Nakai Y, Isayama H, Sasahira N, Kogure H, Sasaki T, Yamamoto N, et al. Risk factors for post-ERCP pancreatitis in wire-guided cannulation for therapeutic biliary ERCP. Gastrointest Endosc. 2015;81(1):119–26.

54. Williams EJ, Taylor S, Fairclough P, Hamlyn A, Logan RF, Martin D, et al. Are we meeting the standards set for endoscopy? Results of a large-scale prospective survey of endoscopic retrograde cholangio-pancreatograph practice. Gut. 2007;56(6):821–9.

55. Cennamo V, Fuccio L, Zagari RM, Eusebi LH, Ceroni L, Laterza L, et al. Can early precut implementation reduce endoscopic retrograde cholangiopancreatography-related complication risk? Meta-analysis of randomized controlled trials. Endoscopy. 2010;42(5):381–8.

56. Bailey AA, Bourke MJ, Kaffes AJ, Byth K, Lee EY, Williams SJ. Needle-knife sphincterotomy: factors predicting its use and the relationship with post-ERCP pancreatitis (with video). Gastrointest Endosc. 2010;71(2):266–71.

57. Choudhary A, Winn J, Siddique S, Arif M, Arif Z, Hammoud GM, et al. Effect of precut sphincterotomy on post-endoscopic retrograde cholangiopancreatography pancreatitis: a systematic review and meta-analysis. World J Gastroenterol. 2014;20(14):4093–101.

58. Katsinelos P, Gkagkalis S, Chatzimavroudis G, Beltsis A, Terzoudis S, Zavos C, et al. Comparison of three types of precut technique to achieve common bile duct cannulation: a retrospective analysis of 274 cases. Dig Dis Sci. 2012;57(12):3286–92.

59. Yasuda I, Tomita E, Enya M, Kato T, Moriwaki H. Can endoscopic papillary balloon dilation really preserve sphincter of Oddi function? Gut. 2001;49(5):686–91.

60. Jang HW, Lee KJ, Jung MJ, Jung JW, Park JY, Park SW, et al. Endoscopic papillary large balloon dilatation alone is safe and effective for the treatment of difficult choledocholithiasis in cases of Billroth II gastrectomy: a single center experience. Dig Dis Sci. 2013;58(6):1737–43.

61. Disario JA, Freeman ML, Bjorkman DJ, Macmathuna P, Petersen BT, Jaffe PE, et al. Endoscopic balloon dilation compared with sphincterotomy for extraction of bile duct stones. Gastroenterology. 2004;127(5):1291–9.

62. Watanabe H, Yoneda M, Tominaga K, Monma T, Kanke K, Shimada T, et al. Comparison between endoscopic papillary balloon dilatation and endoscopic sphincterotomy for the treatment of common bile duct stones. J Gastroenterol. 2007;42(1):56–62.

63. Baron TH, Harewood GC. Endoscopic balloon dilation of the biliary sphincter compared to endoscopic biliary sphincterotomy for removal of common bile duct stones during ERCP: a meta-analysis of randomized, controlled trials. Am J Gastroenterol. 2004;99(8):1455–60.

64. Weinberg BM, Shindy W, Lo S. Endoscopic balloon sphincter dilation (sphincteroplasty) versus sphincterotomy for common bile duct stones. Cochrane Database Syst Rev. 2006;4, CD004890.

65. Liao WC, Tu YK, Wu MS, Wang HP, Lin JT, Leung JW, et al. Balloon dilation with adequate duration is safer than sphincterotomy for extracting bile duct stones: a systematic review and meta-analyses. Clin Gastroenterol Hepatol. 2012;10(10):1101–9.

66. Feng Y, Zhu H, Chen X, Xu S, Cheng W, Ni J, et al. Comparison of endoscopic papillary large balloon dilation and endoscopic sphincterotomy for retrieval of choledocholithiasis: a meta-analysis of randomized controlled trials. J Gastroenterol. 2012;47(6):655–63.

67. Madhoun MF, Wani S, Hong S, Tierney WM, Maple JT. Endoscopic papillary large balloon dilation reduces the need for mechanical lithotripsy in patients with large bile duct stones: a systematic review and meta-analysis. Diagn Ther Endosc. 2014;2014:309618.

68. Sherman S, Hawes RH, Troiano FP, Lehman GA. Pancreatitis following bile duct sphincter of Oddi manometry: utility of the aspirating catheter. Gastrointest Endosc. 1992;38(3):347–50.

69. Kawakubo K, Isayama H, Nakai Y, Togawa O, Sasahira N, Kogure H, et al. Risk factors for pancreatitis following transpapillary self-expandable metal stent placement. Surg Endosc. 2011;26(3):771–6.

70. Terruzzi V, Radaelli F, Meucci G, Minoli G. Is the supine position as safe and effective as the prone position for endoscopic retrograde cholangiopancreatography? A prospective randomized study. Endoscopy. 2005;37(12):1211–4.

71. Tringali A, Mutignani M, Milano A, Perri V, Costamagna G. No difference between supine and prone position for ERCP in conscious sedated patients: a prospective randomized study. Endoscopy. 2008;40(2):93–7.

72. Lee SJ, Lee TH, Park SH, Lee YN, Jung Y, Choi HJ, et al. Efficacy of carbon dioxide versus air insufflation according to different sedation protocols during therapeutic endoscopic retrograde cholangiopancreatography: prospective, randomized, double-blind study. Dig Endosc. 2015;27:512–21.

73. Cheng Y, Xiong XZ, Wu SJ, Lu J, Lin YX, Cheng NS, et al. Carbon dioxide insufflation for endoscopic retrograde cholangiopancreatography: a meta-analysis and systematic review. World J Gastroenterol. 2012;18(39):5622–31.

74. Rey JF, Beilenhoff U, Neumann CS, Dumonceau JM. European Society of Gastrointestinal Endoscopy (ESGE) guideline: the use of electrosurgical units. Endoscopy. 2010;42(9):764–72.

75. Verma D, Kapadia A, Adler DG. Pure versus mixed electrosurgical current for endoscopic biliary sphincterotomy: a meta-analysis of adverse outcomes. Gastrointest Endosc. 2007;66(2):283–90.

76. Moon JH, Cho YD, Cha SW, Cheon YK, Ahn HC, Kim YS, et al. The detection of bile duct stones in suspected biliary pancreatitis: comparison of MRCP, ERCP, and intraductal US. Am J Gastroenterol. 2005;100(5):1051–7.

77. Textor HJ, Flacke S, Pauleit D, Keller E, Neubrand M, Terjung B, et al. Three-dimensional magnetic resonance cholangiopancreatography with respiratory triggering in the diagnosis of primary sclerosing cholangitis: comparison with endoscopic retrograde cholangiography. Endoscopy. 2002;34(12):984–90.

78. Ueno K, Ajiki T, Sawa H, Matsumoto I, Fukumoto T, Ku Y. Role of intraoperative cholangiography in patients whose biliary tree was evaluated preoperatively by magnetic resonance cholangiopancreatography. World J Surg. 2012;36(11):2661–5.

79. Vazquez-Sequeiros E, Gonzalez-Panizo Tamargo F, Boixeda-Miquel D, Milicua JM. Diagnostic accuracy and therapeutic impact of endoscopic ultrasonography in patients with intermediate suspicion of choledocholithiasis and absence of findings in magnetic resonance cholangiography. Rev Esp Enferm Dig. 2011;103(9):464–71.

80. van der Gaag NA, Rauws EA, van Eijck CH, Bruno MJ, van der Harst E, Kubben FJ, et al. Preoperative biliary drainage for cancer of the head of the pancreas. N Engl J Med. 2010;362(2):129–37.

81. Cotton PB, Durkalski V, Romagnuolo J, Pauls Q, Fogel E, Tarnasky P, et al. Effect of endoscopic sphincterotomy for suspected sphincter of Oddi dysfunction on pain-related disability following cholecystectomy: the EPISOD randomized clinical trial. JAMA. 2014;311(20):2101–9.

82. Tenner S, Baillie J, DeWitt J, Vege SS. American College of Gastroenterology guideline: management of acute pancreatitis. Am J Gastroenterol. 2013;108(9):1400–15. 16.

83. Mentula P, Leppaniemi A. Position paper: timely interventions in severe acute pancreatitis are crucial for survival. World J Emerg Surg. 2014;9(1):15.

84. Gardner TB, Vege SS, Pearson RK, Chari ST. Fluid resuscitation in acute pancreatitis. Clin Gastroenterol Hepatol. 2008;6(10):1070–6.

85. Wu BU, Hwang JQ, Gardner TH, Repas K, Delee R, Yu S, et al. Lactated Ringer's solution reduces systemic inflammation compared with saline in patients with acute pancreatitis. Clin Gastroenterol Hepatol. 2011;9(8):710–7.e1.

86. Bhoomagoud M, Jung T, Atladottir J, Kolodecik TR, Shugrue C, Chaudhuri A, et al. Reducing extracellular pH sensitizes the acinar cell to secretagogue-induced pancreatitis responses in rats. Gastroenterology. 2009;137(3):1083–92.

87. Noble MD, Romac J, Vigna SR, Liddle RA. A pH-sensitive, neurogenic pathway mediates disease severity in a model of post-ERCP pancreatitis. Gut. 2008;57(11):1566–71.

88. Sagi SV, Schmidt S, Fogel E, Lehman GA, McHenry L, Sherman S, et al. Association of greater intravenous volume infusion with shorter hospitalization for patients with post-ERCP pancreatitis. J Gastroenterol Hepatol. 2014;29(6):1316–20.

89. DiMagno MJ, Wamsteker EJ, Maratt J, Rivera MA, Spaete JP, Ballard DD, et al. Do larger periprocedural fluid volumes reduce the severity of post-endoscopic retrograde cholangiopancreatography pancreatitis? Pancreas. 2014;43(4):642–7.

90. Choudhary A, Bechtold ML, Arif M, Szary NM, Puli SR, Othman MO, et al. Pancreatic stents for prophylaxis against post-ERCP pancreatitis: a meta-analysis and systematic review. Gastrointest Endosc. 2011;73(2):275–82.

91. Singh P, Das A, Isenberg G, Wong RC, Sivak Jr MV, Agrawal D, et al. Does prophylactic pancreatic stent placement reduce the risk of post-ERCP acute pancreatitis? A meta-analysis of controlled trials. Gastrointest Endosc. 2004;60(4):544–50.

92. Mazaki T, Masuda H, Takayama T. Prophylactic pancreatic stent placement and post-ERCP pancreatitis: a systematic review and meta-analysis. Endoscopy. 2010;42(10):842–53.

93. Mazaki T, Mado K, Masuda H, Shiono M. Prophylactic pancreatic stent placement and post-ERCP pancreatitis: an updated meta-analysis. J Gastroenterol. 2014;49(2):343–55.

94. Fogel EL, Eversman D, Jamidar P, Sherman S, Lehman GA. Sphincter of Oddi dysfunction: pancreaticobiliary sphincterotomy with pancreatic stent placement has a lower rate of pancreatitis than biliary sphincterotomy alone. Endoscopy. 2002;34(4):280–5.

95. Tarnasky PR. Mechanical prevention of post-ERCP pancreatitis by pancreatic stents: results, techniques, and indications. JOP. 2003;4(1):58–67.

96. Tarnasky PR, Palesch YY, Cunningham JT, Mauldin PD, Cotton PB, Hawes RH. Pancreatic stenting prevents pancreatitis after biliary sphincterotomy in patients with sphincter of Oddi dysfunction. Gastroenterology. 1998;115(6):1518–24.

97. Sherman E, Bucksot B, Gottlieb L. Does leaving a main pancreatic duct stent in place reduce the incidence of precut biliary sphincterotomy (ES)-induced pancreatitis? A final analysis of a randomized prospective study. Gastrointest Endosc. 1996;43(4):413.

98. Harewood GC, Pochron NL, Gostout CJ. Prospective, randomized, controlled trial of prophylactic pancreatic stent placement for endoscopic snare excision of the duodenal ampulla. Gastrointest Endosc. 2005;62(3):367–70.

99. Afghani E, Akshintala VS, Khashab MA, Law JK, Hutfless SM, Kim KJ, et al. 5-Fr vs. 3-Fr pancreatic stents for the prevention of post-ERCP pancreatitis in high-risk patients: a systematic review and network meta-analysis. Endoscopy. 2014;46(7):573–80.

100. Freeman ML, Overby C, Qi D. Pancreatic stent insertion: consequences of failure and results of a modified technique to maximize success. Gastrointest Endosc. 2004;59(1):8–14.

101. Bakman YG, Safdar K, Freeman ML. Significant clinical implications of prophylactic pancreatic stent placement in previously normal pancreatic ducts. Endoscopy. 2009;41(12):1095–8.

102. Elmunzer BJ, Scheiman JM, Lehman GA, Chak A, Mosler P, Higgins PD, et al. A randomized trial of rectal indomethacin to prevent post-ERCP pancreatitis. N Engl J Med. 2012;366(15):1414–22.

103. Choksi NS, Fogel EL, Cote GA, Romagnuolo J, Elta GH, Scheiman JM, et al. The risk of post-ERCP pancreatitis and the protective effect of rectal indomethacin in cases of attempted but unsuccessful prophylactic pancreatic stent placement. Gastrointest Endosc. 2015;81(1):150–5.

104. Ohuchida J, Chijiiwa K, Imamura N, Nagano M, Hiyoshi M. Randomized controlled trial for efficacy of nafamostat mesilate in preventing post-endoscopic retrograde cholangiopancreatography pancreatitis. Pancreas. 2015;44(3):415–21.

105. Park JY, Jeon TJ, Hwang MW, Sinn DH, Oh TH, Shin WC, et al. Comparison between ulinastatin and nafamostat for prevention of post-endoscopic retrograde cholangiopancreatography complications: a prospective, randomized trial. Pancreatology. 2014;14(4):263–7.

106. Yuhara H, Ogawa M, Kawaguchi Y, Igarashi M, Shimosegawa T, Mine T. Pharmacologic prophylaxis of post-endoscopic retrograde cholangiopancreatography pancreatitis: protease inhibitors and NSAIDs in a meta-analysis. J Gastroenterol. 2014;49(3):388–99.

107. Bai Y, Ren X, Zhang XF, Lv NH, Guo XG, Wan XJ, et al. Prophylactic somatostatin can reduce incidence of post-ERCP pancreatitis: multicenter randomized controlled trial. Endoscopy. 2015;45:415–20.

108. Omata F, Deshpande G, Tokuda Y, Takahashi O, Ohde S, Carr-Locke DL, et al. Meta-analysis: somatostatin or its long-acting analogue, octreotide, for prophylaxis against post-ERCP pancreatitis. J Gastroenterol. 2010;45(8):885–95.

109. Shao LM, Chen QY, Chen MY, Cai JT. Nitroglycerin in the prevention of post-ERCP pancreatitis: a meta-analysis. Dig Dis Sci. 2010;55(1):1–7.

110. Prat F, Amaris J, Ducot B, Bocquentin M, Fritsch J, Choury AD, et al. Nifedipine for prevention of post-ERCP pancreatitis: a prospective, double-blind randomized study. Gastrointest Endosc. 2002;56(2):202–8.

111. Oh HC, Cheon YK, Cho YD, Do JH. Use of udenafil is not associated with a reduction in post-ERCP pancreatitis: results of a randomized, placebo-controlled, multicenter trial. Gastrointest Endosc. 2011;74(3):556–62.

112. Nojgaard C, Hornum M, Elkjaer M, Hjalmarsson C, Heyries L, Hauge T, et al. Does glyceryl nitrate prevent post-ERCP pancreatitis? A prospective, randomized, double-blind, placebo-controlled multicenter trial. Gastrointest Endosc. 2009;69(6):e31–7.

113. Bai Y, Gao J, Shi X, Zou D, Li Z. Prophylactic corticosteroids do not prevent post-ERCP pancreatitis: a meta-analysis of randomized controlled trials. Pancreatology. 2008;8(4–5):504–9.

114. Bai Y, Gao J, Zhang W, Zou D, Li Z. Meta-analysis: allopurinol in the prevention of postendoscopic retrograde cholangiopancreatography pancreatitis. Aliment Pharmacol Ther. 2008;28(5):557–64.

115. Cao WL, Yan WS, Xiang XH, Chen K, Xia SH. Prevention effect of allopurinol on post-endoscopic retrograde cholangiopancreatography pancreatitis: a meta-analysis of prospective randomized controlled trials. PLoS One. 2014;9(9):e107350.

116. Elmunzer BJ, Higgins PD, Saini SD, Scheiman JM, Parker RA, Chak A, et al. Does rectal indomethacin eliminate the need for prophylactic pancreatic stent placement in patients undergoing high-risk ERCP? Post hoc efficacy and cost-benefit analyses using prospective clinical trial data. Am J Gastroenterol. 2013;108(3):410–5.

117. Katsinelos P, Kountouras J, Paroutoglou G, Beltsis A, Mimidis K, Zavos C. Intravenous N-acetylcysteine does not prevent post-ERCP pancreatitis. Gastrointest Endosc. 2005;62(1):105–11.

118. Li S, Cao G, Chen X, Wu T. Low-dose heparin in the prevention of post endoscopic retrograde cholangiopancreatography pancreatitis: a systematic review and meta-analysis. Eur J Gastroenterol Hepatol. 2012;24(5):477–81.

119. Lua GW, Muthukaruppan R, Menon J. Can rectal diclofenac prevent post endoscopic retrograde cholangiopancreatography pancreatitis? Dig Dis Sci. 2015;60(10):3118–23.

120. Rabenstein T, Fischer B, Wiessner V, Schmidt H, Radespiel-Troger M, Hochberger J, et al. Low-molecular-weight heparin does not prevent acute post-ERCP pancreatitis. Gastrointest Endosc. 2004;59(6):606–13.

121. Dai HF, Wang XW, Zhao K. Role of nonsteroidal anti-inflammatory drugs in the prevention of post-ERCP pancreatitis: a meta-analysis. Hepatobiliary Pancreat Dis Int. 2009;8(1):11–6.

122. Ding X, Chen M, Huang S, Zhang S, Zou X. Nonsteroidal anti-inflammatory drugs for prevention of post-ERCP pancreatitis: a meta-analysis. Gastrointest Endosc. 2012;76(6):1152–9.

123. Elmunzer BJ, Waljee AK, Elta GH, Taylor JR, Fehmi SM, Higgins PD. A meta-analysis of rectal NSAIDs in the prevention of post-ERCP pancreatitis. Gut. 2008;57(9):1262–7.

124. Kubiliun NM, Adams MA, Akshintala VS, Conte ML, Cote GA, Cotton PB, et al. Evaluation of pharmacologic prevention of pancreatitis after endoscopic retrograde cholangiopancreatography: a systematic review. Clin Gastroenterol Hepatol. 2015;13(7):1231–9.

125. Li X, Tao LP, Wang CH. Effectiveness of nonsteroidal anti-inflammatory drugs in prevention of post-ERCP pancreatitis: a meta-analysis. World J Gastroenterol. 2014;20(34):12322–9.

126. Sethi S, Sethi N, Wadhwa V, Garud S, Brown A. A meta-analysis on the role of rectal diclofenac and indomethacin in the prevention of post-endoscopic retrograde cholangiopancreatography pancreatitis. Pancreas. 2014;43(2):190–7.

127. Sun HL, Han B, Zhai HP, Cheng XH, Ma K. Rectal NSAIDs for the prevention of post-ERCP pancreatitis: a meta-analysis of randomized controlled trials. Surgeon. 2012;12(3):141–7.

128. Yaghoobi M, Rolland S, Waschke KA, McNabb-Baltar J, Martel M, Bijarchi R, et al. Meta-analysis: rectal indomethacin for the prevention of post-ERCP pancreatitis. Aliment Pharmacol Ther. 2013;38(9):995–1001.

129. Sotoudehmanesh R, Eloubeidi MA, Asgari AA, Farsinejad M, Khatibian M. A randomized trial of rectal indomethacin and sublingual nitrates to prevent post-ERCP pancreatitis. Am J Gastroenterol. 2014;109(6):903–9.

130. Akbar A, Abu Dayyeh BK, Baron TH, Wang Z, Altayar O, Murad MH. Rectal nonsteroidal anti-inflammatory drugs are superior to pancreatic duct stents in preventing pancreatitis after endoscopic retrograde cholangiopancreatography: a network meta-analysis. Clin Gastroenterol Hepatol. 2013;11(7):778–83.

131. Nicolas-Perez D, Castilla-Rodriguez I, Gimeno-Garcia AZ, Romero-Garcia R, Nunez-Diaz V, Quintero E. Prevention of post-endoscopic retrograde cholangiopancreatography pancreatitis: a cost-effectiveness analysis. Pancreas. 2015;44(2):204–10.

EUS for Pancreaticobiliary Duct Access and Drainage

13

Norio Fukami

Abbreviations

ERCP   Endoscopic retrograde cholangiopancreatography
ERP   Endoscopic retrograde pancreatography
EUS   Endoscopic ultrasound
FNA   Fine-needle aspiration
IR   Interventional radiology
PJ   Pancreaticojejunostomy
PTC   Percutaneous transhepatic cholangiogram
SEMS   Self-expandable metal stent

Introduction

Endoscopic ultrasound (EUS) was originally developed to obtain information about invasion depth and staging for cancers, and identification and evaluation for subepithelial tumors, and to evaluate the pancreas and bile ducts in detail, where air interference, the enemy of ultrasonic imaging, would be minimal. After the curvilinear echoendoscope (linear probe) was introduced and became widely available, sampling from within and outside of the intestinal wall by EUS fine-needle aspiration (FNA) under ultrasound guidance became a popular and frequently used sampling modality. Large-bore needles (19G) enabled passage of commonly used biliary guidewires, and this added the next dimension to the capability of EUS. The progression was natural, from

Electronic supplementary material: The online version of this chapter (doi:10.1007/978-3-319-26854-5_13) contains supplementary material, which is available to authorized users. Videos can also be accessed at http://link.springer.com/chapter/10.1007/978-3-319-26854-5_13.

N. Fukami, M.D., A.G.A.F., F.A.C.G. (✉)
Division of Gastroenterology and Hepatology,
Mayo Clinic Arizona, Scottsdale, AZ, USA
e-mail: fukami.norio@mayo.edu

staging and sampling, to accessing neighboring structures. Subsequebtly, EUS-guided access was initially reported in the early 1990s by Weiserma et al. for cholangiogram [1], and progressed to creation of a fistula from the stomach to pancreas pseudocysts and/or pancreas [2].

This chapter is aimed to guide readers on when and how to use this useful but challenging technique of pancreaticobiliary access and drainage.

When to Use EUS-Guided Access and EUS-Guided Drainage

Endoscopic retrograde cholangiopancreatography (ERCP) remains the primary modality for endoscopic intervention in the biliary and pancreatic ductal systems. A wide variety of equipment and devices are available to make the access mostly successful. However, there is a small percentage (3–10 %) of failure experienced in general practice, with this being even less common at tertiary referral centers [3]. This is usually not due to operator technique, but due to patient conditions, such as difficult stricture, tumor involvement at orifice, or surgically altered anatomy. A repeat trial of ERCP is often recommended at a later date, by the same or a different operator (at the same institution or a tertiary referral center), to improve cannulation success. If failed after appropriate attempts and exhaustion of available equipment and techniques, traditionally, percutaneous transhepatic cholangiogram (PTC) by interventional radiologists (IR) or an experienced gastroenterologist who performs *percutaneous access* is performed (PTC-ERCP rendezvous) to establish access to the target bile duct. Pancreas duct access is very difficult to achieve percutaneously due to its deep-seated location in the body and the smaller size of the target duct. Once access is achieved, however, wire passage through the orifice or stricture is performed from the proximal side (i.e., antegrade wire passage), which guides the retrograde approach. EUS-guided access achieves by the same principle, albeit from with the intestinal lumen, and a wire passed in an antegrade fashion guides the retrograde approach (EUS-ERCP rendezvous). PTC has the benefit of a high success rate for duct access when the duct is dilated and allows easy re-intervention as needed, however, it is associated with a relatively high morbidity rate and the discomfort caused by percutaneous drainage tube to the patient is not insignificant [4]. The site of access for the bile duct by EUS is limited to the left lobe and hepatic hilum, although recently Ogura et al. reported access to the right intrahepatic duct near the confluence to treat a stricture at right main intrahepatic duct [5].

Furthermore, EUS-guided access has enabled direct endoscopic therapy using the same echoendoscope, and, now, the new technique of direct EUS-guided intervention is utilized more often for drainage procedures (e.g., choledochoduodenostomy and hepaticogastrostomy) where retrograde completion with an ERCP scope tends to be difficult, pose risks losing access/wire, and be cumbersome with the need to exchange endoscopes.

EUS has the advantage of easy accessibility to any part of the pancreas duct, and EUS-guided pancreatography and pancreaticogastrostomy or pancreaticoduodenostomy have been uniquely developed. Indications for these special procedures are summarized in Table 13.1.

The technical aspect of the abovementioned procedures is discussed in the later section.

EUS-guided pancreaticobiliary duct access has a higher risk for complications, and these risks should be well discussed prior to the procedure (Table 13.1). Often, an EUS-guided approach is planned day(s) after the initial ERCP attempt so that patients understand risks and benefits, limitations, and alternative methods (e.g., IR or surgical approach). Biliary duct access is less complex and less risky than pancreas duct access, and in each case procedural complexity and the operator's experience should be taken into account.

Biliary Access

Access to the bile duct is feasible from the duodenum, targeting the extrahepatic bile duct, or from the stomach, targeting the intrahepatic duct in the left lobe. Depending on the reason for an EUS-guided approach, completion of the proce-

Table 13.1 Summary: Indication and complications of EUS guided bile duct and pancreas duct access

	Indication	Complications

Bile duct access	Inability to cannulate
	– Torturous distal bile duct
	– Tumor infiltration (peri-ampullary tumor)
	– Tight stricture at orifice
	– Inability to identify the biliary orifice
	– Peri-ampullary diverticulum
		Hepaticocholedochostomy—15–16 %
		  Bile leak—peritonitis—biloma
		  Bleeding
		  Pneumoperitoneum
		  Peritonitis
		  Stent migration
		  Nausea
		  Aspiration pneumonia

	Inability to access ampulla
	– Duodenal stenosis
	– Tumor infiltration
	– Altered anatomy
	  • Gastric bypass
	  • Choledochojejunostomy
	  • Surgical complication	

	Inability to pass the wire through the ductal stricture
	– Complex duct stricture
	– Significant angulation
	– Tight stricture
		Choledochoduodenostomy—14–16 %
		  Bile leak-peritonitis
		  Perforation
		  Pneumoperitoneum
		  Stent migration
		  Cholangitis
		  Cholecystitis
		  Pancreatitis
		  Pneumonia

Pancreas duct access	Inability to access the duct orifice
	Inability to identify the duct orifice
	Inability to pass the wire through the orifice
	Inability to pass the wire through the stricture
	– Complex stricture
	– Disconnected pancreatic duct syndrome
		6–16.5 % (up to 64 %)
		  Bleeding
		  Perforation
		  Pancreas juice leak
		  Pancreatitis
		  Abscess formation
		  Abdominal pain

References: [7, 10–13]

dure can be rendezvous with ERCP or direct EUS-guided therapy. When access to the ampulla is limited due to a malignant stricture in the duodenum, direct drainage (hepaticogastrostomy or choledochoduodenostomy) becomes the intervention of choice for palliation of biliary obstruction.

Planning the route and the method to establish access prior to the needle puncture is extremely important since preparation of the necessary equipment, procedural steps, and briefing assistants with anticipated procedure steps are key elements to a successful procedure, shortening procedure time, reducing the chance of error and loss of guidewire access, and thus reducing complications.

Pancreas

The pancreas is best imaged by EUS owing to its physical proximity to the stomach and the duodenum. Pancreatic duct access is achievable if duct can be visualized at 6–8 o'clock when viewed with the linear EUS scope. Dilated pancreas ducts are more commonly a target for EUS-guided intervention, however, non-dilated pancreatic ducts can also be accessed, although this is, in general, more technically challenging. It is important to assess the proximity of the duct from the gastric wall, the degree of fibrosis in the parenchyma, and the presence or absence of any intervening vessels before attempting EUS-guided access. There is no defined distance between the gastric wall and the pancreas duct that makes transgastric EUS-guided access impossible. It is more difficult to create pancreaticogastrostomy as the distance becomes longer and as more fibrosis becomes present in the parenchyma.

Another consideration is the direction of the needle puncture and the pancreas duct length between the puncture site and the stricture. Needle puncture should be directed towards the pancreas duct stricture or the target area for intervention since wire advancement is significantly dependent upon needle direction. Directing the wire to the other direction causes significant angulation and much friction between the wire and the tip of the needle. If a regular needle is utilized (with a sharp needle tip as compared to a blunt-ended access needle), the wire surface can sometimes be sheared by the needle tip and the wire may be caught by the needle tip, necessitating termination of the access attempt and withdrawal of needle and the wire, forcing the endoscopist to restart the process all over again. If the pancreatic duct decompresses after the initial puncture, it may make repeat attempts even more difficult.

How to Use EUS Guidance

Rendezvous-Retrograde (EUS-Rendezvous ERCP)

The traditional approach is to use the EUS access technique with retrograde rendezvous completion by conventional ERCP. EUS guidance is used to establish access by antegrade wire passage through the biliary or pancreatic ducts through the area of stricture or the ampulla where retrograde access was previously unsuccessful. EUS-guided wire passage is established after needle puncture of the target duct, and aspiration of bile or pancreatic juice to confirm the intraductal position, and to decompress the duct prior to contrast injection. Contrast injection is typically performed to visualize the ductal system fluoroscopically. Wire passage through the stricture should be carefully done, and, finally, the wire is passed through the stricture/anastomosis/ampulla out into the intestinal lumen.

Needle gauge is important since the size of the needle dictates the gauge of the wire. Nineteen-gauge (19G) needles will accept up to 0.035-inch guidewires; however, manipulation tends to be difficult. 0.025-inch guidewires are more easily maneuverable; however, inadequate stiffness may make the negotiation through a tight stricture more difficult. A recently introduced stiff 0.025-inch wire (Visiglide, Olympus, USA) has partially overcome this issue, and more products are on the horizon with different levels of stiffness to ease the maneuver. A 22G needle only accommodates 0.018- or 0.021-inch wire, and maneuverability and negotiation through the tight stricture with these wires are somewhat limited. If available, a stiffer wire is desired with 0.018–0.021 inch size for better maneuverability and tractability.

The choice of either an angled wire or a straight wire is a matter of preference and selected by the anatomy accessed by EUS guidance. Choledochoduodenostomy is rather straightforward and rarely needs aggressive or complex wire manipulation, and thus any stiff wire would work regardless of the wire tip. However, if one wishes to achieve retrograde placement of a stent (EUS-rendezvous ERCP), an angled wire is desirable when accessing the extrahepatic bile duct via the duodenal bulb, since the needle direction is often towards the hepatic hilum, not towards the ampulla, especially if the endoscope is in the "long position" along the greater curvature of the stomach.

The long position of endoscope is ideal for choledochoduodenostomy from the duodenal bulb since this position gives the endoscopist much more stability and a lesser chance of losing access. Short endoscope position with natural needle direction towards the ampulla is ideal for a planned rendezvous procedure. However, stability of the endoscope position needs to be carefully assessed prior to puncture since needle advancement frequently displaces the endoscope back into the stomach if the access attempt is started in the duodenum. It should be stressed that one is always at risk of losing optimal endoscopic position even after achieving access to the duct. The straight endoscope position is ideal for pancreas duct access whenever possible, and left intrahepatic duct access usually requires an upward angle with a curved endoscope tip and is also often not stable from an endoscopic positioning point of view.

Retrograde access can be accomplished in two ways: wire retrieval with over-the-wire cannulation or cannulation alongside the existing antegrade wire. Traditionally, the EUS-guided wire passed into the intestinal lumen is retrieved by an accessory device (e.g., forceps, snare, and basket) and retrieved through the accessory channel of the endoscope. A regular cannula is inserted through the stricture over the retrieved wire. This technique is slow and requires a long wire. Also, the stiff end of the wire needs to go through the patient's body when it is removed. The latter technique (cannulation alongside the antegrade wire) uses this first wire as a visual guide and achieves regular retrograde cannulation and wire passage easily and efficiently, and is the author's preferred method. Once retrograde access is achieved, then EUS guidewire can be removed from patient's mouth with the elastic side of the wire tip coming through the patient [6, 7].

Direct Transmural Drainage and Antegrade Intervention

Direct intervention using EUS-guided access is divided into two categories: EUS-guided transmural drainage and antegrade intervention. The access achieved by EUS needle puncture and wire passage through the needle is used to perform all procedures. The benefits are an elimination of endoscope exchange, reducing the chance for lost wire, and shorter procedure time.

Considerations for selecting the needle, wire and other equipment, and scope position are similar to the rendezvous technique.

Creation of the tract is the critical component of the procedure and frequently is responsible for failure or resultant complications related to the procedure. Simple dilation with a passage dilator may work, however, in some cases tissue is so resistant that passage dilation may not be advanced adequately to dilate the tract. A balloon dilator or tapered catheter may also be used to dilate the tract. If passage dilation is not effective, a needle knife is often used and is effective for this purpose; however, Park et al. cautioned

the use of a needle knife, as their research showed it to be a risk factor for complication [8]. An over-the-wire diathermic catheter is available in some countries that helps creating a tract easier (6, 8.5, 10Fr Cysto-Gastro-Set; Endo-Flex, GmbH, Germany).

To overcome the risk of postoperative bile leak when performing transmural biliary access procedures, fully covered metal stents have gained popularity over time. Self-expandable metal stents (SEMS), especially covered SEMS, can be placed with certain theoretical benefits. Expansion of the covered stent will help to seal the freshly created fistula between the intestinal lumen and the bile duct, reducing the risk for bleeding, biliary, and gastrointestinal leaks and reducing the risk for postoperative peritonitis. SEMS are currently the preferred stent for choledochoduodenostomy. Yet, 10Fr delivery system of SEMS still requires pre-dilation of the tract before insertion. SEMS have also used for hepaticogastrostomy. In this setting, SEMS have the advantage of sealing the tract; however, foreshortening and resultant inward migration out of the stomach into the peritoneal cavity are a much-feared complication, universally causing bile peritonitis and usually requiring surgery. At least one fatality has been reported in this context [9]. For hepaticogastrostomy, the drainage method is still not optimized and adequately compared to make any recommendations, and thus, each endoscopist has to pay careful attention to prevent this severe complication when fully covered SEMS is used.

If a biliary or pancreatic duct can be accessed but the target stricture cannot be crossed with a guidewire, creating a fistulous tract by temporary placement of a stent would serve as an access route to treat the stricture at next visit and allow interval ductal decompression. It is recommended to wait for about 4 weeks for the tract to mature before removing the stent and re-attempting intervention. A mature tract significantly reduces the leak complications and allows for use of a variety of cannulas or balloons with maneuverable stiff wire (0.025–0.035 inch), often resulting in successful intervention and treatment.

The following case studies are presented to demonstrate the aforementioned techniques.

A. Biliary system access
  1. Trans-gastric approach—EUS-rendezvous ERCP (Case 1—Fig. 13.1 and Video 13.1)
  2. Trans-duodenal approach—EUS-guided direct choledochoduodenostomy (Case 2—Fig. 13.2)
B. Pancreas
  1. Trans-gastric approach—EUS-guided antegrade intervention with stent placement and dilation of stricture (Case 3—Fig. 13.3)
  2. Trans-duodenal approach—EUS-guided direct stent therapy and subsequent dilation of stricture (Case 4—Video 13.2)

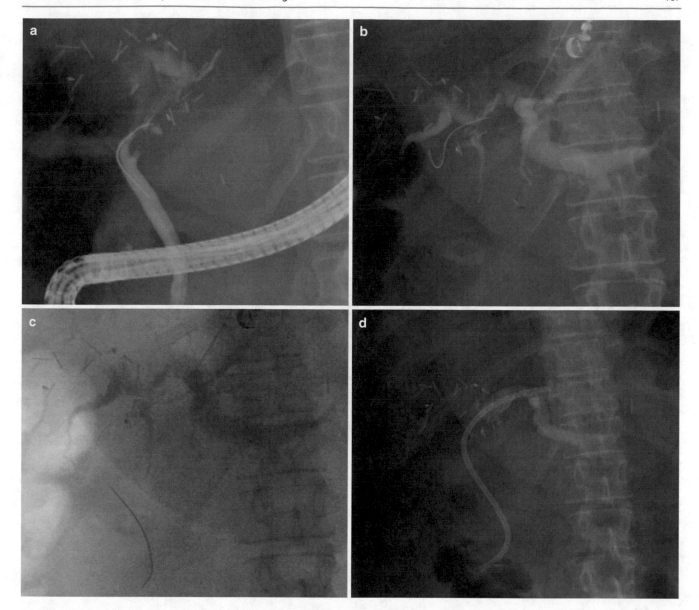

Fig. 13.1 Case 1: 52 y.o. female who underwent right hepatectomy and cholecystectomy for intrahepatic cholangiocarcinoma. Patient developed jaundice postoperatively and intrahepatic ductal dilation was noted on CT scan without biloma. ERCP was performed, showing tight stricture and acute angulation at bifurcation where surgical transection of right main intrahepatic duct was previously performed. Multiple attempts of wire passage through the stenosis failed despite the use of several different catheters and wires. (**a**) EUS-guided left intrahepatic duct access was performed with 19G needle. Cholangiogram confirmed severe dilation of intrahepatic ducts and stenosis near the left main intrahepatic duct. (**b**) Angled 0.025 in wire was manipulated to pass through the stricture (**c**) (Video 13.1). Rendezvous procedure was performed, completing the stent placement in usual retrograde fashion after exchange of endoscope to a duodenoscope (**d**)

Summary

EUS-guided access to the pancreaticobiliary tract provides endoscopists an opportunity to salvage patients from ERCP failure and subsequent percutaneous and surgical intervention. EUS-guided access and intervention are reported to be highly successful at tertiary referral centers. While the higher complication rates of this technique need to be improved, refinement of the technique as well as further development of dedicated equipment for EUS-guided access and drainage would improve outcomes and are expected in near future.

Video Legends

Video 13.1 Case 1: From the stomach, the left lobe of the liver was visualized with a linear echoendoscope. The left lateral segment bile duct was accessed with a 19G needle and contrast was injected. Excessive contrast injection was avoided to minimize leakage. A 0.025 in angled wire was passed through the needle and carefully manipulated to pass through the stricture. The wire was torqued as needed to direct towards the predicted confluence and then towards the extrahepatic duct. Withdrawal of the wire was done very carefully to avoid stripping the wire covering. Smooth

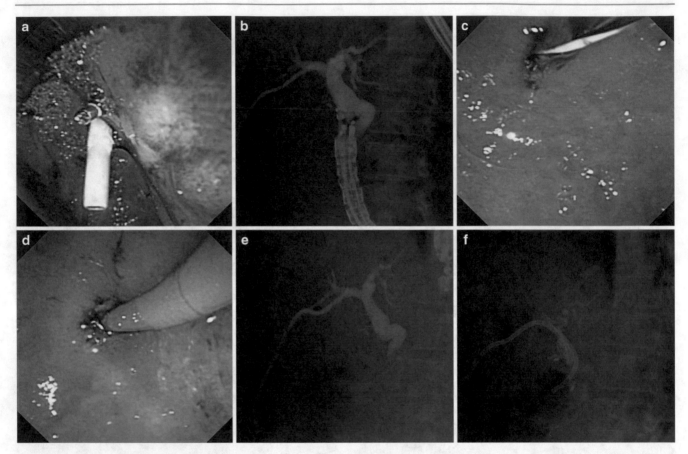

Fig. 13.2 Case 2: 54 y.o. female suffered biliary obstruction after pancreas sparing duodenectomy for duodenal GIST. PTC tube was placed for biliary drainage while unclear of the etiology of biliary obstruction. Later, it was discovered that the major ampulla was resected during the surgery. Contrast was injected via PTC tube and distal bile duct obstruction was confirmed. (**e**) EUS-guided access to extrahepatic duct was performed using 19G needle through the duodenal bulb in long position of endoscope. (**b**) 0.035-G guidewire was passed via 19G needle to right intrahepatic duct. (**c**) Passage dilation was performed. (**d**) 7Fr biliary stent was successfully placed. (**a**) Post-film showed proper position of internal stent with proximal end of stent at right main intrahepatic duct (**f**)

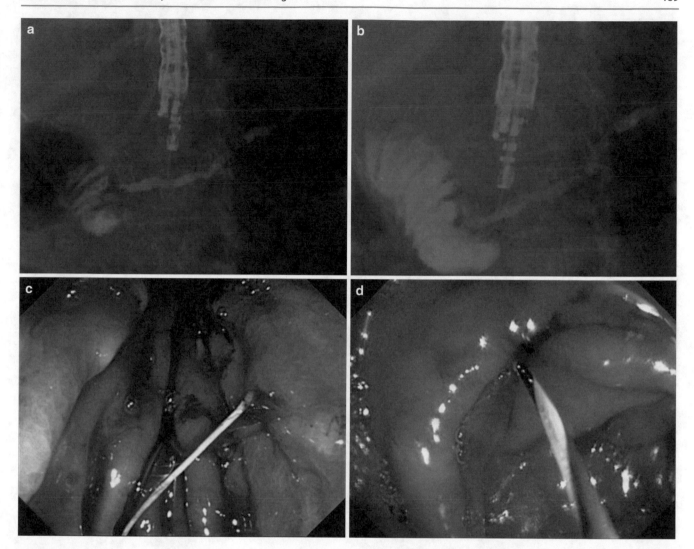

Fig. 13.3 Case 3: 56 y.o. female underwent pancreaticoduodenectomy for symptomatic insulinoma in the head of pancreas. Patient had acute pancreatitis within 1 year of surgery and continued to have recurrent attacks. CT identified postsurgical change but failed to reveal any cause. MRCP showed dilated pancreas duct in the remaining pancreas and suggested anastomotic stricture. Endoscopic retrograde pancreatography (ERP) was attempted but the site of pancreaticojejunostomy (PJ) was not located. EUS-guided pancreatogram was performed. Successful pancreatogram using 22G needle confirmed severe PJ stricture. (**a**) Attempt of 0.018-in guidewire antegrade passage via 22G needle failed. After surgical consultation, patient decided for nonsurgical approach rather than re-operation. EUS-guided transgastric pancreatogram using 19G needle. (**b**) Dilation of the pancreas duct with narrowed segment near the PJ anastomosis was clearly seen with slow contrast outflow into jejunum. Wire (0.025G) was passed through the 19G needle into the jejunum across the stricture. EUS-ERCP rendezvous procedure was performed. Carefully leaving the wire in position, the endoscope was exchanged for ERP to straight view endoscope. (**c**) PJ anastomosis was identified by the exiting wire. (**d**) Wire was grasped and pulled through the endoscope. Catheter was advanced and its intraductal position was confirmed by contrast injection. (**e**) Wire was advanced to the tail in retrograde fashion to ensure proper wire position. Passage dilation was performed. (**f**) Stent was successfully placed in retrograde fashion. (**g**) Final fluoroscopic imaging. (**h**) Patient improved clinically with resolution of postprandial abdominal pain after the procedure

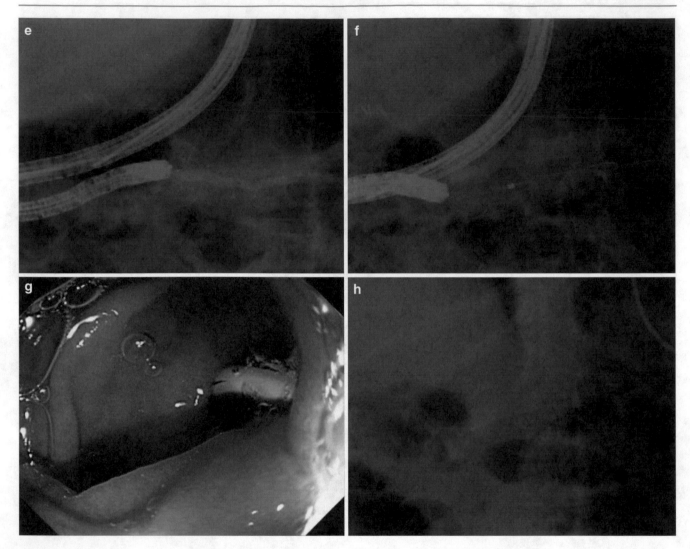

Fig. 13.3 (continued)

advancement of the wire is seen towards the ampulla, and the wire was further advanced to loop inside the duodenum. The wire was successfully passed into the duodenum via the major papilla. The wire was seen with the exchanged duodenoscope. The wire tip was captured into the snare and carefully pulled into the channel to complete retrograde stent placement (MP4 93854 kb).

Video 13.2 Case 4: 47 y.o. male with a history of FAP underwent pancreas-sparing duodenectomy and creation of a neo-ampulla for a fully circumferential large duodenal adenoma. This was complicated with persistent pancreas ascites. ERCP was performed and the biliary orifice was easily identified; however, pancreas duct access failed, suggesting stenosis at the orifice. EUS-guided intervention was planned after thorough discussion (MP4 83553 kb).

References

1. Wiersema M, Sandusky D, Carr R, et al. Endosonography-guided cholangiopancreatography. Gastrointest Endosc. 1996;43:5.
2. François E, Kahaleh M, Giovanni M, et al. EUS-guided pancreaticogastrostomy. Gastrointest Endosc. 2001;53:AB57.
3. Artifon E, Okawa L, Takada J, et al. EUS-guided choledochoantrostomy: an alternative for biliary drainage in unresectable pancreatic cancer with duodenal invasion. Gastrointest Endosc. 2011;73:4.
4. Born P, Rösch T, Triptrap A, et al. Long-term results of percutaneous transhepatic biliary drainage for benign and malignant bile duct strictures. Scand J Gastroenterol. 1998;33:6.
5. Ogura T, Higuchi K. Does endoscopic ultrasound-guided biliary drainage really have clinical impact? World J Gastroenterol. 2015;21:4.
6. Itoi T, Yasuda I, Kurihara T, et al. Technique of endoscopic ultrasonography-guided pancreatic duct intervention (with videos). J Hepatobiliary Pancreat Sci. 2014;21:6.
7. Isayama H, Nakai Y, Kawakubo K, et al. The endoscopic ultrasonography-guided rendezvous technique for biliary cannulation: a technical review. J Hepatobiliary Pancreat Sci. 2013;20:8.
8. Park D, Jang J, Lee S, et al. EUS-guided biliary drainage with transluminal stunting after failed ERCP: predictors of adverse events and long-term results. Gastrointest Endosc. 2011;74:9.
9. Martins F, Rossini L, Ferrari A. Migration of a covered metallic stent following endoscopic ultrasound-guided hepaticogastrostomy: fatal complication. Endoscopy. 2010;42:2.
10. Kahaleh M, Artifon E, Perez-Miranda M, et al. Endoscopic ultrasonography guided drainage: summary of consortium meeting, May 21, 2012, San Diego, California. World J Gastroenterol. 2015;21:16.
11. Fujii L, Topazian M, Dayyeh B, et al. EUS-guided pancreatic duct intervention: outcomes of a single tertiary-care referral center experience. Gastrointest Endosc. 2013;78:11.
12. Itoi T, Kasuya K, Sofuni A, et al. Endoscopic ultrasonography-guided pancreatic duct access: techniques and literature review of pancreatography, transmural drainage and rendezvous techniques. Dig Endosc. 2013;25:12.
13. Iqbal S, Friedel D, Grendell J, et al. Outcomes of endoscopic-ultrasound-guided cholangiopancreatography: a literature review. Gastroenterol Res Pract. 2013;869214:9.

Endoscopic Drainage of Pancreatic Fluid Collections

Natalie Danielle Cosgrove, Pushpak Taunk,
Haroon Shahid, and Ali Ahmed Siddiqui

Classification of Pancreatic Fluid Collections

Pancreatic and peripancreatic fluid collections (PFC) are fluid-filled cavities that develop and evolve in the setting of acute and chronic pancreatitis, pancreatic necrosis, abdominal trauma, pancreatic ductal obstruction, or pancreatic ductal leak. These collections are classified as acute peripancreatic fluid collections (APFC), acute necrotic collections (ANC), pancreatic pseudocysts, and walled-off necrosis (WON) according to their components and level of maturation/organization as per the revised Atlanta classification [1]. The term pancreatic abscess is no longer used and fluid collections are instead described as either infected or sterile [1]. APFC and ANC are immature fluid collections that lack encapsulation with a well-defined wall. An APFC forms in the setting of interstitial edematous pancreatitis and contains only fluid, while an ANC forms in the setting of necrotizing pancreatitis and contains both solid and liquid debris. These immature collections may evolve over several weeks into more organized collections with a radiologically visualized non-epithelial lined capsule, after which they are referred to as pancreatic pseudocysts and WON, respectively. Encapsulation may occur as early as 1 week following an episode of acute pancreatitis but typically requires at least 4 weeks to develop [2].

Electronic supplementary material: The online version of this chapter (doi:10.1007/978-3-319-26854-5_14) contains supplementary material, which is available to authorized users. Videos can also be accessed at http://link.springer.com/chapter/10.1007/978-3-319-26854-5_14.

N.D. Cosgrove, M.D.
Thomas Jefferson University, Philadelphia, PA, USA

P. Taunk, M.D.
University of South Florida, Tampa, FL, USA

H. Shahid, M.D.
Thomas Jefferson University Hospital, Philadelphia, PA, USA

A.A. Siddiqui, M.D. (✉)
Department of Gastroenterology, Thomas Jefferson University Hospital, Philadelphia, PA, USA
e-mail: ali.siddiqui@jefferson.edu

Pseudocysts contain primarily liquid debris while WON contains variable amounts of both solid and liquid debris (Fig. 14.1). While pancreatic fluid collections without mature encapsulation or collections that contain any degree of solid components are often incorrectly referred to as pseudocysts, establishing the correct classification of a fluid collection is an important first step in directing its management [3], although in practice it can sometimes be difficult to distinguish pseudocysts from true WON.

Initial Diagnostic Evaluation

Cross-sectional imaging is useful in establishing the presence, location, type, and extent of pancreatic fluid collections, and may also help to establish the presence of an underlying malignancy, pancreatic duct obstruction, or pancreatic duct disruption. Contrast-enhanced CT (CECT) is less sensitive than MRI, endosonographic ultrasound (EUS), and trans-abdominal ultrasound for detecting the presence of solid necrotic debris but is able to differentiate pseudocysts from WON in most cases [1, 2, 4]. Radiological findings that favor a diagnosis of a WON include larger fluid collection size, extension into a paracolic or retrocolic space, an irregular border with the presence of fat attenuation and debris, presence of pancreatic parenchymal deformity and discontinuity, and absence of main pancreatic duct dilation. Main pancreatic duct dilation (>4 mm) on the other hand favors a diagnosis of pseudocyst [2]. Magnetic resonance cholangio-pancreatography (MRCP) and endoscopic retrograde cholangio-pancreatography (ERCP) are superior to CECT in establishing the presence of a communication between the pancreatic duct (PD) and the presence of a pancreatic duct disruption and should be performed in cases of high clinical suspicion [3, 4].

Additional work-up is needed for patients without any risk factors for PFC, such as a history of acute pancreatitis or evidence of chronic pancreatitis. This is necessary to establish a definitive diagnosis and differentiate PFC from benign and malignant pancreatic cystic neoplasia, pseudoaneurysms, duplication

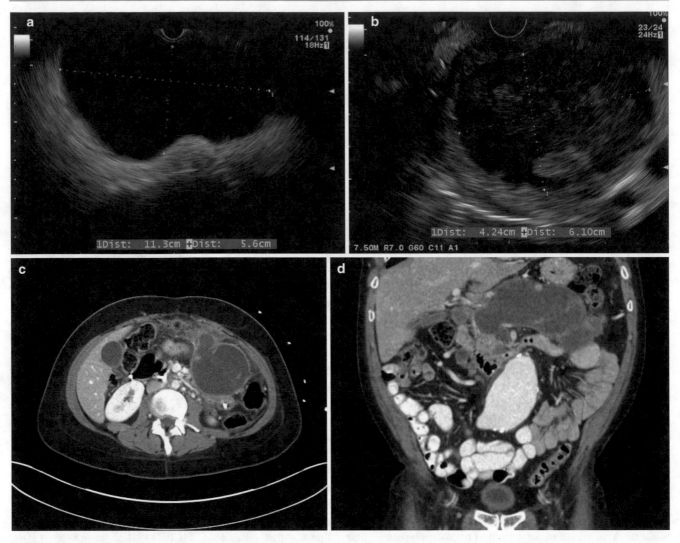

Fig. 14.1 Pancreatic fluid collections. (**a**) EUS image of a large pseudocyst with almost entirely liquid contents. (**b**) EUS image of walled-off necrosis showing solid debris within the cyst cavity. (**c**) CT image of a large pancreatic fluid collection. EUS revealed the lesion to be a pseu- docyst (image courtesy Douglas G. Adler MD). (**d**) CT image of a large pancreatic fluid collection. EUS revealed the lesion to be WON (image courtesy Douglas G Adler MD)

cysts, and other non-inflammatory fluid collections. Contrast-enhanced ultrasound or EUS along with biochemical analysis should be performed in these cases and, in most but not all cases, can distinguish between pancreatic fluid collections and true pancreatic neoplasms. The presence of vascularized internal septae, solid nodules in the cyst wall, positive staining for mucin, and high cystic fluid CEA levels are indicative of cystic neoplasia, while high amylase, low CEA levels, and negative staining for mucin are suggestive of a PFC [5, 6].

Indications for Intervention for PFCs and Optimal Timing

Most pancreatic fluid collections resolve spontaneously without any intervention [5, 7–9]. Historically, pancreatic pseudocysts larger than 6 cm or persisting beyond 6 weeks

were felt to warrant drainage; current indications for intervention for PFC are now symptom driven [5, 10]. Infected or symptomatic pseudocysts (abdominal pain, compression of biliary, intestinal, or vascular structures, or malnutrition) are indications for drainage. Likewise, indications for intervention for necrotizing pancreatitis include suspected or documented infection with clinical deterioration (preferably when the necrosis has become walled-off), ongoing organ failure for several weeks after the onset of acute pancreatitis (in the absence of documented infection), ongoing gastric outlet, intestinal or biliary obstruction due to mass effect (arbitrarily greater than 4–8 weeks after onset), persistent symptoms such as pain or persistent unwellness in patients without signs of infection (>8 weeks after onset), and disconnected duct syndrome with persisting symptomatic collections (>8 weeks after onset) without signs of infection (Table 14.1) [4]. Distinguishing infected from non-infected fluid collections

Table 14.1 Indications for intervention (either endoscopic, radiological, or surgical) in infected or sterile necrotizing pancreatitis [4]

	Infected	Sterile
Early		
<4 weeks	1. Clinical suspicion of or documented infection with clinical deterioration (preferably when necrosis walled-off) 2. In the absence of documented infected necrotizing pancreatitis, ongoing organ failure for several weeks after onset (preferably when walled-off)	1. Abdominal compartment syndrome 2. Ongoing acute bleeding not amenable to endoscopic control 3. Bowel ischemia 4. Bowel perforation
Late		
>4–8 weeks	See above	1. Ongoing gastric outlet, intestinal, or biliary obstruction due to mass effect
>8 weeks	See above	1. Persistent symptoms (i.e.: pain, persistent unwellness) 2. Disconnected duct syndrome with persisting symptomatic (i.e.: pain, obstruction) collections

may be difficult, especially early on in the disease course when the presence of systemic inflammatory response syndrome is nearly universal [3]. Infection of a PFC may be diagnosed based on clinical suspicion, persistent fever, worsening inflammatory markers, and/or imaging findings (i.e., extraluminal gas in the pancreatic and/or peripancreatic tissue) [3, 4]. Routine percutaneous fine-needle aspiration and culture of fluid collections to assess for infection are not recommended due to the risk of introducing infection and the occurrence of false-negative cultures [4].

Conservative management (i.e., without any radiologic, endoscopic, or surgical intervention) may be performed successfully in as many as 62 % of patients with pancreatic or peripancreatic necrosis [11] and 39 % of patients with pancreatic pseudocysts [7]. For symptomatic collections, interventions should be delayed as long as possible to allow for fluid demarcation, necrotic liquefaction of cyst contents, and encapsulation of the fluid collection [4]. Interventions performed prior to encapsulation are often technically difficult, significantly less successful [12, 13], and are associated with significantly higher mortality [11]. When required, early interventions (before fluid collection maturation/encapsulation) should be minimally invasive and should avoid the lesser sac to decrease the risk of procedure-related infection and bleeding [14, 15]. Early collections that require drainage in the setting of acute pancreatitis are often addressed surgically or by interventional radiology approaches.

Endoscopic Interventions for Pancreatic Pseudocysts

Overview of Management Approaches

Surgical drainage was previously the standard management of pancreatic pseudocysts; however less invasive endoscopic approaches are now the preferred intervention in most centers [16]. In a recent randomized trial comparing endoscopic

and surgical pancreatic pseudocyst drainage, endoscopic drainage resulted in significantly better physical and mental health component scores, lower mean cost, and shorter hospital stays [17]. Endoscopic approaches to pancreatic pseudocyst drainage include transpapillary, transmural, and combined transpapillary and transmural drainage. The chosen endoscopic approach should be based on the anatomical relationship of the fluid collection to the gastric and duodenal lumen and the presence or absence of a pancreatic duct communication/duct disruption [6]. Endoscopic drainage results in successful pseudocyst resolution in 74–100 % of patients with low recurrence rates [13, 17, 18]. Percutaneous drainage is associated with the development of pancreaticocutaneous fistulas, and significantly higher rates of reintervention, and should be reserved for pseudocysts that are inaccessible by endoscopic methods [19]. Although not always possible before intervening, differentiating pseudocysts from WON is important prior to attempting any drainage, as performing drainage alone in fluid collections that contain solid debris may cause infection and should be avoided [20]. As stated previously, the presence of any amount of solid debris classifies an encapsulated fluid collection as WON, the management of which will be discussed later in this chapter.

Endoscopic Transmural Drainage

Endoscopic transmural drainage (ETD) involves placing large-bore stents through either the gastric or the duodenal wall and into a cyst cavity to create a cystenterostomy. ETD may be performed with or without EUS guidance. For the conventional (non-EUS guided) method, the location of puncture is determined by endoscopically identifying an area with maximal extraluminal compression, usually in the stomach or the duodenum, which represents an area of external compression by the pseudocyst. Pre-procedure cross-sectional imaging may be used for reference. The initial

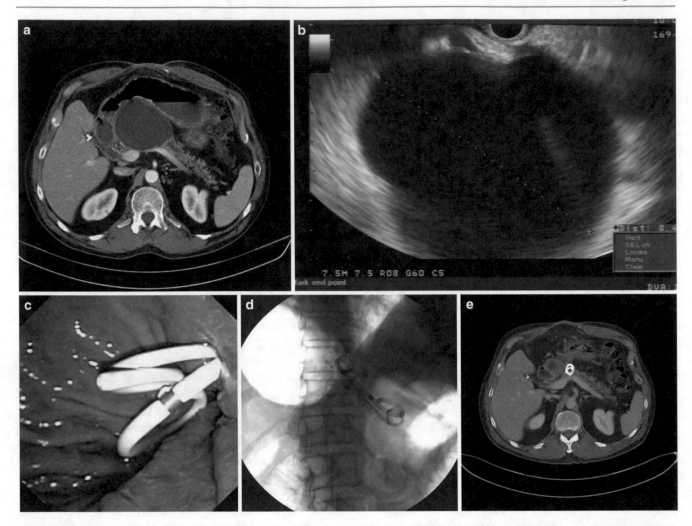

Fig. 14.2 Transmural drainage of a pancreatic pseudocyst with plastic pigtail stents. (**a**) Large pancreatic fluid collection on CT scan. Note the dilated pancreatic duct. (**b**) EUS appearance of the fluid-filled cyst. Note the lack of solid debris. (**c**) Endoscopic appearance of two double-pigtail stents placed across EUS-created cystogastrostomy. (**d**) Fluoroscopic appearance of two double-pigtail stents placed across EUS-created cystogastrostomy. (**e**) CT scan of same patient 6 weeks later. Note that the cyst has completely collapsed and only the pigtail stents remain in place. The pigtail stents were then removed endoscopically (images courtesy Douglas G Adler MD)

endoscopy may be performed with a large-channel therapeutic gastroscope or a side-viewing duodenoscope. When EUS guidance is used, a therapeutic linear echoendoscope may help to identify the optimal site of puncture. A distance of 1 cm or less from the gut lumen to fluid collection is generally considered has been suggested to be the maximum safe distance to perform ETD [15], but in practice this distance can often be somewhat exceeded.

Once the target area has been identified, cyst puncture may be performed using a variety of instruments, including large-caliber aspiration needle, needle-knife electrocautery, precut sphincterotome, exposed end of a polypectomy snare, laser, and a double-channel fistulatome [21]. Aspiration of cystic contents and/or contrast injection into the cyst cavity under fluoroscopy confirms successful puncture into the cyst cavity [22]. Following cyst puncture, a biliary guidewire is advanced into the cyst until stabilizing loops are formed in

the cyst cavity. If needed, the tract can be enlarged using electrocautery to extend the initial incision or using the sheath of a 19-gauge FNA needle. A balloon dilator is then passed over the guidewire to further dilate the tract as needed [13]. Large-bore stents are then placed over the guidewire and are positioned to extend from the gastric or duodenal lumen into the cyst cavity. Freely flowing fluid through the stents and into the gastrointestinal cavity indicates successful stent placement. Plastic double-pigtail stents are commonly used in this setting, but metal biliary stents or dedicated transluminal stents can be used as well to good effect [5] (Fig. 14.2). When multiple plastic stents are placed into a cyst cavity, several guidewires should be placed into the cyst prior to insertion of the first stent to facilitate easier stent placement. Alternatively, metal biliary fully covered self-expanding metal stents (FCSEMS) or a new fully covered lumen-opposing self-expanding metal stent (LASEMS) has recently been demonstrated to be safe and effective for pseudocyst drainage. Prophylactic antibiotics are typically given pre-procedure and for several days following the procedure, although no formal studies have been done to support this [23]. Most patients may be immediately discharged home from the endoscopy suite without hospital admission. Repeat cross-sectional imaging should be performed 4–6 weeks following the procedure. Additional transmural stents may be placed in subsequent sessions as needed. Following successful pseudocyst resolution, transmural stents that do not migrate spontaneously should be removed 1–2 weeks after cyst resolution. In patients with pancreatic duct disruption, however, transmural stents may be left indefinitely to provide a second route for drainage of pancreatic secretions and reduce the risk of recurrence [6, 24].

The routine use of EUS during ETD has been advocated for identifying the optimal puncture site for drainage and stent placement [3]. Advantages of EUS-guided ETD include the ability to perform endoscopic drainage in the absence of external luminal compression, avoidance of vascular structures during cyst puncture using Doppler flow, and easier identification of a site with the appropriate distance from the lumen [5]. EUS may also help to differentiate pancreatic fluid collections from cystic neoplasia, identify occult underlying malignancy [5, 25, 26], and differentiate pseudocysts from WON by establishing the presence of solid cavity debris.

EUS-guided ETD has significantly higher technical success than conventional drainage with reported success rates of up to 100 % [27, 28]. Conventional ETD is successful in only 33–57 % of patients, with procedure failures predominately attributed to the absence of extrinsic luminal compression and the lack of a clear target for endoscopic puncture [26]. While a trend towards fewer complication and bleeding rates has been seen with EUS guidance, this is not statistically significant [27, 28].

An EUS-guided approach should be preferred in patients with a small window of entry on cross-sectional imaging, in the absence of external luminal compression or unusual collection location, indeterminate adherence of the collection to the lumen wall, patients with portal hypertension or known varices, large abdominal arteries, or coagulopathy, after a prior failed conventional approach, and when an alternative diagnosis such as malignancy needs to be ruled out [29, 30]. Conventional drainage may be pursued in patients with a large window of entry based on cross-sectional imaging, external luminal compression, and without evidence of portal hypertension [31].

Transpapillary Drainage

Pseudocysts that are in direct communication with the pancreatic duct are often amenable to transpapillary drain-age [32]. A visualized communication between the PD and a PFC is suggestive of a disconnected or disrupted pancreatic duct. Disconnected pancreatic duct occurs in at least one-third of patients with necrotizing pancreatitis as a result of the destruction of a central portion of the pancreas with viable upstream pancreas draining out of a low-pressure fistula, and may lead to the development of recurrent pancreatitis, fistulae, and PFC [3, 4, 14, 33]. Transpapillary stenting via ERCP across a PD disruption may resolve this disconnection and any fluid collections, pancreatic ascites, and fistulas that communicate with the PD [3, 32, 34, 35] (Fig. 14.3). Transpapillary drainage also allows simultaneous treatment of any downstream pancreatic duct obstruction, stricture, or stenosis. To perform transpapillary drainage, the PD is first visualized with direct pancreatography via ERCP. A pancreatic sphincterotomy can be performed, but is not essential to technical and clinical success. Ductal strictures, if present, are dilated with a 4 or 6 mm dilating balloon catheter or bougie. A PD stent is then inserted over a guidewire into the pancreatic duct branch in contact with the communicating pseudocyst and is positioned with the proximal edge either into the cyst cavity or, preferably, across the site of ductal disruption [34, 36].

Large case series of transpapillary pseudocyst drainage report high success rates of >90 % [31, 32]. Factors associated with improved outcomes include successfully bridging the PD disruption, longer duration of PD stent placement (approximately 6 weeks), and partial (as opposed to complete) duct disruption [31, 37]. Large pseudocysts (>5 cm) that communicate with the PD are often treated by a combination of transpapillary and transmural drainage, but transpapillary drainage may be acceptable in some patients with large cysts [32]. Retrospective studies have drawn mixed conclusions regarding the benefits of combined drainage versus ETD alone [34, 38, 39]. In selected cases of refractory disconnected duct syndrome with persistent fistulae or recurrent collections, internal drainage via EUS-guided pancreatoenterostomy or combined percutaneous and endoscopic internal drainage may be performed [40].

Whether or not to routinely perform direct pancreatography via ERCP at the time of initial pseudocyst drainage to assess for disconnected PD is unclear. PD integrity may be assessed pre-procedure using CECT, MRCP, or EUS, although the presence of a disconnected pancreatic duct may be underestimated by CECT [3]. In ill patients with infected necrosis, some say that ERCP should be avoided before first containing the infection, although a counterargument to this notion is that the ERCP itself may help to control or drain an infection [15]. When done as part of preoperative planning, ERCP should be done shortly before surgery due to a risk of causing PFC infection.

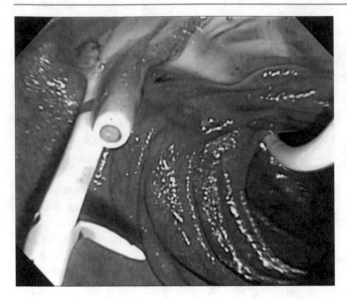

Fig. 14.3 Endoscopic image of transpapillary drainage of an infected pancreatic fluid collection. Note purulent drainage through the pancreatic duct stent lumen into the duodenum. There is also a biliary stent in place as well as a feeding tube (image courtesy Douglas G. Adler MD)

Procedure Adverse Events

Complications for ETD and transpapillary pseudocyst drainage occur in 5.2–19 % of patients and include bleeding, infection, perforation, pancreatitis, aspiration, perforation, and stent occlusion or migration. Patient mortality is low [13, 17, 18]. Overall complication rates for transgastric, transduodenal, and transpapillary drainage are similar [13]. However, pancreatic duct stents placed during transpapillary drainage may cause ductal changes and scarring [41] if left in place for an excessively long amount of time, although in some patients with symptomatic lesions that improve slowly this is an acceptable trade-off.

Interventions for Walled-Off Pancreatic Necrosis

Overview of Management Approaches

WON contains varying amounts of solid debris and liquefied necrosis. Primary management was historically achieved by open or laparoscopic surgical debridement, drainage, and lavage [42, 43]. Endoscopic transmural drainage entails initial access into the WON cavity under EUS guidance and placement of stents (plastic or metal) for drainage of the cavity. Endoscopic transmural drainage is often followed several days or weeks later with repeated endoscopic transmural necrosectomy (ETN) as needed, in which the endoscope is advanced through the previously created cyst-enterostomy tract followed by debridement by a variety of measures.

Endoscopic transmural drainage or image-guided percutaneous drainage (preferably with a retroperitoneal approach) is now recommended as a first-line treatment for WON, with endoscopic transmural necrosectomy (ETN) and, ultimately, minimally invasive surgical necrosectomy reserved as last resort therapies [3, 4]. This "step-up" approach to management has been shown to decrease patient morbidity and mortality and obviates the need for necrosectomy in up to 55 % of patients [11, 44–46]. While a recent small matched cohort study demonstrated superiority of direct ETN versus percutaneous drainage followed by surgical necrosectomy [47], a randomized multicenter trial specifically comparing the surgical "step-up" approach to an endoscopic "step-up" approach for WON therapy is currently under way [48]. Endoscopic necrosectomy is ideal for necrosis that is closely adhered to either the gastric or the duodenal wall with a walled-off partially liquefied collection. Surgery is often indicated for WON that extends into the pelvis or is not in good approximation to the stomach or duodenum. Surgery remains an important salvage therapy in the treatment of complications that arise from endoscopic or percutaneous drainage [49]. Ultimately, the chosen management approach to necrotizing pancreatitis will vary on a case-by-case basis, based on a patient's clinical course, local and regional expertise, and the goal of treatment, and requires a well-thought-out and multidisciplinary approach [15].

Endoscopic Transmural Drainage of WON

Endoscopic transmural drainage (ETD) of pancreatic necrosis is performed in a similar method to that of pseudocysts with EUS-guided transmural puncture into either the gastric or the duodenal luminal wall, tract dilation, and placement of one or several large-bore plastic or self-expandable metal stents into the cavity to create a cystenterostomy. However, tract dilation for WON can be done to a larger size if needed, at typically up to 15–20 mm unless contraindicated, to facilitate drainage of solid debris and any future necrosectomies [50].

As with pseudocyst drainage, EUS guidance may be used to identify the optimal site of puncture and to avoid vascular structures and is strongly advocated in patients without an extraluminal bulge, in the presence of large vessels or varices, and for patients with coagulopathy for reasons stated previously [3, 15]. Pre- and post-procedure antibiotics are generally given for this procedure [23].

The success rate of endoscopic therapy for pancreatic necrosis is significantly lower than for pancreatic pseudocysts (72 %) along with higher recurrence rates (29 %) [13]. This reflects the more complex nature of WON and the overall more ill state of the patient. The presence of solid necrotic debris poses an added challenge to the endoscopic management of WON. Endoscopic drainage alone is sometimes inadequate [50, 51], can convert sterile necrosis into infected necrosis [36], and can be limited by stent occlusion with debris [52]. Vigorous cavity irrigation may be performed by flushing normal saline through either a pigtail nasobiliary tube or a catheter placed through a PEG tube with an extension tube placed endoscopically into the necrosis cavity. Saline irrigation has been shown in trials to decrease stent occlusion and improve WON resolution [52–54]. There is no consensus for the use of or frequency and duration of endoscopic irrigation. Recently, newer techniques for enhanced transluminal drainage and irrigation have been described. The multiple transluminal gateway technique (MTGT) involves creating two or three transmural drainage tracts under EUS guidance, with one tract serving as a portal for vigorous nasocystic tube irrigation and the remaining tracts acting as large conduits to drainage [55]. This technique presupposes that multiple sites for stents or drains can be placed—a situation not encountered in all patients. Single transluminal gateway transcystic multiple drainage technique (SGTMD) has been proposed as a method to obtain sufficient drainage and irrigation in "sub-cavities" than are inaccessible to EUS-guided puncture by using an ERCP catheter and soft guidewire to place multiple double-pigtail stents and nasobiliary tubes into these cavities through a single transmural entry [56]. Small retrospective studies of these newer techniques are promising with clinical success reported at over 90 % [55, 56].

Endoscopic Transmural Necrosectomy

Endoscopic transmural necrosectomy (ETN) was first described in 2000 [57]. A small randomized trial comparing ETN to video-assisted retroperitoneal debridement (VARD) and laparotomy noted significantly improved inflammatory markers mortality and major complications for patients who received ETN [43]. The success of WON resolution via ETN is 80–90 % [12, 58]. ETN may be performed either immediately following ETD or during a subsequent procedure several days to weeks later. To perform ETN, a forward-viewing gastroscope is inserted into the cavity through a previously created cystenterostomy. Various endoscopic accessories are then used to aspirate fluid contents, irrigate the cavity, and extract devitalized tissue and debris (Figs. 14.4 and 14.5) (Video 14.1). These accessories include, but are not limited to, biliary-stone retrieval balloons, baskets, forceps, snares, and nets [3], based on availability and endoscopist preference. It should be noted that the use of these devices is widespread and non-standardized. No consensus exists on the endpoint of each ETN session, but in general all liquid debris and any easily removable devitalized tissue should be removed, revealing pink granulation tissue. Following

debridement, multiple large-bore (10 F) pigtail catheters or covered SEMS are left in the tract to hold open the fistula for continued drainage and to act as a conduit for repeat endoscopic necrosectomy sessions [59]. As with ETD, pre- and post-procedure antibiotics are generally given for this procedure [23]. CO_2 should be used for endoscopic insufflation to reduce the risk of air embolism or pneumoperitoneum. If pneumoperitoneum develops in the absence of true soiling of the abdominal cavity, it can usually be managed conservatively [3, 60].

The optimal timing of ETN, the ideal interval between treatment sessions, optimal tract size, and procedure end points have not been definitively established. These decisions should be based on patient's clinical course, the indication for intervention, and endoscopist expertise and preference. In general, a "step-up" method of delaying ETN until after ETD is recommended [3]. ETN may be repeated either as clinically indicated or on an interval basis, with 3–6 sessions typically required for complete debridement [14]. Serial abdominal CT scans can be used to monitor necrosis resolution. After complete resolution, transmural stents may be removed endoscopically.

Procedure Complications

Endoscopic treatment of WON represents a high-risk procedure. Complication rates for endotherapy for WON vary between 10 and 37 % [13, 52]. Complications of ETN range from 14 to 77 % [58], and include bleeding, perforation, pancreatitis, aspiration, infection of sterile undrained necrosis, pancreatic fistula formation, stent migration/occlusion, and rarely air embolism. The most common complication is bleeding, which occurs in about 18 % of patients [12, 58]. Bleeding may be managed endoscopically in most cases; however it can be severe due to injury to large vessels that may traverse the cavity. Achieving hemostasis in such patients can be difficult and may warrant emergent surgical or interventional radiology intervention [58]. Mean mortality is low at 6 % [58].

Combined Approaches

Most patients with pancreatic fluid collections (over 80 %) will be successfully treated with endotherapy alone [58]. For cases where endoscopic management is not technically feasible, or for patients who fail to respond to endoscopic treatment, minimally invasive retroperitoneal necrosectomy, sinus tract endoscopy using a flexible endoscope, or VARD may be performed [3]. Early aggressive adjuvant therapy should also be performed, in addition to endoscopic treatment, in cases with extensive necrotic debris or deep retroperitoneal extension [3, 61].

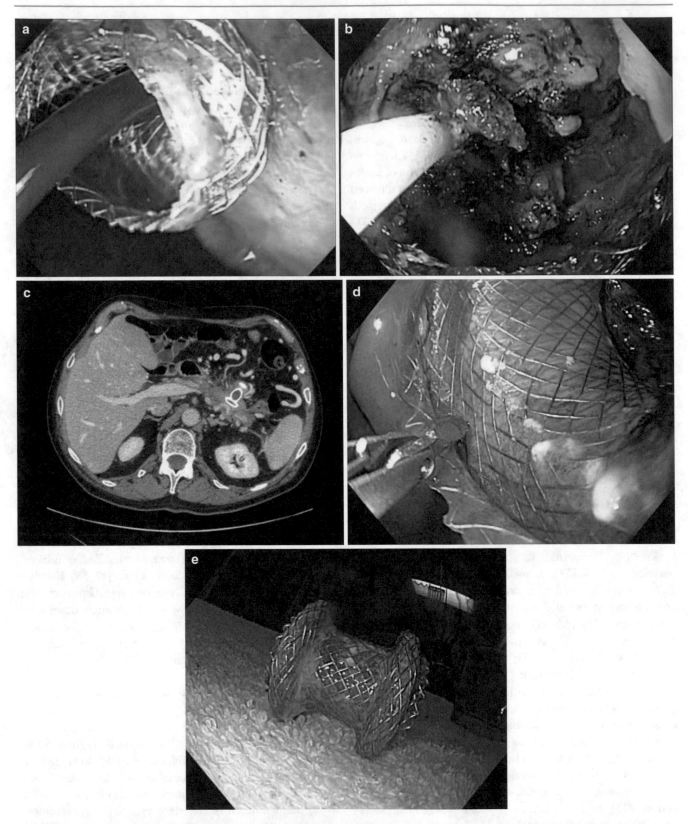

Fig. 14.4 Endoscopic necrosectomy through a metal stent. This procedure was performed in the patient previously shown in Fig. 14.1d. (**a**) Endoscopic view of a lumen-apposing self-expanding metal stent (LASEMS) in a patient with pancreatic necrosis at the time of deployment. Note jet of cyst fluid draining into stomach. (**b**) Endoscopic necrosectomy performed 1 week later. Note removal of necrotic tissue with a snare. (**c**) CT scan image of same patient after three endoscopic necrosectomy treatments. The necrotic cavity has been completely debrided as has resolved. Note that the LASEMS is still in place. (**d**) Removal of LASEMS. The stent is grasped with a rat-tooth forceps. (**e**) LASEMS ex vivo after removal (images courtesy Douglas G Adler MD)

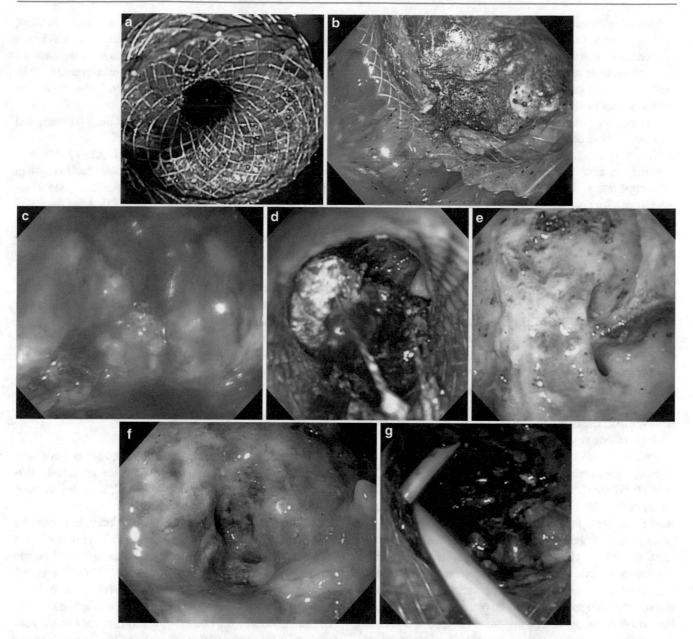

Fig. 14.5 Endoscopic necrosectomy progression. (**a**) Transmural placement of an AXIOS LASEMS stent placed across a cystenterostomy. (**b**) LASEMS appearance 1 week later. Note necrotic debris in stent lumen. (**c**) Necrotic debris in stent lumen is cleared and the endoscope is advanced into the cyst cavity. Necrotic contents are seen. (**d**) Removal of solid necrotic debris with biliary stone retrieval basket. (**e**) Cyst cavity containing purulent solid debris and pink granulation tissue after one session of endoscopic necrosectomy. (**f**) Cyst cavity containing healthy pink granulation tissue after several sessions of ETN. (**g**) Double-pigtail stent catheter placed through AXIOS stent following ETN to promote drainage prior to final stent removal

Primary percutaneous catheter drainage sometimes results in the development of internal and external pancreatic fistulas [46]. However, a hybrid technique of combined percutaneous drainage and ETD prevents the formation of pancreatic-cutaneous fistulas, in addition to hastening WON resolution [62–64]. A hybrid technique of combined endoscopic necrosectomy via large-bore self-expandable metal stents placed through percutaneous tracts has also been described and may be beneficial in select patients [59, 65].

New Devices for Therapy of PFCs

Forward-Viewing Echoendoscope

Current therapeutic echoendoscopes are oblique-viewing with endoscopic accessories deployed at a 45° angle, which can limit visualization and technical success of needle puncture and stent placement. A novel forward-viewing echoendoscope (Olympus Medical Systems, Center Valley, PA) offers a perpendicular approach, allowing transition from endoscopic to ultrasonographic view without reorientation and easier passage of accessories due to its relatively straight tip [66]. Although it lacks an elevator and its scanning range is only 90° (versus 180° for a linear echoendoscope), tip angulation may be performed for up to 180°. A prospective multicenter randomized trial comparing EUS-guided drainage with oblique- versus forward-viewing echoendoscopes reported similar procedure ease, complications, and clinical success rates. While the time to initial puncture was longer with the forward-viewing echoendoscope due to a smaller scanning range, the time to stent placement after puncture was shorter [67]. This device has not been released to widespread commercial availability.

Advances in Stents

PFC drainage was traditionally performed using two double-pigtail plastic stents, and this is still widely performed. The use of larger biliary fully covered self-expanding metal stents (FCSEMS) for transenteric drainage of PFCs is safe and effective but these stents are often too narrow to facilitate endoscope passage for direct endoscopic necrosectomy [68]. Larger diameter esophageal FCSEMS may be successfully used [3, 69, 70]; however their use is limited by the risk of stent migration and inadequate tissue apposition. Newer LASEMS with anti-migration features have been specifically designed for improved PFC drainage and cavity access, including the Nagi stent (TaeWoong Medical Co, Gyeonggi-do, South Korea), the Aixstent (Leufen Medical, Aachen, Germany), BCF Hanaro stent (M.I. Tech, Seoul, South Korea), and the AXIOS stent (Xlumena, Mountain View, California). These fully covered metal stents have a diameter of 10–15 mm and are available in a variety of lengths. Wide flares at both ends help to anchor the stent and prevent migration while providing good tissue apposition. Double-pigtail stents may be placed through these metal stents to theoretically reduce migration rates, but it is unclear if they are truly needed with these devices. Metal stents cost significantly more than plastic stents but provide a much greater tract diameter for drainage and endoscopic necrosectomy [71].

Combination Devices

While the endoscopic management of PFCs requires multiple steps, devices, and exchanges for cyst access and stent placement, the development of new combination devices has reduced the complexity and duration of this procedure. The Cystotome (Cook, Winston-Salem, NC) is a through-the-scope device made of an inner 5 F retractable needle-knife catheter and an outer 10 F sheath with a distal metal cauterizing diathermic ring. A needle-knife is used to make the initial incision after which an electrocautery ring on the outer sheath allows immediate tract enlargement. After the needle-knife is withdrawn, a guidewire is placed into the PFC for access [66, 72].

The NAVIX access device (Xlumena Inc, Mountain View, California) consists of a 19-gauge trocar with a 3.5 mm extendable "switchblade" knife, an 8 mm anchoring balloon, a 10 mm dilation balloon, and two guidewire ports [15, 66]. The trocar is used to make an initial incision, while the "switchblade" knife creates an enterostomy at the initial puncture site. An anchoring balloon, dilating balloon, and guidewires are then advanced into the cyst.

The Giovannini Needle Wire system (Cook, Winston-Salem, NC) is an effective all-in-one stent introduction system consisting of a needle-wire, a 5.5 F dilator catheter, and a pre-loaded straight plastic 8.5 F or 10 F stent [5]. After the 0.035 needle-wire is introduced into the PFC under EUS guidance using cutting current, the rigid internal portion of the needle-wire is then removed, allowing the wire to curl in the collection into stabilizing loops. A guiding and dilation catheter and straight plastic stent are then placed over wire [73].

Recently, a "Hot AXIOS System" (Xlumena, Mountain View, California) has been developed that combines a cautery-enabled access catheter with a pre-loaded therapeutic AXIOS stent for an exchange-free procedure that, in theory, does not even require the use of a guidewire.

Accessories

A variety of endoscopic tools may be used for debridement during direct endoscopic necrosectomy as previously discussed. Several case reports and small case series have described novel methods of debridement.

Irrigation with hydrogen peroxide may facilitate debris dislodgement and extraction of necrotic tissue, but noted adverse events including pneumoperitoneum, bacteremia, and gastric perforation in 28 % of patients in one study [74]. The use of endoscopic vacuum-assisted therapy (EVAT) for an infected pseudocyst has also been described using an Endo-SPONGE (B. Braun, Melsungen, Germany) that is inserted into the cavity after DEN for several days of suction [75]. The endoscopic submucosal dissection (ESD) device Clutch Cutter (Fujifilm, Tokyo, Japan) has been proposed as a method to grasp and dissect necrotic tissue into pieces using an electrosurgical current and may help to achieve hemostasis when needed [76].

Conclusion

Patients with symptomatic pancreatic fluid collection represent high-risk cohorts who are often in need of endoscopic drainage procedures. Pseudocysts and walled-off necrosis can be treated endoscopically in most cases. Transpapillary and transmural techniques to drain pancreatic fluid collections exist and can be used alone or in combination. Endoscopic drainage of pancreatic fluid collections is an area of active research and development, and we can expect continued development in this area to be ongoing.

Video Legend

Video 14.1 The accompanying video demonstrates Dr. Adler performing an endoscopic transluminal necrosectomy using a lumen-apposing stent (WMV 59561 kb).

References

1. Banks PA, Bollen TL, Dervenis C, Gooszen HG, Johnson CD, Sarr MG, et al. Classification of acute pancreatitis—2012: revision of the Atlanta classification and definitions by international consensus. Gut. 2013;62(1):102–11.
2. Takahashi N, Papachristou GI, Schmit GD, Chahal P, LeRoy AJ, Sarr MG, et al. CT findings of walled-off pancreatic necrosis (WOPN): differentiation from pseudocyst and prediction of outcome after endoscopic therapy. Eur Radiol. 2008;18(11):2522–9.
3. Trikudanathan G, Attam R, Arain MA, Mallery S, Freeman ML. Endoscopic interventions for necrotizing pancreatitis. Am J Gastroenterol. 2014;109(7):969–81. quiz 82.
4. Working Group IAPAPAAPG. IAP/APA evidence-based guidelines for the management of acute pancreatitis. Pancreatology. 2013;13(4 Suppl 2):e1–15.
5. Braden B, Dietrich CF. Endoscopic ultrasonography-guided endoscopic treatment of pancreatic pseudocysts and walled-off necrosis: new technical developments. World J Gastroenterol. 2014;20(43):16191–6.
6. Jacobson BC, Baron TH, Adler DG, Davila RE, Egan J, Hirota WK, et al. ASGE guideline: the role of endoscopy in the diagnosis and the management of cystic lesions and inflammatory fluid collections of the pancreas. Gastrointest Endosc. 2005;61(3):363–70.
7. Cheruvu CV, Clarke MG, Prentice M, Eyre-Brook IA. Conservative treatment as an option in the management of pancreatic pseudocyst. Ann R Coll Surg Engl. 2003;85(5):313–6.
8. Barthet M, Bugallo M, Moreira LS, Bastid C, Sastre B, Sahel J. Management of cysts and pseudocysts complicating chronic pancreatitis. A retrospective study of 143 patients. Gastroenterol Clin Biol. 1993;17(4):270–6.
9. Cui ML, Kim KH, Kim HG, Han J, Kim H, Cho KB, et al. Incidence, risk factors and clinical course of pancreatic fluid collections in acute pancreatitis. Dig Dis Sci. 2014;59(5):1055–62.
10. Kim KO, Kim TN. Acute pancreatic pseudocyst: incidence, risk factors, and clinical outcomes. Pancreas. 2012;41(4):577–81.
11. van Santvoort HC, Bakker OJ, Bollen TL, Besselink MG, Ahmed Ali U, Schrijver AM, et al. A conservative and minimally invasive approach to necrotizing pancreatitis improves outcome. Gastroenterology. 2011;141(4):1254–63.
12. Gardner TB, Coelho-Prabhu N, Gordon SR, Gelrud A, Maple JT, Papachristou GI, et al. Direct endoscopic necrosectomy for the treatment of walled-off pancreatic necrosis: results from a multicenter U.S. series. Gastrointest Endosc. 2011;73(4):718–26.
13. Baron TH, Harewood GC, Morgan DE, Yates MR. Outcome differences after endoscopic drainage of pancreatic necrosis, acute pancreatic pseudocysts, and chronic pancreatic pseudocysts. Gastrointest Endosc. 2002;56(1):7–17.
14. Freeman ML, Werner J, van Santvoort HC, Baron TH, Besselink MG, Windsor JA, et al. Interventions for necrotizing pancreatitis: summary of a multidisciplinary consensus conference. Pancreas. 2012;41(8):1176–94.
15. Gardner TB. Endoscopic management of necrotizing pancreatitis. Gastrointest Endosc. 2012;76(6):1214–23.
16. Chauhan SS, Forsmark CE. Evidence-based treatment of pancreatic pseudocysts. Gastroenterology. 2013;145(3):511–3.
17. Varadarajulu S, Bang JY, Sutton BS, Trevino JM, Christein JD, Wilcox CM. Equal efficacy of endoscopic and surgical cystogastrostomy for pancreatic pseudocyst drainage in a randomized trial. Gastroenterology. 2013;145(3):583–90. e1.

18. Varadarajulu S, Bang JY, Phadnis MA, Christein JD, Wilcox CM. Endoscopic transmural drainage of peripancreatic fluid collections: outcomes and predictors of treatment success in 211 consecutive patients. J Gastrointest Surg. 2011;15(11):2080–8.
19. Akshintala VS, Saxena P, Zaheer A, Rana U, Hutfless SM, Lennon AM, et al. A comparative evaluation of outcomes of endoscopic versus percutaneous drainage for symptomatic pancreatic pseudocysts. Gastrointest Endosc. 2014;79(6):921–8. quiz 83 e2, 83 e5.
20. Hariri M, Slivka A, Carr-Locke DL, Banks PA. Pseudocyst drainage predisposes to infection when pancreatic necrosis is unrecognized. Am J Gastroenterol. 1994;89(10):1781–4.
21. Monkemuller KE, Baron TH, Morgan DE. Transmural drainage of pancreatic fluid collections without electrocautery using the Seldinger technique. Gastrointest Endosc. 1998;48(2):195–200.
22. Yusuf TE, Baron TH. Endoscopic transmural drainage of pancreatic pseudocysts: results of a national and an international survey of ASGE members. Gastrointest Endosc. 2006;63(2):223–7.
23. Committee ASoP, Khashab MA, Chithadi KV, Acosta RD, Bruining DH, Chandrasekhara V, et al. Antibiotic prophylaxis for GI endoscopy. Gastrointest Endosc. 2015;81(1):81–9.
24. Arvanitakis M, Delhaye M, Bali MA, Matos C, De Maertelaer V, Le Moine O, et al. Pancreatic-fluid collections: a randomized controlled trial regarding stent removal after endoscopic transmural drainage. Gastrointest Endosc. 2007;65(4):609–19.
25. Holt BA, Varadarajulu S. EUS-guided drainage: beware of the pancreatic fluid collection (with videos). Gastrointest Endosc. 2014;80(6):1199–202.
26. Varadarajulu S, Wilcox CM, Tamhane A, Eloubeidi MA, Blakely J, Canon CL. Role of EUS in drainage of peripancreatic fluid collections not amenable for endoscopic transmural drainage. Gastrointest Endosc. 2007;66(6):1107–19.
27. Panamonta N, Ngamruengphong S, Kijsiricharoenchai K, Nugent K, Rakvit A. Endoscopic ultrasound-guided versus conventional transmural techniques have comparable treatment outcomes in draining pancreatic pseudocysts. Eur J Gastroenterol Hepatol. 2012;24(12):1355–62.
28. Varadarajulu S, Christein JD, Tamhane A, Drelichman ER, Wilcox CM. Prospective randomized trial comparing EUS and EGD for transmural drainage of pancreatic pseudocysts (with videos). Gastrointest Endosc. 2008;68(6):1102–11.
29. Baron TH. Drainage of pancreatic fluid collections: is EUS really necessary? Gastrointest Endosc. 2007;66(6):1123–5.
30. Singhal S, Rotman SR, Gaidhane M, Kahaleh M. Pancreatic fluid collection drainage by endoscopic ultrasound: an update. Clin Endosc. 2013;46(5):506–14.
31. Adler DG, Baron TH, Davila RE, Egan J, Hirota WK, Leighton JA, et al. ASGE guideline: the role of ERCP in diseases of the biliary tract and the pancreas. Gastrointest Endosc. 2005;62(1):1–8.
32. Barthet M, Lamblin G, Gasmi M, Vitton V, Desjeux A, Grimaud JC. Clinical usefulness of a treatment algorithm for pancreatic pseudocysts. Gastrointest Endosc. 2008;67(2):245–52.
33. Varadarajulu S, Wilcox CM. Endoscopic placement of permanent indwelling transmural stents in disconnected pancreatic duct syndrome: does benefit outweigh the risks? Gastrointest Endosc. 2011;74(6):1408–12.
34. Barthet M, Sahel J, Bodiou-Bertei C, Bernard JP. Endoscopic transpapillary drainage of pancreatic pseudocysts. Gastrointest Endosc. 1995;42(3):208–13.
35. Bakker OJ, van Baal MC, van Santvoort HC, Besselink MG, Poley JW, Heisterkamp J, et al. Endoscopic transpapillary stenting or conservative treatment for pancreatic fistulas in necrotizing pancreatitis: multicenter series and literature review. Ann Surg. 2011;253(5):961–7.
36. Telford JJ, Farrell JJ, Saltzman JR, Shields SJ, Banks PA, Lichtenstein DR, et al. Pancreatic stent placement for duct disruption. Gastrointest Endosc. 2002;56(1):18–24.
37. Varadarajulu S, Noone TC, Tutuian R, Hawes RH, Cotton PB. Predictors of outcome in pancreatic duct disruption managed by endoscopic transpapillary stent placement. Gastrointest Endosc. 2005;61(4):568–75.

38. Trevino JM, Tamhane A, Varadarajulu S. Successful stenting in ductal disruption favorably impacts treatment outcomes in patients undergoing transmural drainage of peripancreatic fluid collections. J Gastroenterol Hepatol. 2010;25(3):526–31.

39. Hookey LC, Debroux S, Delhaye M, Arvanitakis M, Le Moine O, Deviere J. Endoscopic drainage of pancreatic-fluid collections in 116 patients: a comparison of etiologies, drainage techniques, and outcomes. Gastrointest Endosc. 2006;63(4):635–43.

40. Irani S, Gluck M, Ross A, Gan SI, Crane R, Brandabur JJ, et al. Resolving external pancreatic fistulas in patients with disconnected pancreatic duct syndrome: using rendezvous techniques to avoid surgery (with video). Gastrointest Endosc. 2012;76(3):586–93. e1–3.

41. Kozarek RA. Pancreatic stents can induce ductal changes consistent with chronic pancreatitis. Gastrointest Endosc. 1990;36(2):93–5.

42. D'Egidio A, Schein M. Surgical strategies in the treatment of pancreatic necrosis and infection. Br J Surg. 1991;78(2):133–7.

43. Bakker OJ, van Santvoort HC, van Brunschot S, Geskus RB, Besselink MG, Bollen TL, et al. Endoscopic transgastric vs surgical necrosectomy for infected necrotizing pancreatitis: a randomized trial. JAMA. 2012;307(10):1053–61.

44. van Santvoort HC, Besselink MG, Bakker OJ, Hofker HS, Boermeester MA, Dejong CH, et al. A step-up approach or open necrosectomy for necrotizing pancreatitis. N Engl J Med. 2010;362(16):1491–502.

45. Tong Z, Li W, Yu W, Geng Y, Ke L, Nie Y, et al. Percutaneous catheter drainage for infective pancreatic necrosis: is it always the first choice for all patients? Pancreas. 2012;41(2):302–5.

46. van Baal MC, van Santvoort HC, Bollen TL, Bakker OJ, Besselink MG, Gooszen HG, et al. Systematic review of percutaneous catheter drainage as primary treatment for necrotizing pancreatitis. Br J Surg. 2011;98(1):18–27.

47. Kumar N, Conwell DL, Thompson CC. Direct endoscopic necrosectomy versus step-up approach for walled-off pancreatic necrosis: comparison of clinical outcome and health care utilization. Pancreas. 2014;43(8):1334–9.

48. van Brunschot S, van Grinsven J, Voermans RP, Bakker OJ, Besselink MG, Boermeester MA, et al. Transluminal endoscopic step-up approach versus minimally invasive surgical step-up approach in patients with infected necrotising pancreatitis (TENSION trial): design and rationale of a randomised controlled multicenter trial [ISRCTN09186711]. BMC Gastroenterol. 2013;13:161.

49. Seewald S, Ang TL, Kida M, Teng KY, Soehendra N, Group EUSW. EUS 2008 Working Group document: evaluation of EUS-guided drainage of pancreatic-fluid collections (with video). Gastrointest Endosc. 2009;69(2 Suppl):S13–21.

50. Baron TH. Endoscopic drainage of pancreatic fluid collections and pancreatic necrosis. Gastrointest Endosc Clin N Am. 2003;13(4):743–64.

51. Gardner TB, Chahal P, Papachristou GI, Vege SS, Petersen BT, Gostout CJ, et al. A comparison of direct endoscopic necrosectomy with transmural endoscopic drainage for the treatment of walled-off pancreatic necrosis. Gastrointest Endosc. 2009;69(6):1085–94.

52. Siddiqui AA, Dewitt JM, Strongin A, Singh H, Jordan S, Loren DE, et al. Outcomes of EUS-guided drainage of debris-containing pancreatic pseudocysts by using combined endoprosthesis and a nasocystic drain. Gastrointest Endosc. 2013;78(4):589–95.

53. Baron TH, Thaggard WG, Morgan DE, Stanley RJ. Endoscopic therapy for organized pancreatic necrosis. Gastroenterology. 1996;111(3):755–64.

54. Baron TH, Morgan DE. Endoscopic transgastric irrigation tube placement via PEG for debridement of organized pancreatic necrosis. Gastrointest Endosc. 1999;50(4):574–7.

55. Varadarajulu S, Phadnis MA, Christein JD, Wilcox CM. Multiple transluminal gateway technique for EUS-guided drainage of symptomatic walled-off pancreatic necrosis. Gastrointest Endosc. 2011;74(1):74–80.

56. Mukai S, Itoi T, Sofuni A, Itokawa F, Kurihara T, Tsuchiya T, et al. Expanding endoscopic interventions for pancreatic pseudocyst and walled-off necrosis. J Gastroenterol. 2014.

57. Seifert H, Wehrmann T, Schmitt T, Zeuzem S, Caspary WF. Retroperitoneal endoscopic debridement for infected peripancreatic necrosis. Lancet. 2000;356(9230):653–5.

58. van Brunschot S, Fockens P, Bakker OJ, Besselink MG, Voermans RP, Poley JW, et al. Endoscopic transluminal necrosectomy in necrotising pancreatitis: a systematic review. Surg Endosc. 2014;28(5):1425–38.

59. Baron TH, Kozarek RA. Endotherapy for organized pancreatic necrosis: perspectives after 20 years. Clin Gastroenterol Hepatol. 2012;10(11):1202–7.

60. Seewald S, Ang TL, Teng KC, Soehendra N. EUS-guided drainage of pancreatic pseudocysts, abscesses and infected necrosis. Dig Endosc. 2009;21 Suppl 1:S61–5.

61. Papachristou GI, Takahashi N, Chahal P, Sarr MG, Baron TH. Peroral endoscopic drainage/debridement of walled-off pancreatic necrosis. Ann Surg. 2007;245(6):943–51.

62. Gluck M, Ross A, Irani S, Lin O, Hauptmann E, Siegal J, et al. Endoscopic and percutaneous drainage of symptomatic walled-off pancreatic necrosis reduces hospital stay and radiographic resources. Clin Gastroenterol Hepatol. 2010;8(12):1083–8.

63. Gluck M, Ross A, Irani S, Lin O, Gan SI, Fotoohi M, et al. Dual modality drainage for symptomatic walled-off pancreatic necrosis reduces length of hospitalization, radiological procedures, and number of endoscopies compared to standard percutaneous drainage. J Gastrointest Surg. 2012;16(2):248–56. discussion 56-7.

64. Ross AS, Irani S, Gan SI, Rocha F, Siegal J, Fotoohi M, et al. Dual-modality drainage of infected and symptomatic walled-off pancreatic necrosis: long-term clinical outcomes. Gastrointest Endosc. 2014;79(6):929–35.

65. Navarrete C, Castillo C, Caracci M, Vargas P, Gobelet J, Robles I. Wide percutaneous access to pancreatic necrosis with self-expandable stent: new application (with video). Gastrointest Endosc. 2011;73(3):609–10.

66. Committee AT, Desilets DJ, Banerjee S, Barth BA, Bhat YM, Gottlieb KT, et al. New devices and techniques for management of pancreatic fluid collections. Gastrointest Endosc. 2013;77(6):835–8.

67. Voermans RP, Ponchon T, Schumacher B, Fumex F, Bergman JJ, Larghi A, et al. Forward-viewing versus oblique-viewing echoendoscopes in transluminal drainage of pancreatic fluid collections: a multicenter, randomized, controlled trial. Gastrointest Endosc. 2011;74(6):1285–93.

68. Talreja JP, Shami VM, Ku J, Morris TD, Ellen K, Kahaleh M. Transenteric drainage of pancreatic-fluid collections with fully covered self-expanding metallic stents (with video). Gastrointest Endosc. 2008;68(6):1199–203.

69. Antillon MR, Bechtold ML, Bartalos CR, Marshall JB. Transgastric endoscopic necrosectomy with temporary metallic esophageal stent placement for the treatment of infected pancreatic necrosis (with video). Gastrointest Endosc. 2009;69(1):178–80.

70. Sarkaria S, Sethi A, Rondon C, Lieberman M, Srinivasan I, Weaver K, et al. Pancreatic necrosectomy using covered esophageal stents: a novel approach. J Clin Gastroenterol. 2014;48(2):145–52.

71. Bang JY, Hawes R, Bartolucci A, Varadarajulu S. Efficacy of metal and plastic stents for transmural drainage of pancreatic fluid collections: A systematic review. Dig Endosc. 2015;7(4):486–98.

72. Ahlawat SK, Charabaty-Pishvaian A, Jackson PG, Haddad NG. Single-step EUS-guided pancreatic pseudocyst drainage using a large channel linear array echoendoscope and cystotome: results in 11 patients. JOP. 2006;7(6):616–24.

73. Kruger M, Schneider AS, Manns MP, Meier PN. Endoscopic management of pancreatic pseudocysts or abscesses after an EUS-guided 1-step procedure for initial access. Gastrointest Endosc. 2006;63(3):409–16.

74. Siddiqui AA, Easler J, Strongin A, Slivka A, Kowalski TE, Muddana V, et al. Hydrogen peroxide-assisted endoscopic necrosectomy for walled-off pancreatic necrosis: a dual center pilot experience. Dig Dis Sci. 2014;59(3):687–90.

75. Wallstabe I, Tiedemann A, Schiefke I. Endoscopic vacuum-assisted therapy of an infected pancreatic pseudocyst. Endoscopy. 2011;43 Suppl 2 UCTN:E312-3.

76. Aso A, Igarashi H, Matsui N, Ihara E, Takaoka T, Osoegawa T, et al. Large area of walled-off pancreatic necrosis successfully treated by endoscopic necrosectomy using a grasping-type scissors forceps. Dig Endosc. 2014;26(3):474–7.

EUS for Pain Control in Chronic Pancreatitis and Pancreatic Cancer

Alexander Lee and Linda S. Lee

Introduction

Chronic abdominal pain is a major component of the morbidity associated with both chronic pancreatitis and pancreatic cancer [1, 2]. Pain can have a significantly detrimental effect on a patient's quality of life, as the pain associated with both of these conditions is often debilitating and may require repeated office and emergency room visits, procedures, and hospitalizations. Particularly in the case of chronic pancreatitis, in which the pain's impact on quality of life endures for many years, the physical, emotional, and financial toll is considerable. A 2014 study estimated that pain due to chronic pancreatitis incurs greater than $600 million in yearly costs [3].

The primary nerve pathway for "pancreatic pain" is the celiac plexus, colloquially referred to as the solar plexus. It is located below and anterior to the diaphragm (anterocrural) in the retroperitoneum, surrounding the celiac trunk at its origin from the aorta. The celiac plexus is comprised of a network of nerve fibers and ganglia including sympathetic fibers (from the greater, lesser, and least splanchnic nerves), parasympathetic fibers from the vagus nerve, and the celiac ganglia at T12–L2 (Fig. 15.1) [4–6]. While the molecular pathophysiology of pancreatic pain—the role of specific neurotransmitters, the relationship between inflammation and nociception, and the drivers of inflammation—is incompletely understood, it is accepted that efferent nerves from the pancreas carry nociceptive signals and travel with the sympathetic chain via the celiac plexus to the brain, wherein the information is perceived as pain [7, 8].

The initial approach to treatment of pain in both pancreatic cancer and chronic pancreatitis is usually analgesic medications, with titration of dosing as needing; however, the use of analgesic medications is often a suboptimal long-term strategy. Non-opioids can have inadequate effect (and are not free of risks), while opioids can cause somnolence, constipation, nausea, and other adverse effects. Opioid medications become even more troublesome as tolerance develops, creating a vicious cycle of ever-increasing opioid requirements and worsening adverse effects [1, 9]. In addition, many patients with chronic pancreatitis have baseline substance abuse issues, and adding chronic opioid medication to this mix can further complicate an already difficult situation.

Given the limitations of analgesic medications, interest in non-pharmacologic treatment for pain relief has led to development of targeted delivery of analgesic/and or cytotoxic agents to the retrogastric space to prevent transmission of pain signals by the celiac plexus, whether for short-term relief (via celiac plexus block (CPB)) or long-term relief (via celiac plexus neurolysis (CPN)). Initially, CPB and CPN were performed by a radiologist (guided by ultrasound, computed tomography, or fluoroscopy), an anesthesiologist, or a surgeon by percutaneous or even open approaches [7, 10]. However, with the rise of endoscopic ultrasound (EUS) in gastroenterology, EUS-guided CPB and CPN have become a commonly performed modality for pain control in pancreatic cancer and chronic pancreatitis.

In this chapter, we provide a comprehensive review of EUS-guided CPB and CPN for pain control in pancreatic cancer and chronic pancreatitis. First, we review the technical aspects of this modality. Second, we examine the data evaluating its efficacy. Third, we highlight the side effects and potential complications. Finally, we examine the newer developments in the technique.

Electronic supplementary material: The online version of this chapter (doi:10.1007/978-3-319-26854-5_15) contains supplementary material, which is available to authorized users. Videos can also be accessed at http://link.springer.com/chapter/10.1007/978-3-319-26854-5_15.

A. Lee, M.D. (✉) • L.S. Lee, M.D.
Division of Gastroenterology, Hepatology and Endoscopy, Brigham and Women's Hospital, Boston, MA, USA
e-mail: alexlee23@gmail.com

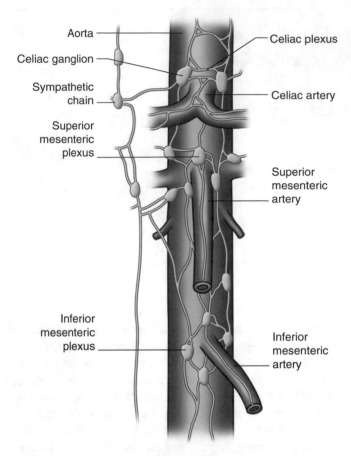

Aorta

Celiac ganglion

Sympathetic
chain

Superior
mesenteric
plexus

Celiac plexus

Celiac artery

Superior
mesenteric
artery

Inferior
mesenteric
plexus

Inferior
mesenteric
artery

Fig. 15.1 Schematic of major abdominal nerve plexuses. Note each of the three major plexuses (celiac, superior mesenteric, inferior mesenteric) in proximity to the corresponding major artery at its origin from the aorta

Traditional Approach to CPB and CPN

Percutaneous CPB/CPN was first described in 1914 and utilizes a percutaneous retrocrural approach [11]. With the patient in prone position, needle puncture is performed near the level of T12 at a 45° angle, bony contact is made between needle and vertebra, needle angle is adjusted, and access to the area at or near the celiac ganglia is judged using tactile cues, directing injection of medication. Usually, the injected solution diffuses over the splanchnic nerves to accomplish celiac plexus block/neurolysis. The procedure was classically performed twice, once into the right and left sides of the vertebral column, respectively. The technique for CPB and CPN is identical, with the only difference being the substances injected—analgesic (typically bupivacaine) followed by steroid or alcohol for CPB or CPN, respectively [7, 11]. As a cytotoxic drug intended to ablate the targeted nerve cells, alcohol functions as the "neurolytic" agent in celiac

plexus neurolysis; by contrast, injected steroid functions as a more temporary "blocking" agent in celiac plexus block, providing effect that is shorter term and does not incur irreversible cell injury [6, 10].

The conceptual foundations of the traditional CPB/CPN technique have remained largely unchanged; modifications have included differing points of percutaneous entry (transaortic, paramedian, transdiscal, anterior) as well as the addition of radiographic guidance (ultrasound, computed tomography, fluoroscopy) (Fig. 15.2) [12]. Potential complications with the percutaneous approach are associated with needle entry and include bleeding, pneumothorax, inadvertent visceral puncture (primarily kidneys), and, rarely, paraplegia (related to injury to the artery of Adamkiewicz), and infection [13].

Technique of EUS-Guided CPB and CPN

The principle driving the introduction of EUS-guided CPB/CPN in the early 2000s was the ability of EUS to guide needle injection into the retrogastric space with an *anterior* approach that theoretically should enhance both the precision and safety of needle visualization, passage, and injection. This requires traversal of fewer nearby structures (compared to the posterior/retrocrural approach) and thereby potentially decreases complications while possibly increasing analgesic effect [14, 15]. In addition, many patients in this population undergo EUS for diagnostic purposes, especially for pancreatic cancer, and as such there is opportunity to administer this therapy without needing additional invasive procedures and additional sedation/anesthesia (i.e., a diagnostic EUS can become a therapeutic EUS if chronic pancreatitis is diagnosed and injection is performed in the same session).

In preparation for the procedure, the patient's history and physical examination are reviewed in the usual manner, with special attention paid to use of anticoagulant medications, allergies to amino-amide anesthetics (including bupivacaine), and/or comorbidities. The primary contraindications to the procedure include coagulopathy, thrombocytopenia, and hemodynamic/respiratory instability. Technical feasibility can also be affected by prior abdominal surgery, a large tumor mass, or atypical vascular anatomy, as these factors can limit visualization of the celiac plexus [10]. Gastroenterologist-administered conscious sedation is generally sufficient to complete EUS with CPB/CPN. However, the chronic pain and associated opiate use in this patient population may necessitate the assistance of an anesthesiologist. Informed consent should be obtained with attention paid to complications specifically associated with CPB/CPN

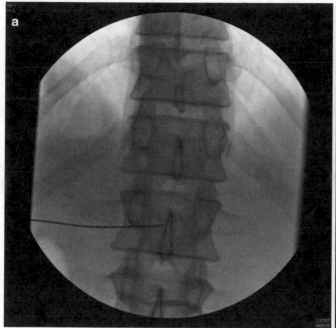 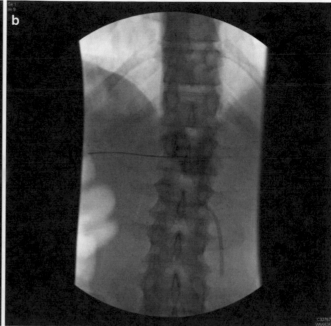

Fig. 15.2 Percutaneous celiac plexus neurolysis. (**a**) Advancement of percutaneous needle under fluoroscopic guidance. (**b**) Injection of a solution containing contrast media and alcohol in the area of the celiac plexus. Previously placed plastic pancreatic duct stent is seen at the lower right area of the image

(described later in this chapter). Some centers prophylactically administer 1 L of isotonic intravenous fluid to minimize the risk of post-CPB/CPN hypotension, but this practice is not standardized [6, 13, 16].

As with the percutaneous approach, the only differentiating factor between CPB and CPN is the choice of injected solution, and it should be prepared in advance before initiating the procedure. For pain relief in pancreatic cancer, CPN is generally the preferred approach and typically requires a solution containing 10–20 mL of 0.25 % bupivacaine plus 5–10 mL of 98 % dehydrated alcohol, although different centers have different preparations for CPN. For pain relief in chronic pancreatitis, CPB is most commonly used with a typical solution containing 10–20 mL of 0.25 % bupivacaine plus a steroid, typically 5–10 mL of triamcinolone (40 mg/mL). Again, institutional protocols vary. CPN for chronic pancreatitis remains controversial, but some centers administer a combined solution of dehydrated alcohol and steroid along with bupivacaine to provide theoretically longer duration of effect [6, 15, 17].

Procedurally, the linear echoendoscope is advanced to the posterior lesser curve of the stomach. As the area is approached, the aorta is visualized and followed inferiorly to the origin of the celiac artery, the first major subdiaphragmatic vessel taking off from the aorta (Fig. 15.3, Video 15.1). Generally, the area directly adjacent and anterior to the celiac takeoff is used as the injection target. However, with careful inspection and slight rotational movements, it is often, but not always, possible to directly visualize the celiac ganglia for targeting [6]. A fine-needle aspiration (FNA) needle is then usually deployed; at some centers, a 20-gauge "spray" needle is used which has multiple side holes, allowing the injected solution to spread potentially over a larger area [6, 18]. No needle has been accepted as ideal, and the choice of needle size and type is left to the operator.

After priming with saline to remove air within the needle and checking the needle path with color Doppler, the needle tip is positioned anterior and cephalad to the celiac takeoff. Once the needle is in position, aspiration is first performed to make sure that blood vessel penetration has not occurred. Injection is then performed, with one of the two strategies: (a) injection of the entire solution into the area cephalad to the celiac trunk, or (b) injection into the right and left sides of the celiac artery [16, 19]. An echogenic cloud is often seen in the injected area. Prior to withdrawal, the needle is flushed with at least 3 mL of saline, as alcohol in the needle that is left behind in soft tissue during withdrawal may lead to post-procedure pain. Following completion of the procedure, the patient should be monitored until stable for discharge; at some centers monitored vital signs include supine and erect blood pressures to rule out orthostasis, although this is not mandatory [20–22].

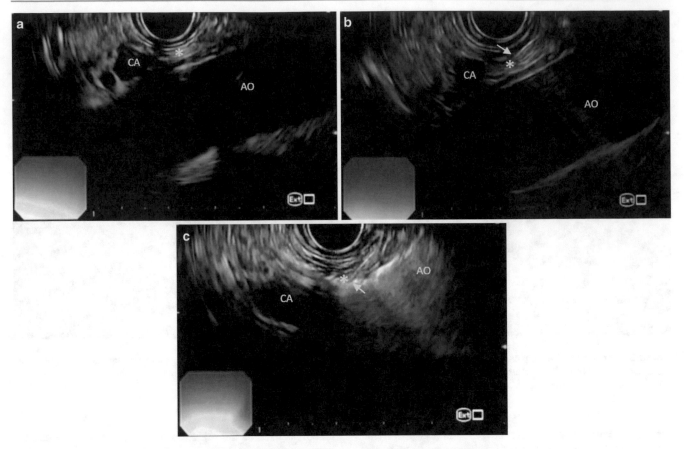

Fig. 15.3 EUS-guided celiac plexus neurolysis. AO, aorta. CA, celiac artery. (**a**) The celiac trunk is visualized at its takeoff from the aorta. The area of the celiac plexus (*yellow asterisk*) is anterior to the celiac trunk. (**b**) The fine-needle aspiration needle is advanced, with the needle tip (*yellow arrow*) positioned in the area of the celiac plexus. Shadowing artifact from the needle is noted in the area of the aorta. (**c**) As injection is performed, the injected alcohol creates an echogenic cloud and additional shadowing artifact

Efficacy of EUS-Guided CPN for Pancreatic Cancer Pain

Wiersema and Wiersema (1996) published one of the earliest series of patients undergoing EUS-guided CPN for cancer pain; this included 30 patients with pain and intra-abdominal malignancy (25 with pancreatic cancer) who underwent EUS-guided CPN using a prototype needle catheter. Over a median follow-up of 10 weeks, 82–91 % required the same or less pain medication and 79–88 % had consistently reduced pain [15]. The first prospective study utilized a cohort of 58 patients with unresectable pancreatic cancer who underwent EUS-guided CPN. Pain scores experienced sustained improvement over the 24-week study period in 78 % of patients; of note, chemotherapy and radiation therapy likely contributed to improvements in pain as well [23].

In a meta-analysis including eight studies of 283 patients with pancreatic cancer, 80 % demonstrated improvement in pain with EUS-guided CPN [24]. A separate meta-analysis of five studies with 119 patients experiencing pancreatic cancer pain noted that EUS-guided CPN alleviated abdominal pain in 73 % of patients [25]. A large study specifically investigating the early use of EUS-guided CPN in pancreatic cancer management included 580 patients who underwent diagnostic EUS, among which 96 patients with confirmed inoperable pancreatic cancer and chronic pain were randomized to early EUS-guided CPN versus conventional pain management. At 3 months, the CPN group reported greater pain relief than the conventional group (mean change in pain score of −60.7 ($P=0.01$)) and trended towards lower opioid consumption, with no difference in quality of life or survival [26]. Similarly, other studies on EUS-guided CPN in pancreatic cancer have shown significant impact on pain, but none have demonstrated an impact on survival as CPN is not a cancer treatment and does not affect underlying disease progression [19, 27].

Although impact on quality of life is uncertain and survival is unaffected, use of EUS-guided CPN in the overall approach to pancreatic cancer pain has been well accepted. Factors predictive of lack of response include (1) direct invasion of the celiac plexus by tumor and (2) injection of only the left side of the celiac artery, according to a multivariate analysis of 47 consecutive patients undergoing EUS-guided CPN for pain associated with upper abdominal cancer [28].

The issue of multiple injection sites has been the subject of significant scrutiny and remains controversial. In a nonrandomized study of 160 consecutive patients who underwent central versus bilateral injection in the area of the celiac trunk, bilateral injection was the only predictor of pain reduction on post-procedure day seven [29]. By contrast, a randomized prospective trial showed no difference in pain relief, safety, or survival between groups receiving a central injection versus bilateral injections during EUS-guided CPN [19].

No large trials have compared EUS-guided CPN to percutaneous CPN for pancreatic cancer pain. However, the preponderance of data regarding CPN for pain relief in pancreatic cancer is based on the percutaneous technique, with efficacy demonstrated to be comparable to the EUS-guided approach. A 1995 meta-analysis of 24 studies including 1124 patients undergoing percutaneous CPN for cancer pain (63 % with pancreatic cancer) demonstrated good-to-excellent pain relief in 89 % within the first 2 weeks and partial-to-complete pain relief in 70–90 % until death; there were no survival differences [30]. A meta-analysis including both percutaneous and intraoperative approaches for CPN demonstrated that among 302 patients in five randomized clinical trials, CPN was associated with decreased pain, opioid usage, and constipation over 8 weeks compared to analgesics alone [14]. A Cochrane systematic review in 2011 of randomized trials also noted significant improvement in pancreatic cancer pain in 358 patients at 4 weeks and 8 weeks posttreatment with the percutaneous or EUS-guided approach [31]. Thus, while some variation in efficacy is reported, overall both percutaneous and EUS-guided CPN are associated with favorable results, and the EUS-guided approach appears at least as effective as its percutaneous counterpart.

Efficacy of EUS-Guided CPB for Chronic Pancreatitis Pain

EUS-guided CPB has also shown efficacy for pain associated with chronic pancreatitis. However, the duration of effect and degree of analgesia is less than that seen in EUS-guided CPN in patients with pancreatic cancer pain, and the role of CPB in the overall management of chronic pancreatitis is not as well defined. One of the largest studies of EUS-guided CPB prospectively evaluated 90 patients with documented ERCP and EUS evidence of chronic pancreatitis and with chronic abdominal pain unresponsive to pharmacologic treatment. Significant pain improvement was seen in 55 % of patients with sustained improvement in 26 % beyond 12 weeks and in 10 % beyond 24 weeks [17]. In a

2010 meta-analysis including 221 patients from six studies who had severe pain from chronic pancreatitis and underwent EUS-guided CPB, pain relief was reported in 51 % of patients [25]. One study comparing unilateral versus bilateral injections for EUS-guided CPB in chronic pancreatitis showed no difference in analgesia, with a median duration of effect of 28 days [19]. Factors predicting efficacy of EUS-guided CPB in chronic pancreatitis patients include older age (greater than 45 years) and no prior history of surgery for chronic pancreatitis [17].

A few studies have compared the traditional percutaneous approach to EUS-guided CPB for chronic pancreatitis pain. One small randomized study of 18 patients demonstrated 30 % with persistent pain relief 24 weeks post-EUS-guided CPB compared with 12 % pain relief 12 weeks post-CT-guided CPB [32]. A more recent and larger randomized prospective trial included an EUS-guided CPB group of 27 patients and a fluoroscopy-guided CPB group of 29 patients; visual analog scale comparisons showed pain improvement in 70 % versus 30 %, respectively ($P=0.044$) [33]. While these studies suffer from relatively small sample sizes and single-center assessments, EUS-guided CPB appears at least equivalent, if not superior, to percutaneous CPB.

The role and cost-effectiveness of EUS-guided CPB in chronic pancreatitis remain an area of ongoing study. Studies with rigorous long-term follow-up over years are lacking. The severity of clinical manifestations (i.e., pain) of chronic pancreatitis does not correlate with its associated radiologic findings, and this makes the decision to pursue EUS-guided CPB difficult to standardize [34–36]. While EUS-guided CPB may not be a first-line approach early in the course of chronic pancreatitis, it remains an option worth consideration when pain has been difficult to manage medically.

Complications of EUS-Guided CPN/CPB

Disruption of signal transmission through injection of the celiac plexus not only reduces pain signals from the pancreas but also blocks sympathetic tone in a diffuse manner. Due to relatively unopposed visceral parasympathetic activity, such sympathetic blockade can manifest as diarrhea and hypotension, and indeed these side effects occur in up to 38 % and 44 %, respectively, although many of these side effects are mild or transient (Table 15.1) [20, 30]. Patients at some centers receive pre- and post-procedural intravenous hydration to help prevent hypotension and orthostasis, and they should be advised of these potential adverse effects, which are self-limited and generally resolve within a few days.

Following CPN/CPB, some patients may experience a temporary increase in abdominal pain, presumably secondary to the trauma of needle access to the celiac plexus, pancreatitis, and/or nerve cell damage and death in those

Table 15.1 Complications of EUS-guided CPN/CPB

Uncommon (5–40 %)	Rare (<1 %)	Very rare (<0.1 %)
Diarrhea (transient)	Infection/abscess	Lower extremity paralysis
Hypotension (transient)	Hemorrhage	Death
Abdominal pain (transient)	Gastroparesis	
	Pneumothorax	

Percentages are approximate ranges of complication rates as reported in the literature

undergoing CPN. In a series of 58 patients undergoing EUS-guided CPN for pancreatic cancer pain, five patients (9 %) experienced transient increased abdominal pain lasting less than 48 h [23]. A larger study of 189 patients undergoing EUS-guided CPN or CPB reported only two patients (1 %) with severe post-procedure pain [22]. Other studies have reported rates of post-procedure pain within this range [17, 37, 38].

Serious complications with EUS-guided injection of the celiac plexus are rare. Infections such as intra-abdominal abscess occur in less than 1 % of cases [20, 22]. One series of 90 patients reported one case of peri-pancreatic abscess [17]. The authors hypothesized that proton pump inhibitor use and small intestinal bacterial overgrowth may have predisposed to infection, leading to the suggestion of peri-procedure antibiotics in patients on proton pump inhibitor undergoing CPB although such practice is not currently standard of care. Infections may be less common with alcohol injection, owing to the bactericidal properties of alcohol. Other serious complications such as significant hemorrhage, persistent diarrhea, and gastroparesis are rare, occurring at an aggregate rate of 1 % of cases [22, 39]. Due to the anterior approach, pneumothorax and renal injury are much less common in EUS-guided CPN/CPB compared to percutaneous CPN/CPB. Perhaps one of the most feared complications specific to CPN is neurologic injury causing lower extremity paralysis, and it is thought to be due to spinal cord ischemia, thrombosis/spasm of the artery of Adamkiewicz, or direct injury to the spinal cord. Although once thought exclusive to the percutaneous posterior approach, paralysis has been reported in one case of EUS-guided CPN [40–42].

Death due to complications of EUS-guided celiac plexus injection is exceedingly rare, although a few cases have been reported. One reported death occurred due to necrotic gastric perforation in a patient with chronic pancreatitis who underwent 13 injections of alcohol over 4 years; laparotomy showed a profusely bleeding necrotic area of aorta superior to the celiac takeoff as well as a large perforation in the posterior wall of the stomach [43]. It should be emphasized that this patient underwent a very atypical treatment regimen. Another fatality followed bilateral EUS-guided CPN in pancreatitis pain due to complete thrombosis of the celiac trunk resulting in multiorgan infarction and bowel pneumatosis [44]. A third fatality occurred with EUS-guided CPN in pancreatic cancer likely due to diffusion of ethanol leading to thrombosis in the celiac artery and vasospasm, which in turn led to embolic infarction of multiple viscera and bowel [45].

EUS-Guided Injection of Celiac Ganglia

With advances in endosonographic imaging and technique, visualization of the celiac ganglia is now feasible in most patients [46, 47]. This has created the possibility of direct injection of the ganglia—celiac ganglia neurolysis (CGN) and celiac ganglia block (CGB)—to provide potentially more precisely targeted analgesic effect.

The celiac ganglia are large clusters of nerve cells located anterior to the aorta, usually on either side of the celiac trunk, and more commonly on the left side (Fig. 15.4). They are part of the sympathetic prevertebral chain and are among the largest ganglia in the autonomic nervous system, transmitting and receiving signals to and from nearby plexuses, including the celiac plexus [4]. Endosonographically, the celiac ganglia are typically oval shaped with irregular borders, hypoechoic with or without internal hyperechoic foci, and can measure from 2 to 3 mm up to approximately 20 mm in maximal width [5, 6, 46]. A celiac ganglion may resemble the adrenal gland, and can be mistaken for an irregularly shaped lymph node. A distinguishing characteristic is the presence of threadlike hyperechoic projections from the celiac ganglia, which are nerve fibers. In a series of 200 consecutive patients undergoing EUS at a single academic center, the celiac ganglia were successfully visualized in 81 % of patients. While identification was less successful with the radial echoendoscope and less experienced endoscopists, patient-related variables including age, body mass index, alcohol consumption, and presence of abdominal malignancy had no impact [47]. Another prospective Korean series of 57 patients reported an even higher rate of celiac ganglia visualization, 89 %, using the radial echoendoscope [48].

In terms of procedural technique, EUS-guided CGN/CGB is largely identical to CPN/CPB, with a few additional technical considerations. If multiple ganglia are visualized, then generally all are injected if possible. For ganglia less than 1 cm, the needle tip should be positioned at the center of the ganglia. For ganglia 1 cm and larger, the needle tip should be advanced to the deepest point, with injection performed slowly as the needle is gradually withdrawn within the ganglia [13, 46].

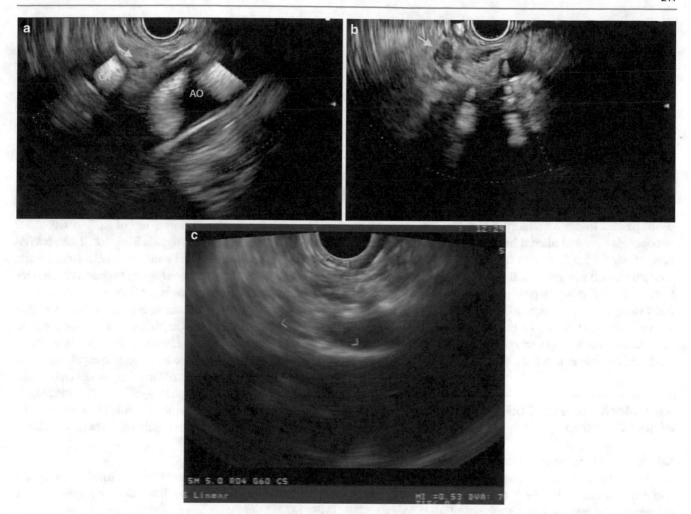

Fig. 15.4 Endosonographic visualization and direct injection of a celiac ganglion. AO, aorta. CA, celiac artery. Note colored portions are Doppler imaging indicating blood vessels. (**a**) A portion of a celiac ganglion (*yellow arrow*) is visualized anterior to the celiac trunk. (**b**) With gentle torque on the echoendoscope, the main portion of the celiac ganglion (*yellow arrow*) is visualized to the left of the celiac trunk. (**c**) An EUS FNA needle is advanced directly into the ganglia prior to celiac plexus neurolysis (image courtesy of Douglas G. Adler MD)

Efficacy of EUS-Guided Injection of Celiac Ganglia

The initial data regarding EUS-guided injection of the celiac ganglia was published in a 2008 retrospective study examining analgesic effect at 2–4 weeks post-procedure in both pancreatic cancer and chronic pancreatitis. In the cancer group, 16/17 (94 %) following CGN experienced pain relief while 0/1 undergoing CGB reported benefit. In the pancreatitis group, pain relief occurred in 4/5 (80 %) following CGN and 5/13 (38 %) after CGB [49]. Similar data supporting EUS-guided CGN was demonstrated in a larger 2011 retrospective study which examined analgesic response in 64 patients undergoing planned EUS-guided CPN or CGN for pancreatic cancer pain; CPN was used if the celiac ganglia were not visualized. Injection of the CGN was the greatest predictor of analgesic response in multivariate analysis, with odds ratio of 15.7 ($P<0.001$) [50]. A recent prospective multicenter trial randomized 68 patients with upper abdominal cancer pain to EUS-guided CPN and EUS-guided CGN. Improvement in pain at 7 days post-procedure was assessed. Pain relief was seen in 46 % with CPN versus 74 % following CGN ($P=0.026$) with no difference in complications [51]. Although EUS-guided CGN appears superior to CPN, the response rate for EUS-guided CPN was much lower than reported in other studies. Furthermore, it is unknown how much of the injected agent *actually gets into the ganglia* and how much simply extravasates and surrounds the nerve as would be seen in standard CPN or CPB. These data suggest that injection of the ganglia is an effective and safe modality for analgesia in chronic pancreatitis and pancreatic cancer, and EUS-guided CGN in particular may be more effective than CPN and CPB.

Complications Specific to EUS-Guided Injection of Celiac Ganglia

Injection of the celiac ganglia sometimes results in immediate increased pain, and when it occurs it is often to a significantly greater degree than that observed with injection of the celiac plexus. Intraprocedurally, this can manifest as sudden patient agitation and altered heart or respiratory rate at the time of needle puncture into the celiac ganglion. Typically this pain resolves very rapidly and appears to be distinct from clinically relevant post-procedure pain. In the initial 2008 study of EUS-guided celiac ganglia injection by Levy and colleagues, 36 % of patients experienced post-procedure pain, and in fact having some degree of post-procedure pain predicted durable pain relief [49].

Novel Techniques in EUS-Guided Celiac Plexus Injection

Sakamoto and colleagues reported a modified technique whereby a 25-gauge needle was used to inject alcohol mixed with contrast into both sides of the superior mesenteric artery to perform "broad plexus neurolysis." Post-procedure CT could then assess the spread of the neurolytic agent around the celiac, superior mesenteric, and inferior mesenteric arteries; greater degree of spread correlated with better response. The study included 67 patients, and the broad plexus neurolysis group exhibited sustained pain relief at 30 days post-procedure [52]. Further studies are necessary to confirm these results, and this technique has not gained widespread use.

EUS-guided brachytherapy, or implantation of radioactive seeds into a malignant neoplasm, has been proposed as a strategy for local ablative therapy in pancreatic cancer. While this has not improved survival, significantly reduced pain has been observed. The largest study included 100 patients, all of whom underwent EUS-guided brachytherapy with iodine-125 seeds, and reductions in mean pain scores were sustained for 3 months [53]. A follow-up study utilized the iodine-125 as the injectate for EUS-guided CGN in 23 patients with pain due to unresectable pancreatic cancer. At 2 weeks, 82 % had reductions in visual analog pain scores, and the effect lasted until the study concluded 5 months post-procedure. No randomized controlled trial has been performed yet, but the authors proposed iodine-125 as a potentially superior neurolytic agent in CPN or CGN, compared to alcohol [54].

Conclusion

Management of chronic pain is a significant clinical challenge, particularly in chronic pancreatitis and pancreatic cancer, and EUS-guided celiac interventions are often able to provide significant analgesic effect with efficacy surpassing traditional pharmacologic management. Furthermore, this benefit is provided in a safe, low-risk procedure that can mitigate the deleterious effects of opioid medications including constipation, somnolence, and tolerance. The progression of endosonographic tools and technique has led to continuing refinements in EUS-guided injection, such as targeting the celiac ganglia.

Areas for future research in the use of EUS in CPN/CPB abound. Heterogeneity in technique is likely inevitable, but further studies in technique should standardize EUS-guided celiac plexus/ganglia injection and perhaps lead to greater consistency in efficacy. Similarly, the integration of EUS-guided therapies in existing care paradigms continues to evolve, and further studies could assist endosonographers in patient selection and prognostication. As with many areas of interventional EUS, the sophistication and breadth of available tools are ever-expanding.

With EUS-guided injection of the celiac plexus and ganglia firmly in the mainstream, our understanding of its potential will continue to grow, and concurrently the role of the endosonographer in the treatment of chronic pain will expand as well.

Video Legend

Video 15.1 EUS-Guided Celiac Plexus Neurolysis. Appropriate technique is demonstrated using live endosonographic imaging (MP4 13293 kb).

References

1. Ventafridda GV, Caraceni AT, Sbanotto AM, et al. Pain treatment in cancer of the pancreas. Eur J Surg Oncol. 1990;16:1–6.
2. Lankisch PG. Natural course of chronic pancreatitis. Pancreatology. 2001;1:3–14.
3. Hall TC, Garcea G, Webb MA, et al. The socio-economic impact of chronic pancreatitis: a systematic review. J Eval Clin Pract. 2014;20(3):203–7.
4. Ward EM, Rorie DK, Nauss LA, et al. The celiac ganglia in man: normal anatomic variations. Anesth Analg. 1979;58:461–5.
5. Netter FH. Atlas of human anatomy. Philadelphia, PA: Saunders; 2014.
6. Brugge WR. EUS-guided ablation therapy and celiac plexus interventions. In: Hawes RH, Fockens P, editors. Endosonography. Philadelphia, PA: Elsevier Press; 2011. p. 281–2.
7. Plancarte R, Velasquez R, Patt RB. Neurolytic blocks of the sympathetic axis. In: Patt RB, editor. Cancer pain. Philadelphia: Lippincott; 1993. p. 377–425.
8. Gebhardt GF. Visceral pain mechanisms. In: Chapman CR, Foley KM, editors. Current and emerging issues in cancer pain. New York, NY: Raven Press; 1993. p. 99.
9. Nusrat S, Yadav D, Bielefeldt K. Pain and opioid use in chronic pancreatitis. Pancreas. 2012;41(2):264–70.

10. Penman ID, Gilbert D. Basic technique for celiac plexus block/neurolysis. Gastrointest Endosc. 2009;69:S163–5.

11. Kappis M. Erfahrungen mit local anasthesie bie bauchoperationen. Vehr Dtsch Gesellsch Chir. 1914;43:87–9.

12. Wang PJ, Shang MY, Qian Z, et al. CT-guided percutaneous neurolytic celiac plexus block technique. Abdom Imaging. 2006;31(6):710–8.

13. Luz LP, Al-Haddad MA, DeWitt JA. EUS-guided celiac plexus interventions in pancreatic cancer pain: an update and controversies for the endonographer. Endosc Ultrasound. 2014;3(4):213–20.

14. Yan BM, Myers RP. Neurolytic celiac plexus block for pain control in unresectable pancreatic cancer. Am J Gastroenterol. 2007;102:430–8.

15. Wiersema MJ, Wiersema LM. Endosonography-guided celiac plexus neurolysis. Gastrointest Endosc. 1996;44:656–62.

16. LeBlanc JK, Dewitt JA, Johnson C, et al. A prospective randomized trial of 1 versus 2 injections during EUS-guided celiac plexus block for chronic pancreatitis pain. Gastrointest Endosc. 2009;69(4):835–42.

17. Gress F, Schmitt C, Sherman S, et al. Endoscopic ultrasound-guided celiac plexus block for managing abdominal pain associated with chronic pancreatitis: a prospective single center experience. Am J Gastroenterol. 2001;96:409–16.

18. Wiersema MJ, Wong GY, Croghan GA. Endoscopic technique with ultrasound imaging for neurolytic celiac plexus block. Reg Anesth Pain Med. 2001;26:159–63.

19. LeBlanc JK, Al-Haddad M, McHenry L, et al. A prospective, randomized study of EUS-guided celiac plexus neurolysis for pancreatic cancer: one injection or two? Gastrointest Endosc. 2011;74(6):1300–7.

20. ASGE Standards of Practice Committee. Adverse events associated with EUS and EUS with FNA. Gastrointest Endosc. 2013;77(6):839–43.

21. Alvarez-Sanchez MV, Jenssen C, Faiss S, et al. Interventional endoscopic ultrasonography: an overview of safety and complications. Surg Endosc. 2014;28:712–34.

22. O'Toole TM, Schmulewitz N. Complication rates of EUS-guided celiac plexus blockade and neurolysis: results of a large case series. Endoscopy. 2009;41:593–7.

23. Gunaratnam NT, Sarma AV, Norton ID, Wiersema MJ. A prospective study of EUS-guided celiac plexus neurolysis for pancreatic cancer pain. Gastrointest Endosc. 2001;54:316–24.

24. Puli SR, Reddy JB, Bechtold ML, et al. EUS-guided celiac plexus neurolysis for pain due to chronic pancreatitis or pancreatic cancer pain: a meta-analysis and systematic review. Dig Dis Sci. 2009;54:2330–7.

25. Kaufman M, Singh G, Das S, et al. Efficacy of endoscopic ultrasound-guided celiac plexus block and celiac plexus neurolysis for managing abdominal pain associated with chronic pancreatitis and pancreatic cancer. J Clin Gastroenterol. 2010;44:127–34.

26. Wyse JM, Carone M, Paquin SC, et al. Randomized, double-blind, controlled trial of early endoscopic ultrasound-guided celiac plexus neurolysis to prevent pain progression in patients with newly diagnosed, painful, inoperable pancreatic cancer. J Clin Oncol. 2011;29:3541–6.

27. Wiechowska-Kozlowska A, Boer K, Wojcicki M, Milkiewicz P. The efficacy and safety of endoscopic ultrasound-guided celiac plexus neurolysis for treatment of pain in patients with pancreatic cancer. Gastroenterol Res Pract 2012; epub Feb 7.

28. Iwata K, Yasuda I, Enya M, et al. Predictive factors for pain relief after endoscopic ultrasound-guided celiac plexus neurolysis. Dig Endosc. 2011;23:140–5.

29. Sahai AV, Lemelin V, Lam E, Paquin SC. Central vs. bilateral endoscopic ultrasound-guided celiac plexus block or neurolysis: a comparative study of short-term effectiveness. Am J Gastroenterol. 2009;104:326–9.

30. Eisenberg E, Carr DB, Chalmers TC. Neurolytic celiac plexus block for treatment of cancer pain: a meta-analysis. Anesth Analg. 1995;80(2):290–5.

31. Arcidiacono PG, Calori G, Carrara S, et al. Celiac plexus block for pancreatic cancer pain in adults. Cochrane Database Syst Rev. 2011;16(3), CD007519.

32. Gress F, Schmitt C, Sherman S, et al. A prospective randomized comparison of endoscopic ultrasound- and computed tomography-guided celiac plexus block for managing chronic pancreatitis pain. Am J Gastroenterol. 1999;94:900–5.

33. Santosh D, Lakhtakia S, Gupta R, et al. Clinical trial: a randomized trial comparing fluoroscopy guided percutaneous technique vs. endoscopic ultrasound guided technique of coeliac plexus block for treatment of pain in chronic pancreatitis. Aliment Pharmacol Ther. 2009;29(9):979–84.

34. Wilcox CM, Yadav D, Ye T, et al. Chronic pancreatitis pain pattern and severity are independent of abdominal imaging findings. Clin Gastroenterol Hepatol. 2015;13(3):552–60.

35. D'Haese JG, Ceyhan GO, Demir IE, et al. Treatment options in painful chronic pancreatitis: a systematic review. HPB (Oxford). 2014;16(6):512–21.

36. Seicean A, Vultur S. Endoscopic therapy in chronic pancreatitis: current perspectives. Clin Exp Gastroenterol. 2014;8:1–11.

37. Hoffman BJ. EUS-guided celiac plexus block/neurolysis. Gastrointest Endosc. 2002;56(4 Suppl):S26–8.

38. LeBlanc JK, Rawl S, Juan M, et al. Endoscopic ultrasound-guided celiac plexus neurolysis in pancreatic cancer: a prospective pilot study of study using 10 mL versus 20 mL alcohol. Diagn Ther Endosc 2013; Epub 2013 Jan 8.

39. Lillemoe KD, Cameron JL, Kaufman HS, et al. Chemical splanchnicectomy in patients with unresectable pancreatic cancer: a prospective randomized trial. Ann Surg. 1993;217(5):447–55.

40. De Conno F, Caraceni A, Aldrighetti L, et al. Paraplegia following coeliac plexus block. Pain. 1993;55(3):383–5.

41. Fujii L, Clain JE, Morris JM, et al. Anterior spinal cord infarction with permanent paralysis following endoscopic ultrasound celiac plexus neurolysis. Endoscopy. 2012;44(Suppl 2 CTN):E265–6.

42. Mercadante S, Nicosia F. Celiac plexus block: a reappraisal. Reg Anesth Pain Med. 1998;23(1):37–48.

43. Loeve US, Mortensen MB. Lethal necrosis and perforation of the stomach and the aorta after multiple EUS-guided celiac plexus neurolysis procedures in a patient with chronic pancreatitis. Gastrointest Endosc. 2013;77:151–2.

44. Gimeno-Garcia AZ, Elwassief A, Paquin SC, et al. Fatal complication after endoscopic ultrasound-guided celiac plexus neurolysis. Endoscopy. 2012;44(Suppl 2 UCTN):E267.

45. Jang HY, Cha SW, Lee BW, et al. Hepatic and splenic infarction and bowel ischemia following endoscopic ultrasound-guided celiac plexus neurolysis. Clin Endosc. 2013;46:306–9.

46. Levy M, Rajan E, Keeney G, et al. Neural ganglia visualized by endoscopic ultrasound. Am J Gastroenterol. 2006;101:1787–91.

47. Gleeson FC, Levy MJ, Papachristou GI, et al. Frequency of visualization of presumed celiac ganglia by endoscopic ultrasound. Endoscopy. 2007;39(7):620–4.

48. Ha TI, Kim GH, Kang DH, et al. Detection of celiac ganglia with radial scanning endoscopic ultrasonography. Korean J Intern Med. 2008;23(1):5–8.

49. Levy MJ, Topazian MD, Wiersema MJ, et al. Initial evaluation of the efficacy and safety of endoscopic ultrasound-guided direct ganglia neurolysis and block. Am J Gastroenterol. 2008;103:98–103.

50. Ascunce G, Ribeiro A, Reis I, et al. EUS visualization and direct celiac ganglia neurolysis predicts better pain relief in patients with pancreatic malignancy. Gastrointest Endosc. 2011;73(2):267–74.

51. Doi S, Yasuda I, Kawakami H, et al. Endoscopic ultrasound-guided celiac ganglia neurolysis vs. celiac plexus neurolysis: a randomized multicenter trial. Endoscopy. 2013;45:362–9.

52. Sakamoto H, Kitano M, Kamata K, et al. EUS-guided broad plexus neurolysis over the superior mesenteric artery using a 25-gauge needle. Am J Gastroenterol. 2010;105(12):2599–606.

53. Du Y, Jin Z, Meng H, et al. Long-term effect of gemcitabine-combined endoscopic ultrasonography-guided brachytherapy in pancreatic cancer. J Interv Gastroenterol. 2013;3:18–24.

54. Wang KX, Jin ZD, Du YQ, et al. EUS-guided celiac ganglion irradiation with iodine-125 seeds for pain control in pancreatic carcinoma: a prospective pilot study. Gastrointest Endosc. 2012;76:945–52.

Additional Interventions in EUS

Truptesh H. Kothari, Shivangi T. Kothari, and Vivek Kaul

Introduction

With the development of the linear array EUS echoendoscopes and fine-needle aspiration (FNA) techniques, various options have emerged for therapeutic application of EUS in patients with pancreatic cancer, pancreatic cystic lesions, chronic pancreatitis, and even gastrointestinal bleeding. Advanced EUS-guided diagnostic interventions include needle-based confocal laser endomicroscopy (nCLE) and EUS-guided cytobrush sampling. Therapeutic interventions include fiducial placement, ethanol ablation, coil placement, delivery of antitumor agents, and radiofrequency ablation (Table 16.1). While some of these interventions are now mainstream (e.g., fiducial placement, nCLE), others remain investigational and need further study both in animal and human platforms. In this chapter, we discuss the current state of the science as it relates to available literature for each intervention with a look towards what progress needs to be made in each case to make it mainstream.

Electronic supplementary material: The online version of this chapter (doi:10.1007/978-3-319-26854-5_16) contains supplementary material, which is available to authorized users. Videos can also be accessed at http://link.springer.com/chapter/10.1007/978-3-319-26854-5_16.

T.H. Kothari, M.D., M.S. • S.T. Kothari, M.D.
V. Kaul, M.D., F.A.C.G., F.A.S.G.E. (✉)
Division of Gastroenterology and Hepatology, University of Rochester Medical Center & Strong Memorial Hospital, Rochester, NY, USA

Center for Advanced Therapeutic Endoscopy, URMC/Strong Memorial Hospital, 601 Elmwood Ave./Box 646, Rochester, NY 14642, USA
e-mail: vivek_kaul@urmc.rochester.edu

EUS-Guided Diagnostic Interventions

Needle-Based Confocal Laser Endomicroscopy

Pancreatic cystic neoplasms (PCNs) are increasingly being diagnosed given the widespread use of cross-sectional imaging and the ability to evaluate these easily with EUS-FNA. Differentiating mucinous cysts from non-mucinous cysts is important given the malignant potential of mucinous lesions, including intraductal papillary mucinous neoplasms (IPMN), and the need for either surgical intervention or close surveillance. Non-mucinous cysts such as pseudocysts and serous cystadenomas are considered benign and do not require continued surveillance. Although CT/MRCP characteristics, EUS-FNA, fluid analysis (CEA, other markers), cytology, fluid characteristics (viscosity), serum tumor markers (CA 19-9), and change in cyst size/morphology over time are currently used to make an overall clinical diagnosis, this approach is not always diagnostic and is limited at times in allowing an accurate differentiation between the various types of pancreatic cysts. This can lead to patients undergoing repeated procedures for surveillance and also for obtaining definitive diagnosis and cyst characterization. It is for these reasons that additional diagnostic modalities like molecular markers and nCLE imaging have been investigated to help facilitate characterization between mucinous and non-mucinous cysts [1–4].

Confocal laser endomicroscopy has been used for some time now for real-time cellular level imaging in Barrett's esophagus and in the biliary tree [5, 6]. Recently, its application has been extended to the evaluation of pancreatic cystic lesions, using the EUS-FNA platform [1].

Technique

A 19-gauge EUS-FNA needle is used, the stylet is removed, and a proprietary locking device is attached to the needle Luer Lock. The AQ-Flex-19 nCLE probe is inserted into the needle and locked into a predetermined position (extends

Table 16.1 Newer interventions in EUS

1. Diagnostic interventions:
(a) Needle-based confocal laser endomicroscopy (nCLE)
(b) Needle-based cytobrushing
2. Therapeutic interventions:
(a) Fiducial placement
(b) Brachytherapy
(c) Ethanol ablation
(d) Coil placement
(e) Pelvic abscess drainage
(f) Gallbladder drainage
(g) Radio-frequency ablation
(h) Other EUS-guided ablation therapies
(i) Delivery of antitumor agents
(j) Immunotherapy

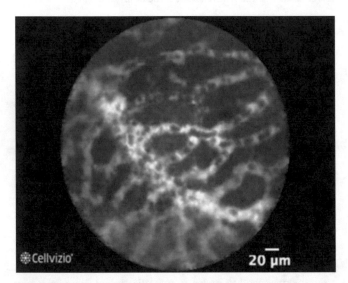

Fig. 16.1 Superficial vessels (seen in serous cystadenoma). Image courtesy of Mauna Kea Technologies

2 mm from the beveled edge). The probe is then retracted 1 cm and the cyst is punctured under real-time EUS guidance. Once the cyst is entered, the probe is pushed back into the needle, and locked in place, and real-time imaging of the cyst wall is begun (Video 16.1). Intravenous injection of fluorescein is done a few minutes prior to the actual imaging.

Diagnostic criteria for various pancreatic cysts as represented by nCLE examination [7].

1. Mucinous cystadenoma—Large white bands with rare vessels. Vessels are deeper in the ovarian-like stroma.
2. Serous cystadenoma—Blood vessels are superficial and closer to the cystic lumen (superficial vascular network) (Fig. 16.1).
3. Intraductal papillary mucinous neoplasm—Fingerlike "papillary" projections, which correspond to the villous changes of the intestinal type IPMN lesion, and presence

of fine caliber vessels characterize benign IPMN (compared to dark clumps with neovascularization and large vessels (>20 μ diameter) which represent malignant IPMN) (Fig. 16.2a, b).

4. Pseudocysts: Three types of structures are noted with nCLE:
   (a) Small black floating particles
   (b) Large, dark, round homogenous floating structures
   (c) Heterogeneous bright particles

Konda et al. performed EUS-FNA with nCLE evaluation of pancreatic cystic lesions in 2011 to evaluate the feasibility of nCLE [8]. Eighteen patients were enrolled in the study (16 cysts and 2 solid masses). Patients received intravenous injection of 2.5 ml of 10 % fluorescein immediately prior to the procedure. The lesion was interrogated with the nCLE probe positioned at the tip of 19 G needle. Technical feasibility to perform nCLE with good imaging was noted in 17 out of 18 cases. Two patients developed post-procedure pancreatitis—first patient with mild pancreatitis requiring short hospitalization and the second patient with moderate pancreatitis requiring a 5-day hospitalization. Out of the 17 patients, 10 patients had very good images, 5 had "moderate" quality images, and 2 had "poor" images. Overall, there were a few technical difficulties with loading of the nCLE probe and performing nCLE via the transduodenal approach.

In 2013, Konda et al. conducted a pilot study (INSPECT trial) to assess both safety and diagnostic potential of nCLE in differentiating pancreatic cystic lesions [1]. 66 patients at eight referral centers underwent nCLE imaging. Images from eight patients were subsequently excluded due to insufficient information for consensus reference diagnosis. Villous structures could be identified in IPMNs as demonstrated by INSPECT trial, which confirmed the preliminary findings of the feasibility trial [8]. Presence of epithelial villous structures on nCLE was strongly associated with PCN (intraductal papillary mucinous neoplasms, mucinous cystic adenoma, or adenocarcinoma) (*P* value—0.04) [1]. Patients identified with villous structures via nCLE may be diagnosed with IPMN despite equivocal fluid analysis and non-diagnostic cytology [1]. This trial demonstrated a sensitivity of 59 %, specificity of 100 %, positive predictive value of 100 %, and a negative predictive value of 50 % in differentiating the different pancreatic cystic lesions. Overall complication rate was 9 %, which included pancreatitis (*n*=2) (one patient developed mild and other patient developed moderate pancreatitis), intracystic bleeding (*n*=3), and transient abdominal pain (*n*=1).

Apart from the potential for complications (although typically mild and self-limited), one limitation with this technology is the inability to image the cyst wall adjacent to the entry point of the FNA needle in the cyst. Also, the ultrathin straight gray bands seen in serous cystadenoma are also seen in adenocarcinoma, representing the desmoplastic fibrous reaction [1].

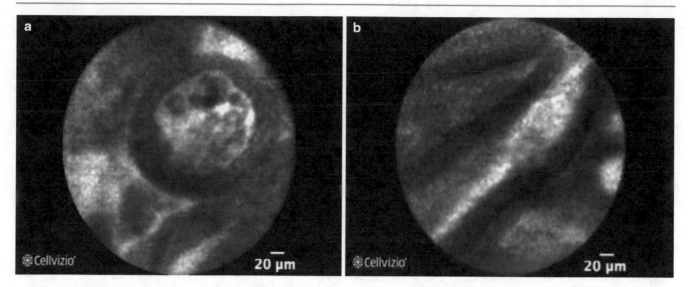

Fig. 16.2 (**a**) Dark ring with white core (seen in IPMN). Image courtesy of Mauna Kea Technologies. (**b**) Fingerlike projection (seen in IPMN). Image courtesy of Mauna Kea Technologies

In 2015, Nakai et al. assessed the feasibility, safety, and diagnostic yield of the combination of cystoscopy (using the spyglass probe) and nCLE in the clinical diagnosis of pancreatic cystic lesions—DETECT study [9]. At a single center, 30 patients with pancreatic cystic lesions underwent dual-modality evaluation as mentioned above. The main outcome measurement was achieving a clinical diagnosis of PCN, using a combination of cystoscopy and nCLE. Clinical diagnoses were established with high probability in 18 patients. The sensitivity of cystoscopy was 90 % (9/10) and that of nCLE was 80 % (8/10), and the combination yielded 100 % sensitivity for diagnosis of PCNs. The procedure was technically successful with the exception of one probe exchange failure. Two patients developed post-procedure pancreatitis requiring 4–5 days of hospitalization without intensive care unit admission or intervention (7 %).

In conclusion, nCLE helps better identify PCNs in patients with pancreatic cysts, and represents a major recent advance in this realm. There are some limitations and there is a learning curve for image interpretation as well as cost associated with the technology. Pancreatitis, albeit mild to moderate, remains a potential risk. Future studies with higher volume of patients and long-term outcomes will help further clarify the role of nCLE in pancreatic cyst evaluation.

EUS-Guided Cytobrush Sampling

Differentiating neoplastic from benign pancreatic cysts remains a challenge in many cases. A "through-the-needle" cytologic brush system (EchoBrush; Cook Endoscopy, Winston-Salem, NC) has been introduced which is FDA approved for cytologic

sampling during EUS evaluation of cystic lesions of the pancreas. The technique of cytobrushing is discussed below.

Technique

The technique for EUS cytobrushing was first described in 2007 by Al-Haddad et al. [10].

After aspirating 50 % of the cyst volume using standard FNA technique using a 19-gauge needle, the EchoBrush (Fig. 16.3) was introduced into the needle and advanced into the cyst under EUS guidance. After ensuring that the needle is in the cyst, the brush is moved back and forth repeatedly for 30 s ensuring adequate tangential contact with the cyst wall. The brush is then removed and final aspirate of the cyst with the needle is performed to collapse the cyst (Video 16.1).

Lozano et al. demonstrated a similar technique in 2011, except that the brush was rotated (on its axis) rather than performing back-and-forth movement in the cyst with an aim to gain maximal contact with the cystic wall in the hope of obtaining the best cytologic specimen [11].

In 2007, Al-Haddad et al. reported their preliminary data using EchoBrush in ten patients with cystic lesions of at least 2 cm in size [10]. They reported a higher yield of epithelial cells compared with standard EUS-FNA. Two patients on anticoagulation had complications of GI bleeding. Warfarin had been discontinued 5 days prior to the procedure in both patients. One patient developed upper GI bleeding 16 days after the procedure, requiring hospitalization (his warfarin was resumed 2 days after the procedure). He received eight units of packed red blood cell transfusion and underwent embolization of the gastroduodenal artery. The second patient reported one melenic bowel movement 12 h after the procedure; no interventions were needed. His warfarin had been resumed 4 days after the procedure.

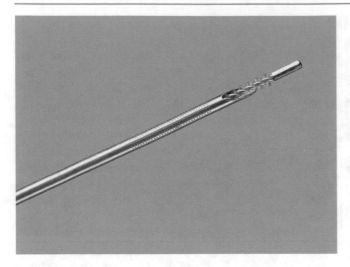

Fig. 16.3 EchoBrush used for cytobrushing. Permission for use granted by Cook Medical Incorporated, Bloomington, Indiana

The same group published another 39-patient controlled study in 2010, which supported their previous findings of EchoBrush being superior to EUS-FNA for cystic lesions of the pancreas, mainly due to the higher yield of epithelial cells with EchoBrush [12].

In 2011, Lozano et al. published their data with a total of 127 cystic lesions of the pancreas from 120 patients [11]. Mean size of the cystic lesions was 23.43 ± 21.67 mm. Diagnostic material was obtained in 85.1 % (40 of 47) cases using EchoBrush and in 66.3 % (53 of 80) with conventional EUS-FNA ($P < 0.05$). Three patients had self-limited intracystic bleeding and were observed in the recovery room postprocedure, and then discharged home. One patient developed perigastric abscess, which required hospitalization.

Despite encouraging results, more studies with larger patient cohorts are required in order to determine the role of EchoBrush in patients with cystic lesions of the pancreas. Patients on anticoagulation may be at higher risk for bleeding. Comparison of different techniques—"back-and-forth" brushing vs. "rotation" of the brush, EchoBrush yield before and after cyst collapse, and randomized comparison with standard FNA are potential areas for future research.

EUS-Guided Therapeutic Interventions

EUS-Guided Fiducial Placement for Image-Guided Radiotherapy

Radiation therapy plays a vital role in the treatment of various cancers. Conventional radiation therapy includes fractional external beam radiation therapy with or without systemic chemotherapy. Newer radiation techniques include interstitial brachytherapy and image-guided stereotactic

radiotherapy. The latter category includes stereotactic body radiotherapy (SBRT) and intensity-modulated radiotherapy (IMRT). These newer techniques are favored due to their precision and accuracy as well as reduced toxicity compared to fractional external beam radiotherapy. Cyberknife frameless radiosurgery system (Accuray, Sunnyvale, CA; USA) revolutionized the practice of treating non-intracranial tumors with the placement of implantable radiographic markers (fiducial markers) as reference/target points.

Before the advent of EUS, these "reference points" (fiducials) were placed through a CT-guided or surgical approach. Fiducial placement using the EUS approach is feasible for any solid lesion that is accessible with a dedicated linear echoendoscope. As such, mediastinal, abdominal, and pelvic lymph nodes, solid organ tumors, and most retroperitoneal and mediastinal malignant lesions are all potential targets for EUS-guided fiducial placement, if stereotactic radiotherapy is planned. The fiducials and needles are FDA approved, commercially available and this procedure is now mainstream.

Endoscopic Technique

Traditionally, EUS-guided fiducial placement was performed using a "re-loadable" standard 22-G or 19-G FNA needle. More recently, a "pre-loaded" fiducial needle has become available that allows for a modified technique. Both are described herein:

Traditional "re-loadable" needle approach: Using a linear array echoendoscope, the lesion is localized; then using sterile forceps, each cylindrical gold fiducial, 0.35 mm–0.5 mm diameter × 10 mm in length, is backloaded into a 22-G or 19-G FNA needle, respectively, after slight retraction of the stylet. The tip of the needle is then sealed using bone wax. The needle is then advanced into the tumor and the stylet is pushed into the needle, deploying the fiducial into the tumor, while slowly retracting the FNA needle. Fluoroscopic visualization can be utilized for confirmation; however fiducial placement can be performed under EUS visualization alone [13, 14]. The needle is withdrawn and reloaded with a new fiducial marker in a similar fashion, for a total of 3 or 4 fiducial placements, ideally 2–3 cm apart, spatially disoriented in 3 dimensions (Fig. 16.4a, b) [14]. Antibiotic prophylaxis during the procedure is used.

Pre-loaded needle approach: More recently (2014) a new 22-G needle with four pre-loaded fiducials has become available, which obviates the need to "reload" fiducials and allows placement of up to four fiducials sequentially in a rapid fashion, potentially reducing the time and tedium associated with the procedure (Video 16.1).

Technical difficulties in the placement of the fiducials could arise due to the stiffness of the 19-G needle, use of larger (5 mm) fiducials, or location of the tumor in an anatomically difficult region (such as in the uncinate process of

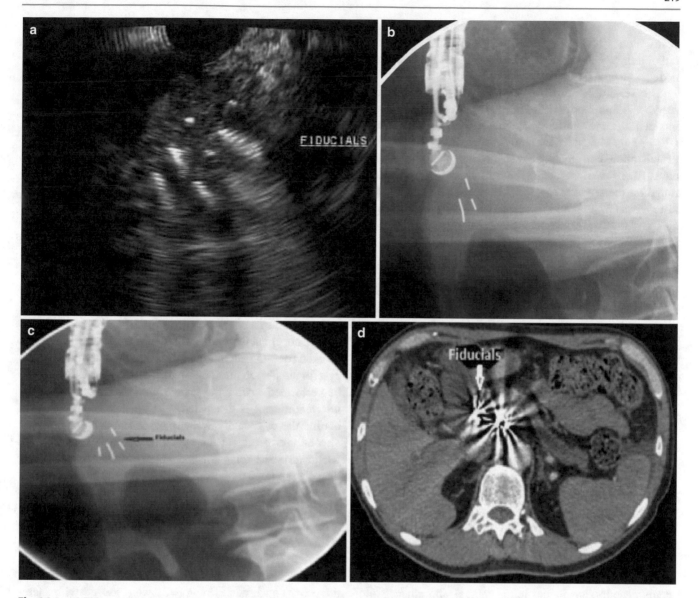

Fig. 16.4 (a) FNA needle in the pancreatic mass. (b) Gold fiducial in pancreatic mass seen on EUS. (c) Gold fiducials seen on fluoroscopy. (d) Gold fiducials seen on CT scan

the pancreas). Some of these can be overcome by straightening of the echoendoscope, using smaller length/diameter fiducial or using a more flexible/smaller gauge needle [15].

In 2006, Pishvaian et al. successfully placed fiducial markers under EUS guidance in six of the seven pancreatic cancer patients without any reported complications [16]. A recent study in 2014 by Choi et al. demonstrated the safety and feasibility of EUS-guided fiducial placement in pancreatic and hepatic tumors [17]. Primary outcome measurements included technical success, fiducial migration rate, and overall complication rates. 32 patients with pancreatic and hepatic malignancies referred for SBRT underwent fiducial placement. 29 patients (90.6 %) underwent successful SBRT and fiducial migration was noted in one patient (3.1 %). One patient (3.1 %) developed mild pancreatitis with

hospitalization for 2 days after fiducial placement. A recent prospective study by Davila Fajardo et al. in 2014 demonstrated the use of 22-gauge needle as a safe and feasible procedure for deploying the fiducial markers in patients with pancreatic carcinoma [15]. In conclusion, larger prospective trials comparing conventional radiotherapy and image-guided radiotherapy will help assess the value of EUS-guided fiducial placement in treatment of malignant tumors.

EUS-Guided Brachytherapy

Interstitial brachytherapy involves placement of radioactive seeds into a tumor, traditionally performed surgically or using a percutaneous approach. The tumor is subjected to local emission of gamma rays with the intention of tissue destruction. Therapeutic effects of EUS-guided interstitial radiotherapy for treatment of pancreatic tumors and lymph node metastasis have been reported [18, 19].

The feasibility of EUS-guided placement of radiation seeds was first reported in 2005 by Sun et al. in a porcine model [20]. The study involved placement of radioactive I-125 seeds (4.5 mm long and 0.85 mm thick) under EUS visualization into six pigs with normal pancreas. After 7 days, EUS revealed heterogeneous hypoechoic lesions surrounding the seeds in all pigs. The median diameter of the lesions was 32 mm and increased to 38 mm on day 14. On autopsy, the hypoechoic lesions were suggestive of local inflammatory response with necrosis and fibrotic tissue surrounding the seeds.

Thereafter, several clinical studies were performed in patients with locally advanced pancreatic cancer. Sun et al. and Jin et al. reported EUS-guided placement of radioactive seeds in 15 patients (8 patients with stage III, 7 with stage IV pancreatic cancer) and 22 patients, respectively [21, 22]. Sun et al. demonstrated "partial" response in 27 % patients, "minimal" response in 20 % patients, and "stable" disease in 33 % patients after a mean follow-up of 10.6 months [21]. Pain reduction was noted in 30 % patients. Complications included pancreatitis, pseudocyst formation, and hematologic toxicity in three patients.

Similarly Jin et al. demonstrated "partial" response in 13.6 % patients and "stable" disease in 45.5 % patients after a mean follow-up of 9.3 months [22]. In addition to the EUS-guided placement of radioactive seeds, all patients received gemcitabine-based 5-fluorouracil chemotherapy 1 week after the brachytherapy. Pain reduction was noted in all patients. No complications were reported in the study.

In conclusion, although EUS-guided brachytherapy seems encouraging in the initial animal and clinical pilot studies with respect to disease progression and pain reduction, there is no survival benefit data reported yet. Randomized clinical trials are needed to clarify the benefit of this technique in this population of patients with advanced pancreatic malignancy where novel therapeutic modalities are desperately needed.

EUS-Guided Ethanol Ablation

Ethanol injection via the percutaneous route has been used to ablate hepatic cysts, renal cysts, and liver and adrenal tumors [23–26]. With the evolution of EUS and EUS FNA since the 1990s, various therapeutic EUS techniques have also developed using EUS-guided fine needle injection (EUS-FNI).

Ethanol injected into a cyst causes cell death by breaking down the cell membrane, causing protein denaturation and vascular occlusion within a few minutes [27, 28]. Pancreatic cystic neoplasms with malignant potential in patients who are deemed poor surgical candidates are a clinical challenge. Surgical resection of pancreatic cysts can involve a morbidity rate of 27.5 % and mortality rate of up to 5 %, with higher morbidity seen in the elderly population (>70 years of age) [29].

For this reason, EUS-guided ethanol ablation of premalignant (or malignant) pancreatic cystic lesions has become an attractive option in patients who are not good surgical candidates or those who refuse to undergo surgery.

Endoscopic Technique

Using the curvilinear-array echoendoscope, the cyst is located and detailed evaluation of the cystic lesion is undertaken for the presence of features like septations, wall thickness, mural nodules, or associated solid mass. The cyst is punctured with a 22-gauge FNA needle. After subtotal evacuation of the cyst contents with aspiration, a bolus of ethanol is injected, equal in volume to the fluid aspirated. The cyst is lavaged for 3–5 min alternating filling and emptying of the cyst (or simple retention of injected ethanol for 3–5 min may be performed). After the lavage process is completed, the injected ethanol is evacuated, just leaving enough fluid to outline the cyst cavity wall. A second ablative agent may also be used to inject the cyst and left in the cavity (e.g., paclitaxel). The total injected volume should not be more than the aspirated fluid from the cyst cavity. After completion of the injection and lavage, the needle is removed from the cavity [30, 31].

Gan et al. reported the first clinical trial of EUS-guided ethanol injection for lavage and ablation of pancreatic cystic lesions [32]. In the pilot trial, 25 patients with pancreatic cysts (MCN = 13, IPMN = 4, serous cystadenoma = 3, pseudocyst = 3, uncertain etiology = 2) were treated with incremental doses of ethanol (5–80 %) for 3–5 min. Patients were followed for 6–12 months. No complications or adverse events were reported with the procedure. 35 % of patients had complete resolution of the cysts. Septated cysts persisted despite ethanol ablation. Five patients who underwent surgical resection had histological evidence of mucinous cystic neoplasm (MCN) and epithelial ablation was observed on surgical pathology.

A multicenter randomized double-blind prospective trial that compared the change in pancreatic cyst size after EUS-guided lavage with 80 % ethanol vs. saline solution reported a greater decrease in size of pancreatic cystic lesions in the ethanol injection group [33]. Overall, there was complete resolution of the pancreatic cystic lesions in 33.3 % of patients. Major complications such as abdominal pain, significant bleeding, and acute pancreatitis were similar in both the groups.

Oh et al. performed EUS-guided ethanol lavage of pancreatic cysts (99 % ethanol) in combination with paclitaxel and found complete resolution of the pancreatic cystic tumors in 11 of 14 patients [34]. The median follow-up of these patients was 20 months. There was no case of acute pancreatitis reported with the procedure.

Dewitt et al. reported complete resolution of cystic lesions in 11 of 22 patients treated with 100 % ethanol injection combined with paclitaxel over a median follow-up of 27 months [35]. Genomic evaluation of post-ablation cyst fluid revealed elimination of all baseline mutations in 8 out of the 11 patients.

Patient selection for alcohol cyst ablation should be based on the specific type of cyst. MCN is the ideal target for EUS-guided ethanol ablation due to its malignant potential and unilocular morphology. Branch duct IPMN may be unilocular but its tortuous septated internal structure decreases the effective contact of the ablative therapy with the epithelial lining, thereby reducing treatment efficacy [36]. Cyst ablation may be considered for macrocystic serous cystadenomas (SCAs) that demonstrate a size increase during follow-up evaluation [37].

Cases of EUS-guided ethanol ablation of insulinoma [38], GIST [39], left adrenal metastasis from non-small-cell lung cancer [40], hepatic metastases [41], and metastatic pelvic lymph nodes in patients after endoscopic resection of polypoid rectal cancer [42] have been reported.

The technique of EUS-FNI with ethanol ablation continues to evolve; however, larger studies are needed to better understand the safety and long-term efficacy of this technique. Several centers have now adopted this intervention as part of their overall pancreatic cyst management algorithm.

EUS-Guided Coil Placement for GI Bleeding

In 1986, Soehendra et al. first described management of gastric variceal hemorrhage (GVH) with bucrylate (glue) [43]. Practice guidelines and expert consensus opinion have recommended cyanoacrylate injection as preferred therapy for GVH based on available evidence [44, 45]. Transjugular intrahepatic portosystemic shunt (TIPS) has remained the first-line treatment in many centers for GVH because of several hurdles to the use of glue, including its off-label use, risk of serious adverse events from glue embolization, and lack of familiarity with the injection technique. Though conventional free-hand injection has proved effective, the risk of embolization has led to alternative treatment modalities, including EUS-guided fine needle injection of coils, glue, or both as well as balloon-occluded retrograde transvenous obliteration (BRTO) [46, 47]. Treatment under EUS guidance may help better visualize and target the varix. In addition, EUS can also confirm the obliteration of the varix by using Doppler [48, 49]. Coil placement in combination with glue injection may reduce the risk of embolization. Coils with attached synthetic fibers (wool coils) may function as a scaffold to retain glue within the varix and help decrease the amount of glue injection needed to achieve complete variceal obliteration.

Technique for EUS-Guided Coil Placement with Glue Injection for Gastric Fundic Varices

All patients should receive prophylactic antibiotics during the procedure. Standard endoscopy is used to locate the varices, followed by EUS examination using a linear echoendoscope to confirm active flow using Doppler. Intraluminal water filling of the gastric fundus helps improve acoustic coupling and visualization of varices. A standard EUS-FNA needle (19-gauge) is inserted into the gastric fundic varices (GFV) using a transesophageal-transcrural approach. The embolization coil (12–20 mm in diameter, MReye Embolization coil; Cook Medical) is delivered into the varix by using the stylet as a pusher. Following this, immediate injection of 1 ml of 2-octyl-CYA (Dermabond; Johnson & Johnson, New Brunswick, NJ) is performed through the same needle over 30 s by using normal saline solution to flush the glue through the catheter [47]. Obliteration of the GFV is confirmed with the help of color Doppler, which demonstrates absence of flow in the varix after the treatment.

In 2008, Levy et al. reported the first case using EUS-guided coil embolization in a patient with refractory bleeding secondary to ectopic anastomotic varices seen at the choledochojejunal anastomosis in a patient who had undergone total pancreatectomy and autologous islet cell transplant for chronic pancreatitis [50].

Binmoeller et al. assessed the feasibility, safety, and outcomes of transesophageal EUS-guided therapy of GFV with combined coil and glue injection [47]. Thirty patients with GFV were treated between March 2009 and January 2011. At index endoscopy, two patients had active bleeding and 14 had stigmata of recent hemorrhage. EUS-guided treatment of GFV was performed with 100 % hemostasis. Among 24 patients with a mean follow-up of 193 days, GFV were obliterated after a single treatment session in 23 patients (96 %). Rebleeding occurred in four patients (16.6 %), from different sites and not the treated GFV sites. No procedure-related complications or glue embolization-related events were reported.

Further studies are required to demonstrate the efficacy and safety of EUS-guided angiotherapy over conventional glue injection treatment. Multicenter trials are required to justify the additional cost associated with EUS and fluoroscopy while using EUS-guided coil treatment over conventional glue injection treatment.

EUS-Guided Pelvic Abscess Drainage

Pelvic abscess drainage not amenable to the traditional interventional radiology approach has been successfully performed via transrectal EUS [51]. Internal drainage of pelvic abscess offers more comfort to the patient and also allows access to anatomically difficult areas that are not easily accessible via the percutaneous approach [52].

EUS-guided internal stent placement along with transrectal drainage catheter placed for flushing has been reported as a successful technique for drainage of pelvic abscess [53].

The advantage of this technique provides shorter hospitalization and less risk of drainage catheter dislodgement. No major complications have been reported in multiple reports of EUS-guided drainage of pelvic abscesses [54, 55].

EUS-Guided Gallbladder Drainage

Percutaneous transhepatic gallbladder drainage (PTGBD) is the established treatment for acute cholecystitis in a patient not deemed suitable for emergent cholecystectomy. Few contraindications to the percutaneous approach where an EUS-guided approach is favorable include large perihepatic abscess, intervening bowel loops between the diaphragm and liver, and patients on anticoagulants/antiplatelet therapy [56–58].

Technique

The gallbladder is imaged using the linear echoendoscope from the distal gastric antrum or the duodenal bulb station. The gallbladder is punctured with a 19-gauge FNA needle, the stylet is removed, and bile may be aspirated to send for cultures. Under fluoroscopic guidance, contrast is injected into the gallbladder to perform cholecystography. A 0.035-inch guidewire is advanced through the needle and coiled into the gallbladder under EUS and fluoroscopic vision. The needle is exchanged out over the wire and the tract is dilated to facilitate stent placement. There have been two different dilation techniques—cautery (cystotome or needle knife) and non-cautery (stepped axial or balloon catheters). Once dilation is achieved, a stent (plastic or fully covered metal SEMS) is placed in the gallbladder under EUS and fluoroscopic vision to establish transluminal drainage [58]. The patient is continued on antibiotics and supportive care.

A review of the cases of EUS-guided gallbladder drainage reported a high overall success rate in 153 patients out of a total of 157 patients (97.45 %) [59]. Causes of failure in the four patients were cobblestone gallbladder—preventing easy advancement of wire and uncontrolled stent release [60] and accidental guidewire loss [56, 58]. Overall, complete resolution of acute cholecystitis was reported in 151 (of 153) patients; only one case did not have resolution leading to death due to sepsis [61]. Overall clinical success rate in patients with acute cholecystitis was 99.34 %. Overall complication rate has been noted to be relatively low. There were 12 adverse events reported from a total of 157 patients (7.64 %) [59].

Plastic stents or metal stents are not specifically designed for EUS-guided gallbladder drainage. Limitations of these stents include technical difficulty in deployment and lack of adequate anchorage/wall apposition leading to bile leak or pneumoperitoneum [62]. Stent migration can also be an issue with self-expanding metal stents. This led to the development of lumen-apposing metal stents (LAMS) that are designed to provide robust anchorage between non-adherent luminal structures and minimize the risk of stent migration. The first such LAMS introduced commercially is the Axios stent (Boston Scientific, MA, USA) and recently the Niti-S Spaxus (Taewoong Medical Seoul, South Korea) stent has also been released [62, 63].

EUS-guided gallbladder drainage is a novel technique; however further studies are needed for establishing the safety and long-term outcomes of this procedure, especially using the newer LAMS.

EUS-Guided Radio-Frequency Ablation for Pancreatic Tumors

Pancreatic cancer is the fourth leading cause of cancer death in the USA with 5-year survival rate of <10 % and a median survival of less than 6 months [64, 65]. Radiofrequency ablation (RFA) has been a widely accepted procedure for unresectable liver tumors. RFA works on the principle of delivering high-frequency alternating current, which in turn causes cellular damage by inducing coagulation necrosis. There is a growing interest and clinical need for RFA treatment of locally advanced pancreatic tumors. Studies have shown that RFA of unresectable pancreatic cancer has been feasible with acceptable mortality but high morbidity [66, 67].

Technique

Under EUS guidance using a transgastric approach, a 19-gauge FNA needle is advanced into the pancreatic tumor and the stylet is removed. The pilot RFA probe (Fig. 16.5a–c) is advanced through the needle into the pancreas. The pilot Habib EUS RFA probe (EMcision Ltd, London, UK) is a 1 Fr filament probe (0.33 mm, 0.013″) and has a working length of 190 cm. RFA is performed using the ERBE generator with bipolar settings of 10 W, effect 2, for 2 min [68] (Video 16.1).

In 1999 Goldberg et al. first reported the application of EUS-guided RFA treatment in a porcine model [69]. In 2014, Sethi et al. published EUS-guided lymph node ablation with

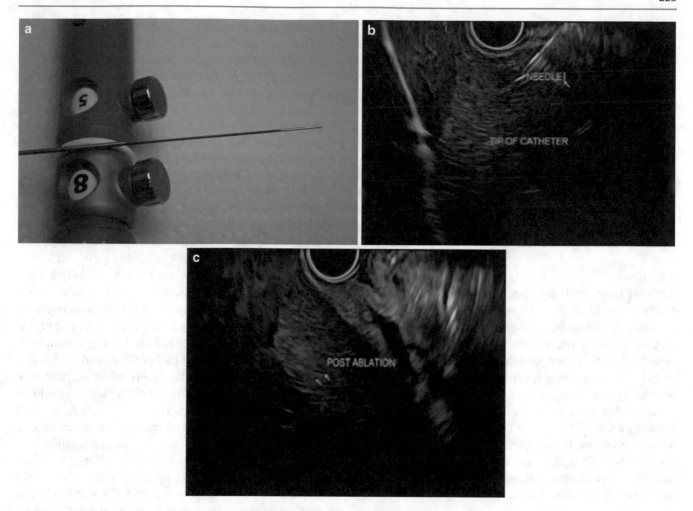

Fig. 16.5 (**a**) RFA probe. Courtesy of EMcision. (**b**) Preablation RFA probe. Courtesy of EMcision. (**c**) Postablation RFA prob

the RFA probe. A total of 18 mediastinal lymph nodes were ablated in a porcine model (mean size 20.8 ± 6.6 mm). The average length of the extended probe was 10 mm ± 3.0 mm. The mean length and diameter of necrosis was 9.8 ± 3.6 mm. No complications were reported with the procedure [68].

Carrara et al. utilized a hybrid cryotherm in a live porcine model combining bipolar RFA with simultaneous cryogenic cooling with carbon dioxide (650 psi). Successful RFA was performed in normal pancreatic body ($n = 14$), demonstrating positive correlation between treatment zone and treatment duration with fewer complications than conventional RFA techniques [70].

In order to evaluate the validity, efficacy, safety, and effect of RFA in normal or malignant pancreatic tissue, further studies are necessary. EUS-guided RFA in the management of unresectable pancreatic tumor is a promising area of research given the technical feasibility of the procedure, minimally invasive approach with the ability to perform the ablation under real-time EUS guidance, and the unmet need for local therapeutic options in pancreatic cancer.

Other EUS-Guided Ablation Therapies

- *Photodynamic therapy (PDT)*—PDT treatment involves ablation of target tissue using cytotoxic oxygen species generated by photosensitizers upon exposure to light of the appropriate wavelength [71]. This modality has been widely used in the past for treatment of dysplastic Barrett's and esophageal neoplasia.

Technique

In 2004, Chan et al. studied the safety and feasibility of EUS-guided PDT in a porcine model. After intravenous injection of a photosensitizer (porfimer sodium), a 19-gauge FNA needle was introduced into the porcine pancreas under EUS guidance followed by delivery of PDT with the help of a quartz optical fiber [72]. Localized areas of coagulation necrosis with low-dose PDT in the normal pancreas were noted ($n = 3$ with 9 applications). No immediate complications were reported. Yusuf et al. investigated the role of verteporfin (a photosensitizer with lower photosensitivity), in EUS-guided PDT using the 19-gauge FNA needle [73]. There was a linear correlation between the diameter of the necrotic tissue and the duration of exposure to the laser light with PDT treatment. No complications were reported with the procedure.

Further studies are warranted to validate the above studies and better understand the efficacy/safety of this technology.

- *Neodymium-yttrium aluminum garnet (Nd:YAG) laser—* It is defined as a solid-state laser which emits light at mid-infrared wavelengths of different pulse, duration, and energy, causing necrosis and phototoxicity of the pancreas. Precise laser-induced tissue necrosis is the main advantage of Nd:YAG laser.

Technique

Nd:YAG laser ablation is performed with an optical laser fiber advanced through a 19-gauge EUS-FNA needle inserted into the pancreas under EUS guidance.

Di Matteo et al. reported this technique in a porcine model in 2010 [74]. No major complications were reported ($n=8$). In 2013, the same group investigated optimal Nd:YAG laser settings by evaluating ablation volume and central carbonization volume, a measure which reveals unintended surrounding thermal injury [75]. They concluded that there was a linear correlation between ablation volume and laser output up to 10 W. Subsequent increase in output power to 20 W was directly associated with larger carbonization volume but no increase in ablation volume.

EUS-Guided Delivery of Antitumor Agents

Another exciting EUS-guided intervention that has been evaluated over the last few years is EUS-guided antitumor therapy. A variety of antitumor agents have been used for local treatment of pancreatic cancer using the EUS-FNI technique. Some of these agents such as activated allogenic mixed lymphocyte culture (cytoimplant), oncolytic attenuated adenovirus (ONYX-015), and replication-deficient adenovirus vector carrying the tumor necrosis factor-α gene are discussed in this section.

Technique

Under real-time EUS guidance the FNA needle is advanced into the tumor and the antitumor agent is delivered by fine needle injection technique. The advantage of this technique is the ability to deliver agents directly into the tumor under real-time EUS guidance, ensuring maximal tissue concentrations and using a minimally invasive technique.

- Cytoimplant (Allogenic Mixed Lymphocyte Culture): Chang et al. reported the feasibility and safety data for injecting cytoimplant conjugates (allogenic mixed lym-

phocyte culture) under EUS guidance directly into locally advanced pancreatic cancer [76]. In this study, eight patients with unresectable pancreatic cancer were given escalating doses of cytoimplants (3, 6, or 9 billion cells) using a single EUS-guided fine needle injection with a 22-gauge FNA needle. No major complications were reported. Seven of eight patients (86 %) experienced low-grade fever that was managed with acetaminophen. Median survival was 13.2 months, with partial response (more than 50 % decrease in cross-sectional tumor area) seen in two patients and minor response seen in one patient. There was no change observed in three patients while two patients had progression of disease. No further studies have been reported to date using this technique.

- Oncolytic Virus Therapy (ONYX-015): Oncolytic viruses such as adenovirus and herpes virus have been studied for antitumor therapy in pancreatic cancer using EUS-FNI technique. ONYX-015 is an oncolytic gene-deleted replication selective adenovirus that preferentially replicates in tumor cells and destroys them leading to cell death. A phase I trial of CT-guided ONYX-015 injection in 22 patients with locally advanced pancreatic cancer was first reported in 2001 [77]. The treatment was well tolerated with a minor response seen in 6 of 22 patients. In 2003, Hecht et al. reported a phase I/II trial of EUS-guided ONYX-015 injection, in combination with gemcitabine, in 21 patients [78]. A total of eight sessions of EUS-guided ONYX-015 injections into the pancreatic tumor were performed over a period of 8 weeks. The last four treatments were given with gemcitabine infusion on the same day. The efficacy of this treatment was inconclusive as only 2 patients (10 %) had objective partial regression of >50 % tumor volume, 2 had minor disease progression, 6 had stable disease, and 11 had progressive disease (or had to be dropped from the study due to treatment toxicity). Median survival time was 7.5 months. Two patients had sepsis leading to institution of prophylactic antibiotic during the procedure and a change in the needle withdrawal technique. Two patients had duodenal perforations (protocol was subsequently changed to transgastric injections only). EUS-guided ONYX-15 therapy remains controversial for the above reasons.

- TNFerade injection: TNFerade is a replication-deficient adenovirus vector, which contains a radiation-inducible promoter (Egr-1, early growth response) carrying the human tumor necrosis factor (TNF) alpha gene. Chang et al. have evaluated EUS-guided TNFerade in patients with locally advanced pancreatic cancer [79, 80]. The advantage of this technique is to maximize local antitumor activity and minimize systemic side effects. A phase I/II trial evaluated the efficacy of TNFerade combined with IV chemotherapy (5-fluorouracil) and radiation therapy [81]. Dose-limiting toxicity was seen in three patients at 1×10^{12} PU in EUS group (two pancreatitis and one cholangitis). Overall grade 3 and 4 toxicities included GI bleeding, deep vein thrombosis (DVT), pulmonary emboli, pancreatitis, and cholangitis. A single complete response was seen in 1 patient (2 %), 3 patients (6 %) had a partial response, 12 patients (24 %) had stable disease, and 19 (38 %) had progressive disease. The median time to tumor progression was 108 days. The overall median survival was 297 days, with the best median survival seen in the 4×10^{11} PU cohort (332 days). Also, patients receiving higher doses were seen to have better loco-regional disease control, longer tumor progression-free survival, and a higher chance of resective surgery after combination treatment.

In 2013 Herman et al. reported a randomized phase III multicenter trial of TNFerade biologic with 5-fluorouracil and radiotherapy for locally advanced pancreatic cancer [82]. This trial included 90 patients who received standard treatment compared to 187 patients who received standard treatment plus TNFerade+5FU+radiotherapy. Median survival was similar in both groups (10 months), suggesting that this approach was ineffective in prolonging survival. A pilot study has confirmed the feasibility of EUS-guided TNFerade intratumoral injection with IV capecitabine and radiation therapy as neoadjuvant therapy followed by surgery in patients with locally advanced rectal cancer [83].

Though EUS-guided antitumor agent injection is feasible, currently no survival advantage has been demonstrated with this approach. However, larger randomized controlled trials with newer agents may reveal more encouraging results.

EUS-Guided Immunotherapy

Immunotherapy against cancer has been studied using different kinds of immune cells; however, dendritic cells (DC) are the most potent antigen-presenting cells that stimulate naïve T-lymphocytes into tumor-specific cytolytic cells. Immunotherapy for pancreatic cancer has been studied using the EUS-guided FNI techniques. A study of DC-based therapy against syngeneic hamster pancreatic cancer showed an 82 % growth inhibition rate [84].

A study of EUS-guided injection of immature dendritic cells in seven patients with advanced pancreatic cancer who had failed chemotherapy previously demonstrated feasibility of this technique and no complications were reported [85].

Technique
Prior to the initial DC injection, five of the seven patients were given radiation to maximize antigen exposure caused from tumor necrosis. Using EUS-FNI technique, patients received intratumoral injection of ten billion or more DC at two to three sites. No complications were associated with the procedures and no toxicity was reported from the DC injection.

Two patients had mixed response, three patients had progressive disease, and two patients had stable disease with a median survival of 9.9 months.

In 2009, Hirooka et al. reported a combination therapy of gemcitabine with immunotherapy for patients with locally advanced pancreatic cancer [86]. Gemcitabine was used to induce apoptosis causing release of tumor antigens that would stimulate the DC. Five patients were treated with IV gemcitabine and EUS-guided intra-tumoral injection of OK-432-pulsed DC. This was followed by infusion of lymphokine-activated killer cells stimulated with anti-CD3 monoclonal antibody. Three of the five patients demonstrated effective response to the treatment, one with partial response and two with stable disease. No treatment complications were reported. Thus combination of chemotherapy and immunotherapy could be considered to be synergistically effective.

A phase I trial reported the feasibility and safety of preoperative intra-tumoral EUS-guided FNI of immature DC with OK-432 in patients with resectable pancreatic cancer [87]. Two of the nine patients treated (one of which was a stage IV cancer patient with distant lymph node metastasis) survived more than 5 years without requiring adjuvant therapy. Further larger studies are needed to demonstrate the efficacy of these techniques.

Summary

The evolution of EUS from a simple diagnostic imaging technology to a diverse platform capable of facilitating a wide range of therapeutic interventions has been quite dramatic and remarkable. Using the FNA technique as the basis, a vast range of complex interventions have emerged allowing advanced imaging and tissue sampling, delivery of agents using the FNI technique, and transluminal therapeutic procedures to help manage even the most challenging of clinical scenarios. In many clinical settings, these newer EUS-based interventions have completely changed the management paradigm and have significantly contributed to the medical-surgical treatment of patients. Even though many interventions remain investigational, several have acquired mainstream status.

The rapid pace at which device development and technology have progressed has enabled the EUS-based interventional endoscopy platform to make huge strides in a relatively short period of time. Future collaborative efforts among interventional endoscopists, surgeons, and industry device development teams will no doubt allow for even greater expansion of the therapeutic capabilities of EUS-based interventions.

Clearly, this is a tremendous area of growth and opportunity in medicine and one which holds tremendous promise in the coming years.

Video Legend

Video 16.1 Additional interventional EUS procedures (MOV 187183 kb).

Acknowledgement The authors wish to thank Glen Hintz, MS, Assoc Prof and Interim Chair of the School of Art, College of Imaging Arts & Sciences, Rochester Institute of Technology (RIT), for his time and effort in creating the animation clips for the video associated with this chapter.

Financial Disclosure The authors have no relevant financial disclosures.

References

1. Konda VJ, Meining A, Jamil LH, Giovannini M, Hwang JH, Wallace MB, Chang KJ, Siddiqui UD, Hart J, Lo SK, et al. A pilot study of in vivo identification of pancreatic cystic neoplasms with needle-based confocal laser endomicroscopy under endosonographic guidance. Endoscopy. 2013;45(12):1006–13.

2. Levy MJ, Clain JE. Evaluation and management of cystic pancreatic tumors: emphasis on the role of EUS FNA. Clin Gastroenterol Hepatol. 2004;2(8):639–53.

3. Hutchins GF, Draganov PV. Cystic neoplasms of the pancreas: a diagnostic challenge. World J Gastroenterol. 2009;15(1):48–54.

4. Attasaranya S, Pais S, LeBlanc J, McHenry L, Sherman S, DeWitt JM. Endoscopic ultrasound-guided fine needle aspiration and cyst fluid analysis for pancreatic cysts. JOP. 2007;8(5):553–63.

5. Meining A, Chen YK, Pleskow D, Stevens P, Shah RJ, Chuttani R, Michalek J, Slivka A. Direct visualization of indeterminate pancreaticobiliary strictures with probe-based confocal laser endomicroscopy: a multicenter experience. Gastrointest Endosc. 2011;74(5): 961–8.

6. Gaddam S, Mathur SC, Singh M, Arora J, Wani SB, Gupta N, Overhiser A, Rastogi A, Singh V, Desai N, et al. Novel probe-based confocal laser endomicroscopy criteria and interobserver agreement for the detection of dysplasia in Barrett's esophagus. Am J Gastroenterol. 2011;106(11):1961–9.

7. Giovannini M, Caillol F, Lemaistre A, et al. Endoscopic ultrasound guided confocal microscopy: Atlas of cystic pancreatic lesions. Endosc Ultrasound. 2014;3:S19–21.

8. Konda VJ, Aslanian HR, Wallace MB, Siddiqui UD, Hart J, Waxman I. First assessment of needle-based confocal laser endomicroscopy during EUS-FNA procedures of the pancreas (with videos). Gastrointest Endosc. 2011;74(5):1049–60.

9. Nakai Y, Iwashita T, Park DH, Samarasena JB, Lee JG, Chang KJ. Diagnosis of pancreatic cysts: EUS-guided, through-the-needle confocal laser-induced endomicroscopy and cystoscopy trial: DETECT study. Gastrointest Endosc. 2015.

10. Al-Haddad M, Raimondo M, Woodward T, Krishna M, Pungpapong S, Noh K, Wallace MB. Safety and efficacy of cytology brushings versus standard FNA in evaluating cystic lesions of the pancreas: a pilot study. Gastrointest Endosc. 2007;65(6):894–8.

11. Lozano MD, Subtil JC, Miravalles TL, Echeveste JI, Prieto C, Betes M, Alvarez Cienfuegos FJ, Idoate MA. EchoBrush may be superior to standard EUS-guided FNA in the evaluation of cystic lesions of the pancreas: preliminary experience. Cancer Cytopathol. 2011;119(3):209–14.

12. Al-Haddad M, Gill KR, Raimondo M, Woodward TA, Krishna M, Crook JE, Skarvinko LN, Jamil LH, Hasan M, Wallace MB. Safety and efficacy of cytology brushings versus standard fine-needle aspiration in evaluating cystic pancreatic lesions: a controlled study. Endoscopy. 2010;42(2):127–32.

13. Al-Haddad M, Eloubeidi MA. Interventional EUS for the diagnosis and treatment of locally advanced pancreatic cancer. JOP. 2010; 11(1):1–7.

14. Majumder S, Berzin TM, Mahadevan A, Pawa R, Ellsmere J, Sepe PS, Larosa SA, Pleskow DK, Chuttani R, Sawhney MS. Endoscopic ultrasound-guided pancreatic fiducial placement: how important is ideal fiducial geometry? Pancreas. 2013;42(4):692–5.

15. Davila Fajardo R, Lekkerkerker SJ, van der Horst A, Lens E, Bergman JJ, Fockens P, Bel A, van Hooft JE. EUS-guided fiducial markers placement with a 22-gauge needle for image-guided radiation therapy in pancreatic cancer. Gastrointest Endosc. 2014; 79(5):851–5.

16. Pishvaian AC, Collins B, Gagnon G, Ahlawat S, Haddad NG. EUS-guided fiducial placement for CyberKnife radiotherapy of mediastinal and abdominal malignancies. Gastrointest Endosc. 2006;64(3): 412–7.

17. Choi JH, Seo DW, Park do H, Lee SK, Kim MH. Fiducial placement for stereotactic body radiation therapy under only endoscopic ultrasonography guidance in pancreatic and hepatic malignancy: practical feasibility and safety. Gut Liver. 2014;8(1):88–93.

18. Zhongmin W, Yu L, Fenju L, Kemin C, Gang H. Clinical efficacy of CT-guided iodine-125 seed implantation therapy in patients with advanced pancreatic cancer. Eur Radiol. 2010;20(7):1786–91.

19. Kishi K, Sonomura T, Shirai S, Noda Y, Sato M, Kawai M, Yamaue H. Brachytherapy reirradiation with hyaluronate gel injection of paraaortic lymphnode metastasis of pancreatic cancer: paravertebral approach—a technical report with a case. J Radiat Res. 2011;52(6):840–4.

20. Sun S, Qingjie L, Qiyong G, Mengchun W, Bo Q, Hong X. EUS-guided interstitial brachytherapy of the pancreas: a feasibility study. Gastrointest Endosc. 2005;62(5):775–9.

21. Sun S, Xu H, Xin J, Liu J, Guo Q, Li S. Endoscopic ultrasound-guided interstitial brachytherapy of unresectable pancreatic cancer: results of a pilot trial. Endoscopy. 2006;38(4):399–403.

22. Jin Z, Du Y, Li Z, Jiang Y, Chen J, Liu Y. Endoscopic ultrasonography-guided interstitial implantation of iodine 125-seeds combined with chemotherapy in the treatment of unresectable pancreatic carcinoma: a prospective pilot study. Endoscopy. 2008;40(4):314–20.

23. Omerovic S, Zerem E. Alcohol sclerotherapy in the treatment of symptomatic simple renal cysts. Bosn J Basic Med Sci. 2008; 8(4):337–40.

24. Larssen TB, Jensen DK, Viste A, Horn A. Single-session alcohol sclerotherapy in symptomatic benign hepatic cysts. Long-term results. Acta Radiol. 1999;40(6):636–8.

25. Livraghi T, Bolondi L, Lazzaroni S, Marin G, Morabito A, Rapaccini GL, Salmi A, Torzilli G. Percutaneous ethanol injection in the treatment of hepatocellular carcinoma in cirrhosis. A study on 207 patients. Cancer. 1992;69(4):925–9.

26. Xiao YY, Tian JL, Li JK, Yang L, Zhang JS. CT-guided percutaneous chemical ablation of adrenal neoplasms. AJR Am J Roentgenol. 2008;190(1):105–10.

27. Bean WJ, Rodan BA. Hepatic cysts: treatment with alcohol. AJR Am J Roentgenol. 1985;144(2):237–41.

28. Gelczer RK, Charboneau JW, Hussain S, Brown DL. Complications of percutaneous ethanol ablation. J Ultrasound Med. 1998;17(8): 531–3.

29. Goh BK, Tan YM, Cheow PC, Chung YF, Chow PK, Wong WK, Ooi LL. Cystic lesions of the pancreas: an appraisal of an aggres-

sive resectional policy adopted at a single institution during 15 years. Am J Surg. 2006;192(2):148–54.

30. Oh HC, Seo DW. Endoscopic ultrasonography-guided pancreatic cyst ablation (with video). J Hepatobiliary Pancreat Sci. 2015;22(1):16–9.

31. Oh HC, Seo DW, Song TJ, Moon SH, Park do H, Soo Lee S, Lee SK, Kim MH, Kim J. Endoscopic ultrasonography-guided ethanol lavage with paclitaxel injection treats patients with pancreatic cysts. Gastroenterology. 2011;140(1):172–9.

32. Gan SI, Thompson CC, Lauwers GY, Bounds BC, Brugge WR. Ethanol lavage of pancreatic cystic lesions: initial pilot study. Gastrointest Endosc. 2005;61(6):746–52.

33. DeWitt J, McGreevy K, Schmidt CM, Brugge WR. EUS-guided ethanol versus saline solution lavage for pancreatic cysts: a randomized, double-blind study. Gastrointest Endosc. 2009;70(4): 710–23.

34. Oh HC, Seo DW, Lee TY, Kim JY, Lee SS, Lee SK, Kim MH. New treatment for cystic tumors of the pancreas: EUS-guided ethanol lavage with paclitaxel injection. Gastrointest Endosc. 2008;67(4): 636–42.

35. DeWitt JM, Al-Haddad M, Sherman S, LeBlanc J, Schmidt CM, Sandrasegaran K, Finkelstein SD. Alterations in cyst fluid genetics following endoscopic ultrasound-guided pancreatic cyst ablation with ethanol and paclitaxel. Endoscopy. 2014;46(6):457–64.

36. DeWitt J. Endoscopic ultrasound-guided pancreatic cyst ablation. Gastrointest Endosc Clin N Am. 2012;22(2):291–302. ix-x.

37. Khashab MA, Shin EJ, Amateau S, Canto MI, Hruban RH, Fishman EK, Cameron JL, Edil BH, Wolfgang CL, Schulick RD, et al. Tumor size and location correlate with behavior of pancreatic serous cystic neoplasms. Am J Gastroenterol. 2011;106(8): 1521–6.

38. Jurgensen C, Schuppan D, Neser F, Ernstberger J, Junghans U, Stolzel U. EUS-guided alcohol ablation of an insulinoma. Gastrointest Endosc. 2006;63(7):1059–62.

39. Gunter E, Lingenfelser T, Eitelbach F, Muller H, Ell C. EUS-guided ethanol injection for treatment of a GI stromal tumor. Gastrointest Endosc. 2003;57(1):113–5.

40. Artifon EL, Lucon AM, Sakai P, Gerhardt R, Srougi M, Takagaki T, Ishioka S, Bhutani MS. EUS-guided alcohol ablation of left adrenal metastasis from non-small-cell lung carcinoma. Gastrointest Endosc. 2007;66(6):1201–5.

41. Barclay RL, Perez-Miranda M, Giovannini M. EUS-guided treatment of a solid hepatic metastasis. Gastrointest Endosc. 2002;55(2):266–70.

42. DeWitt J, Mohamadnejad M. EUS-guided alcohol ablation of metastatic pelvic lymph nodes after endoscopic resection of polypoid rectal cancer: the need for long-term surveillance. Gastrointest Endosc. 2011;74(2):446–7.

43. Soehendra N, Nam VC, Grimm H, Kempeneers I. Endoscopic obliteration of large esophagogastric varices with bucrylate. Endoscopy. 1986;18(1):25–6.

44. Garcia-Tsao G, Sanyal AJ, Grace ND, Carey WD, Practice Guidelines Committee of American Association for Study of Liver D, Practice Parameters Committee of American College of G. Prevention and management of gastroesophageal varices and variceal hemorrhage in cirrhosis. Am J Gastroenterol. 2007;102(9): 2086–102.

45. de Franchis R, Baveno VF. Revising consensus in portal hypertension: report of the Baveno V consensus workshop on methodology of diagnosis and therapy in portal hypertension. J Hepatol. 2010;53(4):762–8.

46. Irani S, Kowdley K, Kozarek R. Gastric varices: an updated review of management. J Clin Gastroenterol. 2011;45(2):133–48.

47. Binmoeller KF, Weilert F, Shah JN, Kim J. EUS-guided transesophageal treatment of gastric fundal varices with combined coiling and cyanoacrylate glue injection (with videos). Gastrointest Endosc. 2011;74(5):1019–25.

48. Lee YT, Chan FK, Ng EK, Leung VK, Law KB, Yung MY, Chung SC, Sung JJ. EUS-guided injection of cyanoacrylate for bleeding gastric varices. Gastrointest Endosc. 2000;52(2):168–74.

49. Romero-Castro R, Pellicer-Bautista FJ, Jimenez-Saenz M, Marcos-Sanchez F, Caunedo-Alvarez A, Ortiz-Moyano C, Gomez-Parra M, Herrerias-Gutierrez JM. EUS-guided injection of cyanoacrylate in perforating feeding veins in gastric varices: results in 5 cases. Gastrointest Endosc. 2007;66(2):402–7.

50. Levy MJ, Wong Kee Song LM, Kendrick ML, Misra S, Gostout CJ. EUS-guided coil embolization for refractory ectopic variceal bleeding (with videos). Gastrointest Endosc. 2008;67(3):572–4.

51. Puri R, Eloubeidi MA, Sud R, Kumar M, Jain P. Endoscopic ultrasound-guided drainage of pelvic abscess without fluoroscopy guidance. J Gastroenterol Hepatol. 2010;25(8):1416–9.

52. Ulla-Rocha JL, Vilar-Cao Z, Sardina-Ferreiro R. EUS-guided drainage and stent placement for postoperative intra-abdominal and pelvic fluid collections in oncological surgery. Therap Adv Gastroenterol. 2012;5(2):95–102.

53. Trevino JM, Drelichman ER, Varadarajulu S. Modified technique for EUS-guided drainage of pelvic abscess (with video). Gastrointest Endosc. 2008;68(6):1215–9.

54. Giovannini M, Bories E, Moutardier V, Pesenti C, Guillemin A, Lelong B, Delpero JR. Drainage of deep pelvic abscesses using therapeutic echo endoscopy. Endoscopy. 2003;35(6):511–4.

55. Varadarajulu S, Drelichman ER. Effectiveness of EUS in drainage of pelvic abscesses in 25 consecutive patients (with video). Gastrointest Endosc. 2009;70(6):1121–7.

56. Jang JW, Lee SS, Song TJ, Hyun YS, Park do H, Seo DW, Lee SK, Kim MH, Yun SC. Endoscopic ultrasound-guided transmural and percutaneous transhepatic gallbladder drainage are comparable for acute cholecystitis. Gastroenterology. 2012;142(4):805–11.

57. Hasan MK, Itoi T, Varadarajulu S. Endoscopic management of acute cholecystitis. Gastrointest Endosc Clin N Am. 2013;23(2): 453–9.

58. Choi JH, Lee SS, Choi JH, Park do H, Seo DW, Lee SK, Kim MH. Long-term outcomes after endoscopic ultrasonography-guided gallbladder drainage for acute cholecystitis. Endoscopy. 2014;46(8):656–61.

59. Penas-Herrero I, de la Serna-Higuera C, Perez-Miranda M. Endoscopic ultrasound-guided gallbladder drainage for the management of acute cholecystitis (with video). J Hepatobiliary Pancreat Sci. 2015;22(1):35–43.

60. de la Serna-Higuera C, Perez-Miranda M, Gil-Simon P, Ruiz-Zorrilla R, Diez-Redondo P, Alcaide N, Sancho-del Val L, Nunez-Rodriguez H. EUS-guided transenteric gallbladder drainage with a new fistula-forming, lumen-apposing metal stent. Gastrointest Endosc. 2013;77(2):303–8.

61. Widmer J, Alvarez P, Gaidhane M, Paddu N, Umrania H, Sharaiha R, Kahaleh M. Endoscopic ultrasonography-guided cholecystogastrostomy in patients with unresectable pancreatic cancer using anti-migratory metal stents: a new approach. Dig Endosc. 2014;26(4): 599–602.

62. Binmoeller KF, Shah J. A novel lumen-apposing stent for transluminal drainage of nonadherent extraintestinal fluid collections. Endoscopy. 2011;43(4):337–42.

63. Moon JH, Choi HJ, Kim DC, Lee YN, Kim HK, Jeong SA, Lee TH, Cha SW, Cho YD, Park SH, et al. A newly designed fully covered metal stent for lumen apposition in EUS-guided drainage and access: a feasibility study (with videos). Gastrointest Endosc. 2014;79(6):990–5.

64. Niederhuber JE, Brennan MF, Menck HR. The National Cancer Data Base report on pancreatic cancer. Cancer. 1995;76(9): 1671–7.

65. Warshaw AL, Fernandez-del Castillo C. Pancreatic carcinoma. N Engl J Med. 1992;326(7):455–65.
66. Wu Y, Tang Z, Fang H, Gao S, Chen J, Wang Y, Yan H. High operative risk of cool-tip radiofrequency ablation for unresectable pancreatic head cancer. J Surg Oncol. 2006;94(5):392–5.
67. Spiliotis JD, Datsis AC, Michalopoulos NV, Kekelos SP, Vaxevanidou A, Rogdakis AG, Christopoulou AN. High operative risk of cool-tip radiofrequency ablation for unresectable pancreatic head cancer. J Surg Oncol. 2007;96(1):89–90.
68. Sethi A, Ellrichmann M, Dhar S, Hadeler KG, Kahle E, Seehusen F, Klapper W, Habib N, Fritscher-Ravens A. Endoscopic ultrasound-guided lymph node ablation with a novel radiofrequency ablation probe: feasibility study in an acute porcine model. Endoscopy. 2014;46(5):411–5.
69. Goldberg SN, Mallery S, Gazelle GS, Brugge WR. EUS-guided radiofrequency ablation in the pancreas: results in a porcine model. Gastrointest Endosc. 1999;50(3):392–401.
70. Carrara S, Arcidiacono PG, Albarello L, Addis A, Enderle MD, Boemo C, Campagnol M, Ambrosi A, Doglioni C, Testoni PA. Endoscopic ultrasound-guided application of a new hybrid cryotherm probe in porcine pancreas: a preliminary study. Endoscopy. 2008;40(4):321–6.
71. Kushibiki T, Hirasawa T, Okawa S, Ishihara M. Responses of cancer cells induced by photodynamic therapy. J healthc Eng. 2013;4(1):87–108.
72. Chan HH, Nishioka NS, Mino M, Lauwers GY, Puricelli WP, Collier KN, Brugge WR. EUS-guided photodynamic therapy of the pancreas: a pilot study. Gastrointest Endosc. 2004;59(1):95–9.
73. Yusuf TE, Matthes K, Brugge WR. EUS-guided photodynamic therapy with verteporfin for ablation of normal pancreatic tissue: a pilot study in a porcine model (with video). Gastrointest Endosc. 2008;67(6):957–61.
74. Di Matteo F, Martino M, Rea R, Pandolfi M, Rabitti C, Masselli GM, Silvestri S, Pacella CM, Papini E, Panzera F, et al. EUS-guided Nd:YAG laser ablation of normal pancreatic tissue: a pilot study in a pig model. Gastrointest Endosc. 2010;72(2):358–63.
75. Di Matteo F, Martino M, Rea R, Pandolfi M, Panzera F, Stigliano E, Schena E, Saccomandi P, Silvestri S, Pacella CM, et al. US-guided application of Nd:YAG laser in porcine pancreatic tissue: an ex vivo study and numerical simulation. Gastrointest Endosc. 2013;78(5):750–5.
76. Chang KJ, Nguyen PT, Thompson JA, Kurosaki TT, Casey LR, Leung EC, Granger GA. Phase I clinical trial of allogeneic mixed lymphocyte culture (cytoimplant) delivered by endoscopic ultrasound-guided fine-needle injection in patients with advanced pancreatic carcinoma. Cancer. 2000;88(6):1325–35.
77. Mulvihill S, Warren R, Venook A, Adler A, Randlev B, Heise C, Kirn D. Safety and feasibility of injection with an E1B-55 kDa

78. gene-deleted, replication-selective adenovirus (ONYX-015) into primary carcinomas of the pancreas: a phase I trial. Gene Ther. 2001;8(4):308–15.
78. Hecht JR, Bedford R, Abbruzzese JL, Lahoti S, Reid TR, Soetikno RM, Kirn DH, Freeman SM. A phase I/II trial of intratumoral endoscopic ultrasound injection of ONYX-015 with intravenous gemcitabine in unresectable pancreatic carcinoma. Clin Cancer Res. 2003;9(2):555–61.
79. Chang KJ, Lee JG, Holcombe RF, Kuo J, Muthusamy R, Wu ML. Endoscopic ultrasound delivery of an antitumor agent to treat a case of pancreatic cancer. Nat Clin Pract Gastroenterol Hepatol. 2008;5(2):107–11.
80. Chang KJ, Irisawa A, Group EUSW. EUS 2008 Working Group document: evaluation of EUS-guided injection therapy for tumors. Gastrointest Endosc. 2009;69(2 Suppl):S54–8.
81. Hecht JR, Farrell JJ, Senzer N, Nemunaitis J, Rosemurgy A, Chung T, Hanna N, Chang KJ, Javle M, Posner M, et al. EUS or percutaneously guided intratumoral TNFerade biologic with 5-fluorouracil and radiotherapy for first-line treatment of locally advanced pancreatic cancer: a phase I/II study. Gastrointest Endosc. 2012;75(2):332–8.
82. Herman JM, Wild AT, Wang H, Tran PT, Chang KJ, Taylor GE, Donehower RC, Pawlik TM, Ziegler MA, Cai H, et al. Randomized phase III multi-institutional study of TNFerade biologic with fluorouracil and radiotherapy for locally advanced pancreatic cancer: final results. Journal Clin Oncol. 2013;31(7):886–94.
83. Citrin D, Camphausen K, Wood BJ, Quezado M, Denobile J, Pingpank JF, Royal RE, Alexander HR, Seidel G, Steinberg SM, et al. A pilot feasibility study of TNFerade biologic with capecitabine and radiation therapy followed by surgical resection for the treatment of rectal cancer. Oncology. 2010;79(5-6):382–8.
84. Akiyama Y, Maruyama K, Nara N, Hojo T, Cheng JY, Mori T, Wiltrout RH, Yamaguchi K. Antitumor effects induced by dendritic cell-based immunotherapy against established pancreatic cancer in hamsters. Cancer Lett. 2002;184(1):37–47.
85. Irisawa A, Takagi T, Kanazawa M, Ogata T, Sato Y, Takenoshita S, Ohto H, Ohira H. Endoscopic ultrasound-guided fine-needle injection of immature dendritic cells into advanced pancreatic cancer refractory to gemcitabine: a pilot study. Pancreas. 2007;35(2):189–90.
86. Hirooka Y, Itoh A, Kawashima H, Hara K, Nonogaki K, Kasugai T, Ohno E, Ishikawa T, Matsubara H, Ishigami M, et al. A combination therapy of gemcitabine with immunotherapy for patients with inoperable locally advanced pancreatic cancer. Pancreas. 2009;38(3):e69–74.
87. Endo H, Saito T, Kenjo A, Hoshino M, Terashima M, Sato T, Anazawa T, Kimura T, Tsuchiya T, Irisawa A, et al. Phase I trial of preoperative intratumoral injection of immature dendritic cells and OK-432 for resectable pancreatic cancer patients. J Hepatobiliary Pancreat Sci. 2012;19(4):465–75.

Index

© Springer International Publishing Switzerland 2016
D.G. Adler (ed.), *Advanced Pancreaticobiliary Endoscopy*, DOI 10.1007/978-3-319-26854-5

Printed in the United States
By Bookmasters